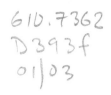

Family Health

A Framework
for Nursing

Sharon A. Denham, RN, DSN

Associate Professor
Ohio University
School of Nursing
Athens, Ohio

D1603208

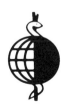

F.A. Davis Publishers
Philadelphia

F. A. Davis Company
1915 Arch Street
Philadelphia, PA 19103
www.fadavis.com

Printed in the United States of America

Last digit indicates print number: 10 9 8 7 6 5 4 3 2 1

Acquisitions Editor: Joanne DaCunha
Developmental Editor: Marilyn Kochman
Production Editor: Nwakaego Fletcher-Perry
Cover Designer: Louis Forgione

As new scientific information becomes available through basic and clinical research, recommended treatments and drug therapies undergo changes. The author(s) and publisher have done everything possible to make this book accurate, up to date, and in accord with accepted standards at the time of publication. The author(s), editors, and publisher are not responsible for errors or omissions or for consequences from application of the book, and make no warranty, expressed or implied, in regard to the contents of the book. Any practice described in this book should be applied by the reader in accordance with professional standards of care used in regard to the unique circumstances that may apply in each situation. The reader is advised always to check product information (package inserts) for changes and new information regarding dose and contraindications before administering any drug. Caution is especially urged when using new or infrequently ordered drugs.

Library of Congress Cataloging-in-Publication Data
Denham, Sharon A., 1945–
     Family health : a framework for nursing / Sharon A. Denham.—
  1st ed.
        p. cm.
     Includes bibliographical references and index.
     ISBN 0-8036-0944-2
     1. Nurse practitioners.   2. Primary care (Medicine)   3. Family—Health and hygiene.
  I. Title.

  RT82.8 .D46   2002
  610.73'06'92—dc21   2002073319

This book is dedicated to the families who were willing to share their family health stories, my own families and friends who have provided me with a personal, lived experience of family health, and to the nurses and others who might use this book in the future to improve family health outcomes.

Preface

The Family Health Model described in this text evolved from a knowledge of current literature, the author's professional nursing practice and life experiences, and findings from a series of three qualitative studies about how Appalachian families defined and practiced family health within their households (Denham, 1997, 1999a, 1999b, 1999c). This research was completed to learn about family health from a household perspective, rather than institutional ones. The aims of the research were to:

- Identify the ways families defined family health.
- Identify the routine family patterns, behaviors and daily activities perceived as part of the family health construction.
- Describe behaviors perceived as deleterious and adjuncts to family health.
- Identify the ways families modified their family health construction.
- Identify the contextual influences that affected family health.

Over a period of five years, three ethnographic studies about family health were completed with Appalachian families in two southeastern Ohio counties. Taped and later transcribed, interviews (n = 125) lasting 1 to 2 hours captured data about 24 families (80 interviews), eight families in each study, and a total of 45 community informants (Denham, 1997, 1999a, 1999b, 1999c). Participants were well families referred by informants at community agencies. A series of semi-structured questions guided the data collection. Approximately 6 to 9 months were spent collecting data for each study. The length of time for the series of interviews to be completed varied (i.e., 6 weeks to 6 months), with either 3 or 4 interviews conducted with multiple members of each family in their homes. Ethnographic methods were used to investigate family health from a community perspective. Data were analyzed using HyperResearch, a qualitative software package. Spradley's ideas (1979, 1980) about domains and Yin's (1994) ideas about continuous comparison and cross-case analysis provided the basis for analysis. Expert checks with those familiar with the Appalachian culture facilitated interpreting cultural inferences and identifying themes.

Participants in two studies were Appalachian families with school age or preschool children (Denham, 1997, 1999a, 1999c) and subjects in the third study were bereaved families who had recently experienced a member's death (Denham, 1999b). Families consisted of individuals who were commited to the general well-being of one another and identified themselves as family (Landesman, Jaccard, & Gunderson, 1991).

The first study, a dissertation research about family health in rural Appalachian families with preschool children, was conducted in a rural southeastern Ohio county where employment was limited and a consistently high poverty rate prevailed for several decades (Denham, 1997, 1999a). The other two studies were conducted in a more urban, but still rural, county within the same region. The dissertation provided findings pertinent to family health, but other dimensions also seemed important to enhance understandings (i.e., family health during change or transition, family health of economically disadvantaged families) and resulted in the follow-up studies.

The second study, funded by the American Nurses Foundation, provided a chance to learn about family health after hospice families had cared for a dying member and were experiencing the losses from deaths (Denham, 1999b). Nurses often work with ill individuals when they seek cure or care from health-care systems, but most have less understandings about the ways families incorporate prescribed care into households to meet members' health needs. Participants were members from different generations, used hospice services while the member was dying, and some were still receiving bereavement support. Findings indicated differences in health patterns and changes in routines as a result of the terminal condition and member's death.

Research is often completed with middle-class white populations and fails to include minorities or vulnerable populations. The third study, funded by the College of Health and Human Services at Ohio University, inquired about the ways economically disadvantaged families defined and practiced family health in their households (Denham, 1999c). These Appalachian families had at least one elementary school age child and received public assistance either when the study was conducted or in the recent past. While all mothers were white, fathers of several children were black, and some families included biracial children. Several households were single-parent families, all families had experienced socioeconomic constraints, and most families had members with chronic health problems or disabilities. Findings identified family health as a dynamic household construction affected by multiple member and contextual stressors. The findings supported much of what is described in the literature about health, but also provided some new knowledge about family health from structural, functional, and contextual perspectives. Findings emphasized the complexity of the variables that comprise family health and suggested ways to conceptualize family health as a household process influenced by family context, family functioning, and daily routines. While socio-demographic factors such as age, employment, economic status, and education were important, some cultural themes related to family health were different from what some have identified about Appalachians (Denham, 1996). For example, fatalism is often identified, but when family health was studied the participants seemed focused on the present as praxis or a way to cope with the stresses and needs of daily life. Rather than living lives directed by future goals, subjects were centered on the present and used it as a positive way to cope with life as it was encountered. While sense of place and strong kin relationships were visible in families, they were not geographically isolated, unaware of the larger world context or unexposed to difference and diversity. Families were apt to consult extended members about non-emergency situations health concerns and often took a "wait and see" attitude prior to actions. While some cultural differences existed, many responses were similar to those identified in non-Appalachian families.

In all three studies, mothers were the key health-care providers and gatekeepers for health resources. Many speak of male dominance as characteristic of Appalachian families, but when family health was the concern mothers played primary roles. The findings provide ways to conceptualize family health from process and system perspectives, provide evidence for contextual, functional, and structural points of view, and define a scope of practice for family-focused care. Contextual perspectives include members and their characteristics, household niches, embedded neighborhoods, situated communities, and larger societal systems. Functional perspectives are the processes members use to care for one another's processes of becoming, health, and well-being. Structural perspectives are related to the socially constructed routines that families use to organize health knowledge and behaviors. The Family Health Model provides a framework to describe, explain, and predict health outcomes and a means to circumscribe the boundaries of household production of health for family-focused care.

The book is divided into five sections. Section I introduces the Family Health Model and describes domains and variables relevant to the schema. Chapter 1 provides an overview about the usefulness of ecological models in considering family health and introduces many ideas used in the Family Health Model. Chapter 2 describes some conceptual ideas relevant to using a model to guide practice. Chapter 3 discusses the family concept and talks about its relevance to nursing and Chapter 4 discusses interpretations of health concepts.

Section II focuses on the contextual aspects of family health. Chapter 5 describes concepts related to family context, Chapter 6 emphasizes the family microsystem, and Chapter 7 provides information about the larger contextual systems that affect family health.

Section III focuses on the functional aspects of family health. Chapter 8 provides an overview about functional processes and the relevance to family health, Chapter 9 describes functional perspectives related to the household production of health, and Chapter 10 targets the core processes members use that are especially pertinent to the household production of health.

Section IV focuses on the structural aspects of family health. Chapter 11 provides arguments for considering family health routines as the structural aspect of family health, Chapter 12 suggests some of the factors pertinent to assessment and interventions related to routines, and Chapter 13 supplies an overview of the family health routine categories.

Section V focuses on family-focused practice. Chapter 14 supplies an overview of relevant family theories, and Chapter 15 discusses findings from the family health research applicable to mother's roles. The final two chapters provide some considerations for conceptualizing and developing family-focused practice for the 21st century.

The book is intended to initiate conversations about family-focused care from nursing perspectives and to suggest a family health model that might be useful for conceptualizing practice and initiating a research agenda that is more central to family care.

Sharon A. Denham, RN, DSN
Ohio University
Athens, Ohio

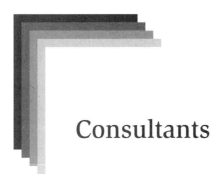

Consultants

Janet Geare Allen, RN, MSN, PHN, CHPN
Full Time Administrator of Hospice and Palliative Care Program
Kaiser Permanente
Downey, California

Jean Krajicek Bartek, PhD, APRN
Associate Professor
University of Nebraska Medical Center
Colleges of Nursing, and Medicine (Pharmacology).
Omaha, Nebraska

Barbara Mathews Blanton, MSN, RN, CARN
Assistant Professor of Nursing
Texas Woman's University
Dallas, Texas

Amy Sedlacek Cooper, MSN, WHNP
Research Nurse Practitioner
Women & Infants' Hospital, Division of Research
Providence, Rhode Island

Brenda Drummond, MSN, CNS, CNP
Instructor II
Mercy College of Northwest Ohio
Owner, Nurse Practitioner
Nurse Practitioner Consultants, LLC
Perrysburg, Ohio

Kelli S. Dunham, RN, BSN
Nurse-Home Visitor in the Nurse Family Partnership Collaborative
MCP-Hahnemann University
Philadelphia, Pennsylvania

Margaret J. Hickman, RN, PhD
Associate Professor
University of Kentucky
Lexington, Kentucky

Melanie Lutenbacher, RN, CS, PhD
Assistant Professor of Nursing
Vanderbilt University
Nashville, Tennessee

Heather J. McKnight, BSN, MSN
Pediatric Nurse Practitioner
Children's Hospital of Philadelphia
Philadelphia, Pennsylvania

Pamela McHugh Schuster, PhD, RN
Professor of Nursing
Youngstown State University
Youngstown, Ohio

Mary Oesterle, EdD, APRN, BC
Associate Professor
Saint Xavier University
Chicago, Illinois

Marilyn Smith-Stoner, RN, PhD
Nursing Faculty
California State University
Fullerton, California

Lynnette Leeseberg Stamler, RN, PhD
Associate Professor and Director
Collaborative BScN Program
Nipissing University
North Bay, ON Canada

Valerie A. Boebel Toly, RN, MSN, CPNP
Instructor of Nursing
Frances Payne Bolton School of Nursing
Case Western Reserve University
Cleveland, Ohio

Patricia M. Woodbery, RN, MSN, ARNP-CS
Professor of Nursing
Valencia Community College
Orlando, Florida

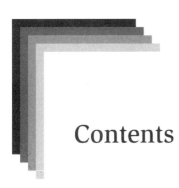

Contents

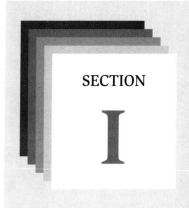

SECTION

I

Introduction
to the Family
Health Model

Chapter

1

An Ecological Model
of Family Health

CHAPTER OBJECTIVES *At the end of this chapter, the reader will be able to:*

- Discuss broad perspectives of the Family Health Model.
- Differentiate between the contextual, functional, and structural aspects of the Family Health Model.
- Explain what is implied by *family-focused care.*

> *Two roads diverged in a wood, and I—*
> *I took the one less traveled by,*
> *And that has made all of the difference.*
> Robert Frost "The Road Not Taken"

This chapter provides an overview of the Family Health Model and introduces the contextual, functional, and structural perspectives related to family health. The author cites implications from her family health research, provides operational definitions for some key concepts used in the model, and draws some conclusions.

As the 21st century evolves, needs exist to develop more universally applicable models for use with diverse populations regardless of where they reside in the global village. Old and new ways of thinking need to be blended. International views often seem contradictory to what many American nurses recognize as health. Focusing on the illness requirements of individuals needs to be better balanced with considerations of prevention, health promotion, and wellness. Although family health includes traditional medical services and concerns about illnesses and disease, the concept extends beyond illness orientations. The Family Health Model encourages nurses and others to move beyond ideas and practices incorporated in the medical model and in Western thinking about health, illness, and disease and to consider potential differences (Table 1–1). The

Table 1–1	Comparing a Medical Model with the Family Health Model
Medical Model	**Family Health Model**
Systems models	Contextually embedded family systems
Focuses on illness and disease	Focuses on well-being and processes of becoming
Aim is treatment and cure	Aim also includes health promotion and prevention
Health as an outcome	Health as an interactive contextual, functional, structural process
Target is the individual	Target is the family
Episodic care	Care over the life course
Care viewed from individual perspectives	Care viewed from contextually embedded perspectives
Client as care seeker	Care provider as collaborator and partner
Individual and environment	Family in embedded context
Individual as the reservoir of health and illness	Household as the reservoir of health and illness
Individual behavior as a threat or initiator of health	Community as a threat or initiator of health
Physicians as the primary health-care providers	Mother as the primary health-care provider
Medical providers as experts	Family as expert
Expert as decision maker	Family as decision maker
Institutional- and agency-based care	Care targeted at family household and context

value of health-care systems and providers are not discounted; rather, they are viewed as part of a large complex rubric that influences health.

Operationalizing the Family Health Model

Clear operational definitions are needed to describe the complex relationships among the biophysical, holistic, and contextual aspects of family health. The value of a conceptual schema or model is enhanced when the terms being used are clear. The lexicon, or language, of a model provides the syntax for understanding its concepts, and explicit definitions provide ways to understand links between related concepts. A glossary that provides definitions used in this model has been included (Appendix A). However, mastery of the Family Health Model requires time spent reflecting and thinking critically about its implications and possibilities.

In the Family Health Model, *health* is defined as an adaptive state that persons experience as they seek opportunities and wrestle with liabilities found within themselves and their families, households, and diverse contexts throughout the course of their lives. Health is experienced when a person can fulfill personal goals and enjoy life. *Family health* suggests the interactions that occur within a household and environment affect members as they seek to obtain, sustain, and regain maximum health. Family health includes the systems, interactions, relationships, and processes that have the potential to maximize processes of becoming, to enhance well-being, and to capitalize on the household production of health. The model emphasizes the biophysical, holistic, and environmental factors that impact health.

Another way to define the term *family health* is the interactions and processes of individuals who identify as family and dwell together in a household niche that is dynamically impacted by complex contextual systems with potentials to affect health. In other words, families use a variety of processes to individually and collectively strive to achieve a state in which they feel good about themselves and one another.

A household is a pivotal point for coping with biophysical needs and the world in which people live. Family health includes the idea of *person-process-context* (Bronfenbrenner, 1986). Family health is less a goal and more a process that includes the complex interactions of individuals, family subsystems, family members, and their context over the life course. A game of tug-of-war is an analogy to understand the balancing and rebalancing that occurs as family systems interact with their embedded contexts. The term *family health* implies a striving to enhance processes of becoming and strive toward individual and family well-being.

The *process of becoming* is a dynamic state through which family members seek opportunities to overcome individual liabilities and potentiate possibilities across the life course. Members form relationships and interact with environmental systems from household perspectives to maximize health opportunities. Processes of becoming include biophysical concerns, but they also address psychological, emotional, and intellectual functioning; social wholeness; interpersonal integrity; personal need fulfillment; tradition keeping; spiritual wholeness; and vocational connectedness. The process of becoming is closely aligned with Parse's (1987) ideas of Man-Living-Health in that developing persons are viewed as "open being(s), more than and different from the sum of his (their) parts in mutual simultaneous interchange with the environment who chooses from options and bears responsibility for choices" (p. 160). Although individuals have some responsibility for the process of becoming as a result of choices they make and lifestyles they choose, embedded contexts have positive and negative effects of great consequence.

Family nursing aims to provide holistic care for individuals and family units. *Holism* is defined as the struggle with complex phenomena and traits that are sometimes dichotomous or ambiguous to attain well-being. Holistic care can be provided in many different realms (e.g., biological, psychological, social, spiritual, vocational, safety). *Well-being* is defined as an optimum health state in which opportunities are realized, liabilities are minimized, and contexts are maximized. Well-being includes many dimensions (e.g., biophysical, psychological, emotional, social, spiritual, vocational) and goals associated with risk reduction, disease prevention, health maintenance, health-care competence, lifestyle, congruence, self-actualization, hardiness, resilience, or other targets.

Families or even some members in the same family may operationalize well-being differently. For some families, the absence of disease and the ability to work may be essential to well-being; however, a family with a dying member may view well-being as a pain-free death, family cohesiveness during the terminal stages of their loved one, or consensus about funeral plans. Another family may view well-being in terms of overcoming obstacles that prevent them from resolving stresses related to an alcoholic family member. Well-being might be viewed in terms of transportation availability for physician appointments or even in terms of parents' ability to cope with an autistic child. Well-being may be an ephemeral or inconstant state, but it may also appear as a state of permanence and constancy. Well-being and the process of becoming are abstract concepts that may be redefined over the life course by individuals and families as problems that seem to conflict with health are encountered.

Person-in-context implies that unique personal characteristics and contextual perspectives impact health (Bronfenbrenner, 1986). Person-in-context implies interactions occurring between the household members as a response to the contextual systems that permeate family life and present ambiguous and contradictory influences integral to health. Thus, a person of Hispanic origin may have much community support if he or she is living in a neighborhood where the majority of people are also Hispanic. However, if this person is Mexican, works as a migrant farmer, travels across the nation, and lives in rural areas for short periods, then his or her community support may be limited. When the migrant worker is residing in his or her own neighborhood, he or she might have support from extended family, the church, and a local clinic. However, when living briefly in rural regions where the people are very different, a migrant worker may not only have far less support available, but he or she may also encounter greater risks. A nurse working

---

Box 1-1 Dimensions and Processes of Nursing Related to Family-Focused Care

Dimensions of care
- Clarifying family meanings related to past, present, and future health orientations
- Synchronizing patterns of nurse–individual, nurse–family, nurse–context interaction
- Transcending past obstacles, validating present potentials, and anticipating future opportunities

Processes of nursing
- Collaborating, partnering, advocating, explaining, guiding, counseling, and teaching
- Moving developing persons toward well-being, maturity, hardiness, individuation, transcendence, and empowerment
- Facilitating family processes, family identity, family resilience, and family development over the life course
- Assisting individuals and families with the processes of becoming, illness occasions, and unpredictable experiences
- Enabling developing persons and families through living and dying and generational processes
- Acting on and in conjunction with the contextual systems affecting family health

Sources: Some ideas originally derived from Parse (1987) Man-Living-Health Model.

---

with migrant workers can use a person-in-context model for assessment, intervention, and evaluation to better understand complex health needs.

The aim of family nursing is to assist persons-in-context achieve well-being and optimize the processes of becoming. *Family-focused care* is aimed at *persons-in-context* to assist developing persons situated within their embedded ecological context to (1) clarify meanings related to the past, present, and future; (2) synchronize patterns of interaction between a nurse and a family; and (3) transcend the past, validate the present, and anticipate the future (Box 1–1). *Family-focused care* implies that the care that is given is appropriate for achieving individual and family health, and uses goals and strategies related to individuals; family subsystems; family processes, behaviors, and interactions; the household production of health; and embedded contextual systems. Family-focused care seeks collaborative or partnering strategies to support, change, facilitate, or alter processes or contexts that affect family goals and potentiate health. Family-focused care helps nurses meet persons-in-context and assists them to adapt, accommodate, or alter processes or contexts that preclude achievement of desired goals or outcomes.

Reflective Thinking

Before delving very far into this chapter, take some time to think about what is meant by *family health*. When you think about the term *family health,* what comes to your mind? How do you describe *family?* How would you describe *health?* Ask your family members how they define these terms. What about your friends or your peers where you work?

Put your definitions in writing considering what you usually mean when you say the words *family* and *health*. Keep these definitions nearby as you study this text so you can identify the ways your ideas may change or stay the same.

In class, break into groups and share your definitions. Develop a consensus definition for each of these three terms. Share your group definitions with the entire class.

Operationalizing Family Health

Although there is strong evidence that health is learned and experienced within a family context (Bomar, 1990; Harkness & Super, 1994; Keltner, 1992; Lasky & Eichelberger, 1985; Lau, Quadrel, & Hartman, 1990; Ross, Mirowsky, & Goldsteen, 1990; Thomas, 1990), few family-focused studies have investigated family health (Backett, 1992; Duffy, 1988; Gillis, 1991a; Ransom, 1986; Thomas, 1990), and little substantive evidence describes how healthy lifestyles are promoted (Blecke, 1990; Campbell, 1986; Kelly, Zyzanski, & Alemagno, 1991; Whall & Loveland-Cherry, 1993; Wierenga, Browning, & Mahn, 1990). Although changes are beginning to occur, family research has predominately emphasized pathology and poorly functioning families (Feetham, 1991). Health has been studied less frequently and is often viewed as curing or caring for individuals rather than being a family characteristic (Pender, 1987). In a review of health research, Reynolds (1988) noted that investigators infrequently provide operational definitions of health and have minimal agreement about the adequacy of techniques or instruments to measure health. In addition, the health concept needs to be explored more thoroughly through qualitative models.

Before formulating a model that describes, explains, or predicts family health, the dilemma of clearly ascertaining what is implied by the construct of family health remains. Throughout the nursing literature, the term *family health* is rarely defined. When the term is defined, single authors are often inconsistent in their usage and loosely slip among concepts of family and the health of its members, healthy family, family functioning, family structure, and family health without clearly differentiating what was intended. "Family scientists and family physicians tend to use inconsistent definitions of family health and to approach the concept primarily from a psychosocial functioning perspective without integrating specific health variables of significance to nursing." (Anderson & Tomlinson, 1992, p. 60). Family descriptions often compare one person's health status with another's through reasoning that suggests that either the structure or the functions of the family are root causes of the condition.

A large body of literature describes complex family relationships and member roles during procreation and caring for members' health and illness needs. Less is known about the ways families teach developing members how to care for health; incorporate health knowledge into family living; promote healthy lifestyles; and prevent disease, illness, and injury. Family models can increase the understanding about roles and socialization processes related to health and illness, coping factors, and interactions related to family needs. However, models do not always provide clear ways to conceptualize family-focused care or promote family health.

An Overview of the Family Health Model

The Family Health Model draws information from the literature about individual and family health, and provides a framework that can be applied to nursing and inquiry into family health. The model identifies the many interacting systems related to the holistic needs of developing persons and families. An ecological model is a way to conceptualize the complex interactive relational systems relevant to families and their health. It is important to note that this is a model of family health, not merely a family model. Thus, the context and variables are more inclusive than merely considering family processes. In other words, family health is influenced by its embedded contextual aspects as well as those related to members, the family as a whole, and family processes. To provide the reader with a clear understanding of some of the underlying premises of the model, foundational assumptions have been stated as succinctly as possible (Box 1-2). Family health involves all members who reside in a household

---

Box 1-2   **Assumptions of the Family Health Model**

1. Developing persons experience individual and family health in relation to the contextual, functional, and structural realms over the life course.

2. Individual and family health are inextricably tied to the household production of health.

3. Individual and family health are affected by the nested contexts of microsystems, mesosystems, exosystems, macrosystems, and chronosystem interactions that create intrapersonal, interpersonal, intrafamilial, and intergenerational interactions.

4. The microsystem includes persons who reside in the household niche named as family and the interactions that occur between the family subsystems and diverse external contexts that have the potential to influence individual and family health.

5. Mesosystems are the multiple external environments (e.g., home, work, school, peer groups) that have the potential to affect individual and family health.

6. Exosystems are diverse contextual settings (e.g., administrative decisions made by a parent's employer, boards that govern school policies) that possess the potential to affect individual and family health even when members do not actively participate.

7. Macrosystems represent the ideologies of the evolving world (e.g., legislation, social policy, culture, media, history) that have the potential to affect individual and family health.

8. Chronosystems affect microsystems, mesosystems, exosystems, and macrosystems and create dynamics that affect developing persons, member relationships, household niches, and contextual systems.

9. The context has an inherent potential to delineate, circumscribe, delimit, potentiate, and negate individual and family health.

10. Family health is composed of the complex interactions of the microsystem and diverse contextual systems that have the potential to maximize or minimize the well-being and the *process of becoming* for individuals and the family as a whole.

11. Family health can be understood through a person-process-context model at specific time points and over the life course.

12. Individuals within a household niche form dyads and triads, internal and external to the household niche, that have the potential to affect individual and family health.

13. Processes, relationships, and interactions alone are not effective predictors of individual or family health.

14. Family health routines provide a way to discuss, describe, assess, intervene, and evaluate interventions and outcomes pertinent to individual and family health.

---

but includes ways relationships and environments affect health over time. Findings from the qualitative research conducted by the author have provided evidence that indicate a need to conceptualize family health from ecological and process perspectives.

Repeated family health studies using similar research methods provided a way to compare and contrast three different family populations. Inductive methods were effective in assisting the investigator to move from abstract to more concrete conclusions and have resulted in some rather explicit statements about the family health phenomenon:

▩ Family health is a complex abstract concept with contextual, functional, and structural domains.

▩ Family health is an evolving multimember interactional process used to attain, maintain, or regain the health of individual members and a family over time.

▩ Family health is a positively viewed health state or ideal that members strive toward even when some members face chronic illness, terminal illness, substance abuse, mental health concerns, or unpredictable life events.

- Family health is a collective experience that is affected by individual and family factors and member processes that are supported and challenged by the values, goals, and resources of the larger embedded society.
- Family health is more greatly influenced by household and member variables, member interactions, and routine behaviors than by occasional medical encounters.
- Family health is positively and negatively influenced by contextually embedded factors that extend beyond individual members and the family household.
- Family health includes the dynamic ways family members holistically care for one another using functional processes to establish individual and family health routines.
- Unique members may view family health differently, but members tend to have greater agreement than disagreement about the defining criteria.
- Mothers play key roles in family health.

Findings from the research implied that educators, practitioners, and researchers should consider the following points when addressing family health:

- Include contextual, functional, and structural domains when proposing variables related to family health.
- Identify family health as more closely related to the household production of health than to brief episodic encounters with medical and health-care providers.
- Determine which contextual factors outside of the control of family members most contribute to or threaten the household production of health.
- Increase knowledge about individual and family health routines as primary ways that health behaviors are learned and practiced within household settings.
- Consider mothers' interactions with family members as a principal means for promoting and protecting family health.
- Identify specific family interventions for measuring, promoting, and evaluating family health from household perspectives.
- Guard against semantic slippage surrounding the family health construct.
- Encourage use of a shared lexicon by family-care providers, legislators, and consumers.

The Family Health Model encourages nurses to consider the daily lived experiences of multiple members embedded within a diverse ecological contexts as factors associated with family health. Although the model has its basis in nursing practice, other practitioners may also find it useful. To understand this model, thinking must move beyond the systems perspectives usually used to describe pathology, illness care, and medical needs based in Western thinking. Family health is best understood from a salutogenic or wellness perspective in which the household is viewed as the primary location where health is produced or negated. The household is where health is learned, lived, and experienced and is the niche where members encounter and respond to disease and illness.

Family Health as Context

Family health has contextual, functional, and structural dimensions or realms (Figure 1–1). The proposed Family Health Model also provides a way to consider the contextual, functional, and structural perspectives of family health (Table 1–2). The contextual domain of family health is affected by the internal environment (i.e., member context, family context, household context) and external environment (i.e., neighborhood context, community context, greater social context, historical context, political

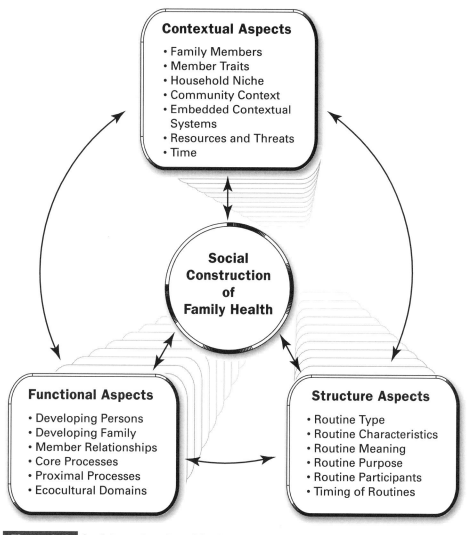

Figure 1–1   Social construction of family health.

context). The context has to do with the diverse environments with the potential to affect individual and family health. Contextual dimensions include all persons identified as family, defining characteristics of the family (e.g., race, culture, age, gender, educational level attained, economic status, extended family), family household, neighborhood, community, and diverse environments relevant to family health.

The *family context* includes all of the environments in which individual members interact or have the potential to interact with them. Context includes family members and household embedded in the larger environment. The *family microsystem* includes (1) the household niche of the developing person, (2) all developing persons residing in the household, (3) relationships with extended family members, (4) intergenerational relationships even when persons are no longer alive or present in the setting, (5) the

Table 1–2	Definition of Family Health from the Three Family Health Studies		
Family Health Domains	**Contextual Aspects of Family Health**	**Functional Aspects of Family Health**	**Structural Aspects of Family Health**
Family health categories	**Internal environment:** ■ Member context ■ Family context ■ Household context	**Individual factors:** ■ Values ■ Perceptions ■ Coping ■ Health knowledge ■ Motivation ■ Education	**Self-care routines:** ■ Dietary ■ Hygiene ■ Sleep–rest ■ Physical activity and exercise ■ Gender and sexuality
	External environment: ■ Neighborhood ■ Community ■ Greater social context ■ Historical context ■ Political context	**Family factors:** ■ Cohesiveness ■ Resilience ■ Shared values or goals ■ Resources and threats ■ Boundaries	**Safety and prevention:** ■ Health protection ■ Disease prevention ■ Smoking ■ Abuse and violence ■ Alcohol and substance abuse
		Member processes: ■ Caregiving ■ Cathexis ■ Celebration ■ Change ■ Communication ■ Connectedness ■ Coordination	**Mental health behaviors:** ■ Self-esteem ■ Personal integrity ■ Work and play ■ Stress levels
			Family care: ■ Family fun (e.g., relaxation activities, hobbies, vacations) ■ Celebrations, traditions, special events ■ Spiritual and religious practices ■ Pets ■ Sense of humor
			Illness care: ■ Decision making related to medical consultation ■ Use of health-care services ■ Follow-up with prescribed medical regimens
			Member caretaking: ■ Health teaching (i.e., health, prevention, illness, disease) ■ Member roles and responsibilities ■ Supportive member actions

immediate neighborhood, and (6) the local community. The *family household* is the domicile maintained and resided in by the developing members; this residence includes (1) the physical structure, (2) the immediate surroundings, (3) material goods, (4) tangible and intangible family resources, and (5) all the developing persons' interactions with the above.

The complexity of family context deepens as one also considers the dynamic interactions that occur over the life course. The family context interacts with diverse external environments that have the potential to potentiate, mediate, and negate individual and family health. The context supports or threatens well-being and processes of becoming.

Family members act on the context that has potential to strengthen, weaken, maintain, sustain, or destroy them. The embedded context includes history, society, policy, law, ethics, traditions, culture, and time pertinent to health. The environment influences the family and tempers behaviors, goals, resources, and experiences. The context is integral to health; pervades all aspects of family life; and influences where persons interact and develop beliefs, gather health information, identify support systems, and establish health routines.

Family Health as Function

Most practitioners view family health from functional perspectives, with the greatest focus on innate personal characteristics or personality traits or in terms of person-to-person interactions. The Family Health Model suggests that the functional interactions should be viewed from bi-directional perspectives. *Family functioning* refers to the individual and cooperative processes used by individual persons to engage with one another and their embedded contextual systems over the life course. These interactive processes can assist individuals, family subsystems, and families as a whole to attain, sustain, maintain, and regain health. Individuals act independently, but they also interact with one another through dyadic and triadic relationships to potentiate, mediate, or negate family health. The core family processes of caregiving, cathexis, celebration, change, communication, connectedness, and coordination especially affect individual and family health over the life course.

These interactions or processes include such things as roles, relationships, power structures, values, beliefs, communication, decision making, socialization, and coping. The functional dimension includes actions that occur within the family relevant to family health.

The functional domain includes individual factors (e.g., values, perceptions, coping, spirituality, motivation, roles), family process factors (e.g., cohesiveness, resilience, individuation, boundaries), and member processes (e.g., communication, coordination, caregiving, control).

Family interactions or processes are powerful socializing mechanisms through which family identity is constructed, deconstructed, and reconstructed. Although *family identity* has ties to family context, it is primarily the dynamic ways developing family members view the microsystem and collectively interpret memories and meanings of unique affiliations and attachments to persons, places, and things. Relationships between family identity and family health may not immediately be clear, but the ways members view themselves and their family ultimately affect values, attitudes, and patterned health behaviors. Some things that affect family identity include new information and experiences with diverse environments, maturation and change, and the character of personal and environmental relationships over the life course. Family identity evolves and affects the well-being, processes of becoming, and health.

Families of origin values influence those of the family of procreation. Individual bonding or failure to bond into dyads and triads influences the opportunities to share, refute, modify, and negotiate health beliefs, knowledge, and behaviors. Prior parental learning about health, illness, and disease is shared and influenced by developing family members. Beliefs, knowledge, and behaviors are modified as members interact with one another and diverse contexts. These interactions result in a fluid, evolving family identity from which the family socially constructs a lived household experience of family health. Social construction can be described as an up-to-date interpretation of all that has gone before. In other words, values, beliefs, attitudes, knowledge, traditions, and behaviors go through many incarnations as they are interpreted into the present family experience. Things such as the effectiveness, potency, type, and length of relationships between family members and contextual systems have the potential to affect health. Things such as biophysical attributes; psychological, emotional, and intellectual functioning; social wholeness; interpersonal integrity; personal needs fulfillment; tradition keeping; spiritual attainment; and vocational direction all have functional and contextual aspects affiliated with health. Families develop unique health paradigms that are aligned with family identity.

The *family health paradigm* is defined as the ways individuals, family subsystems, and families interpret the meaningfulness of complex health factors and collectively engage in patterned health behaviors. As individuals identify behaviors as meaningful, the likelihood of specific actions' being repeated and incorporated into definitions and practices of individual and family health are increased. Although diverse family groups have some commonalities in these definitions and practices, discrete differences occur based on family characteristics (e.g., education, culture, ethnicity, race, economics). Family health paradigms are most resilient when (1) beliefs and practices are viewed as meaningful by family members, (2) new knowledge is supported by values and beliefs, (3) the embedded context provides support for values and beliefs, and (4) family processes are congruent with the embedded contexts. The family health paradigm is the sum of beliefs, attitudes, values, knowledge, and behaviors of member interactions with one another and the embedded context.

Family Health as Structure

Functioning or processes have the potential to affect health routines and are the antecedents for the valued behaviors that are constructed into identifiable patterns of behavior relevant to health outcomes. Structural aspects of family health are the complex habitual patterns used to construct the lived family health experience. This social construction occurs as members interact with one another and with the embedded context. *Family health routines* are dynamic patterns of behavior relevant to health to which members rather consistently adhere and are daily life structures that can be recalled, described, and discussed from individual, family, and diverse environmental perspectives. Structured behaviors have unique qualities and involve all family members within a household even if they are not actively engaging in the behavior. Family health routines are not static; rather, they evolve over time. Although health routines evolve, developing persons strive to maintain the integrity of the routines they view as meaningful. Despite what might initially appear to an outsider as random or chaotic patterns of health behaviors, persons within a family are cognizant of members' routines. The structural dimension provides ways to plan, strategize, and intervene.

The structural domain is composed of six categories of family health routines: self-care, safety and precautions, mental health behaviors, family care, illness care, and taking care of members. Members interact with one another, extended families, peers, friends, others, and the larger society in ways that potentiate and negate individual and family health. These dynamic interactions affect solitary individuals, the family unit as a whole, and the embedded context where they reside. Children initially learn health routines in their family of origin, but these routines can be reinforced or altered as the children develop and mature. For example, a mother may teach her child about hand-washing after using the toilet at home, and this behavior can be positively reinforced if the child's peers also wash their hands after using the toilet or if the preschool teacher monitors this behavior. Family-focused care can target routines for assessing, planning, devising strategies, intervening, and measuring health outcomes.

Health routines tend toward steadfastness, but other persons, information, and availability of support or resources can challenge them. Several needs seem especially applicable to the development and continuance of health routines: (1) avoid illness, disease, and injury; (2) overcome illness, disease, and injury events; and (3) make lifestyle changes related to well-being and the process of becoming. Functional factors that strongly impact the development of health routines include needs to (1) participate in expected family roles and life tasks, (2) balance priorities that impact multiple members' needs, and (3) cope with the inconsistencies between stated health beliefs and actual behaviors. Factors such as gender, values, knowledge, and resources also affect health routines.

Routine rigidity, complexity, and frequency; the present level of participation in behaviors; and internal motivation to participate in the routine are some ways to consider the meaning and usefulness of a particular routine to a family. Lack of valuing and non-availability of needed resources can be impediments to health routines. As individuals engage in peer and social relationships, establish procreating or partnering relationships, become challenged by new information and skills, and encounter unpredictable life events, they often modify their beliefs and practices associated with health.

ᛀᛀᛀᛀᛀᛀᛀ   *Cooperative Learning*

Form groups that each have three members. Group members should choose one of the three dimensions of the family health model: family context, family function, or family structure.

Take turns explaining your chosen dimension to the other two members of your group. After you all have had a turn, each person should write a one- to two-sentence description of the three dimensions. Share your descriptions with each other.

Summary

The field of nursing needs a comprehensive model for discussing family health. The proposed Family Health Model uses an ecological framework to conceptualize this complex construct. Language for describing various aspects of the model is provided so that terms can be defined and operationalized for use in practice and research. Using this model, nurses can historically and developmentally compare and contrast families over the life course. Conceptualizing family health from contextual, functional, and structural viewpoints establishes a frame of reference for understanding multi-member households and the ways various members interact with one another and the environment to realize health, mediate well-being, and cope with illness and disease. This chapter has introduced some basic understandings about this model.

Test Your Knowledge

1. In your own words, explain what is meant by *family health.*
2. Briefly describe what the term *contextual aspects of family health* means.
3. Give two examples of functional aspects of family health.
4. Explain what the term *structural perspective of family health* means.
5. Identify how you might be able to use the Family Health Model in your nursing practice.

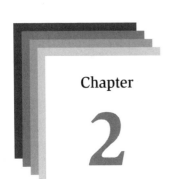

Conceptual Underpinnings of Family Health

CHAPTER OBJECTIVES *At the end of this chapter, the reader will be able to:*

- Discuss the characteristics of conceptual models.
- Understand ways the family health concept may be operationalized.
- Use operational definitions related to family health.

Introducing Conceptual Understandings

> *Heroes are those with courage to leave what they have—their land, their family, their property—and move out, not without fear, but without succumbing to their fear.*
>
> Erich Fromm (1976) "To Have or Be"

Defining *family health* is a difficult task. Although the term is often used, clear understandings about what the term implies are lacking. Different interpretations about ways family should be characterized and difficulties in agreeing about what is meant by health increase the confusion. Failing to clearly define the term results in misinterpretations, with family health meaning almost anything and practically nothing.

Family and *health* are both concepts that lack universally understood and accepted definitions. *Concepts* are defined as basic building blocks related to nursing knowledge, thought, and communication (Waltz, Strickland, & Lenz, 1991); they are formed from observations of particular behaviors (Kerlinger, 1986); and they enable us to categorize, interpret, and structure the phenomenon (Fawcett & Downs, 1992). Concepts are abstract thoughts, ideas, symbols, or notions used to describe phenomena (Polit & Hungler, 1999). "A concept enables us to categorize, interpret, and structure the phenomenon" (Fawcett & Downs, 1992, p. 19). We lack the language to describe what we do for families, so we use language that does not capture the nuances of family phenomena (Gillis, 1991a).

When we use terms without clearly defining the meanings, the result is often conceptual vagueness. *Conceptual vagueness* is the absence of concise meanings or interpretations. A *definition* is a statement that describes the meaning of a word or a concept. When concepts are highly abstract, ambiguity increases and must sometimes be accompanied by a greater tolerance (Chinn & Kramer, 1991). Adding together two obscure or poorly defined concepts results in what might be called *conceptual slippage,* an inability to fully understand or communicate what is implied. Do you remember the childhood game of pin the tail on the donkey? If so, then you probably have some insight about conceptual slippage. After being blindfolded and turned around several times, it was always a strong possibility that even though you were aiming for the donkey's hindmost parts, you could end up pinning the tail almost anywhere! What you needed was some clear direction. Can you recall what an advantage it was in having an adult steer you in the right direction? At least when you took off the blindfold, you found yourself in closer proximity to the target than if you did not have the guidance. Clear definitions are aids; they point us in the right direction and provide some shared understandings about what is intended.

Identifying direction is similar to what is implied when we say a concept needs to be operationalized—making something obscure clearer. Concept use generally assumes that the meanings are implicit and well understood, but unique interpretations may only vaguely resemble what was intended. Although it is important to define concepts, most practitioners or researchers would concede that it is nearly impossible to fully measure all variables that characterize a concept. *Variables* are attributes or objective and subjective criteria that take on different values depending on changing circumstances or environments. Variables can be dichotomous or discrete (e.g., male–female, married–single, child–adult), continuous (e.g., height and weight), and categorical (e.g., religious choice). Whereas concepts are mostly nonobservable, variables are more measurable. For instance, *health* is an abstract concept, but if we discuss cholesterol levels, height and weight, and vital signs, we have identified measurable variables that can assist our understandings about health.

 ## *Reflective Thinking*

Can you think of other nursing terms in which the problem of conceptual slippage occurs? For example, what about the terms *family support, quality of life,* and *family functioning*? When you hear these terms, how do you interpret them? List some terms whose definitions are not always clear and then discuss them with your colleagues or classmates. What can nurses do about conceptual slippage when they are talking to one another? What can nurses do to decrease conceptual slippage when speaking to patients, families, other health professionals, community persons, legislators, and others?

Operationalizing the Family Health Construct

Have you ever played a board game at a friend's house and heard him or her say, "Whenever you are at my house, you play by my rules"? If so, then the friend was operationalizing the way the game was to be played. Although these rules were not necessarily the ones provided by the game's manufacturer, your friend decided on new rules for the game. You may know that all people may not play the game this way. In fact, if you tried to use those rules somewhere else, you might be accused of cheating.

What does it mean to *operationalize* a term or concept? An operational definition is one that defines concepts within the boundaries of what is intended and in terms of what is to be measured. "The operational definition provides the concept with empirical meaning by defining it in terms of observable data, such as the activities necessary to measure the concept or manipulate it" (Fawcett & Downs, 1992, p. 26). An operational definition is the ways a concept is used within particular circumstances or activities. Operationalizing a concept is the process of taking obscure or abstract phenomena and making them measurable. An operational definition bridges comprehension among people who share interests about particular phenomena. An operational definition can be similar to a ruler, microscope, or stethoscope because it enables one to identify what is less obvious and tangible and provide more succinct understanding.

We might call *family* and *health* "fuzzy concepts," terms with blurred boundaries. In earlier decades, Americans mostly identified a family as a multimember unit that included a male and a female parent who shared a household, goods, and resources and gave birth to children that they raised and supported. Today's family definitions often include single parents, blended families, gay and lesbian families, and others with characteristics and boundaries that seem more "fuzzy" than clear. Although *health* is sometimes defined as the absence of sickness, a myriad of other definitions also exist. Hence, the term *family health* presents even greater conceptual vagueness because it is an even more abstract idea. Complex phenomena such as family health need to be operationalized. Although commonalities among perceptions and experiences may exist, differences can be significant and can result in serious barriers to practice, goal accomplishment, and outcome measurement. Variant perceptions and interpretations of concepts can decrease the continuity of care, limit the effects of interventions, and preclude the achievement of intended outcomes.

For example, when you talk to a patient about family health, how can you be sure that you are communicating clearly? It is possible that when you say *family health*, you mean "the physical well-being of all family members residing within a household." However, another nurse might say, "No, family health has to do with the ways household members function and cooperate to meet their goals." Another nurse might say, "Family health has to do with reaching a goal of optimum wellness for each family member" and may view optimum wellness as having emotional, physical, spiritual, and social perspectives. Still another nurse might interpret family health to mean "a family state that exists on a continuum and is dynamically influenced by members' health and illness state, household factors, and the social environment." How might these different views of family health affect nursing practice?

Patients might view the term *family health* from even other perspectives. For example, one patient might say, "Family health has to do with us all being well enough to do what we need to do." Another might say, "Family health means we are all working together, pulling our weight, and getting along with one another." Still another patient might say, "Family health has to do with not getting diseases or being sick." Another interpretation might be "family health has to do with the family history of our diseases" or "family health is when one of us has a need and other persons are there to provide support."

The variant views held by other health-care providers and professionals from various disciplines further complicate the issue. For example, a physician may view family health from only biophysical perspectives. A psychiatrist may view family health from mental health perspectives. A psychologist may want to discuss the developmental perspectives related to family health. A politician may imply that family health has to do with lower taxes or broader access to medical services. A social worker may view family health in relationship to neighborhoods and the availability of support systems. A marketer may see family health as spending money to purchase modern conveniences. An economist may identify family health as the economic well-being of households. A teacher may perceive family health in relation to parental support for children's learning. A pastor or clergy member may view family health from religious or spiritual perspectives. People in each discipline choose different vantage points from which they begin to discuss family health and pitch their ideas.

Critical Thinking Activity

Think about the various ways family health might be interpreted by nurses or patients and then consider the possible outcomes of this case: Mr. James, a 68-year-old, recently widowed man, is about to be discharged from the urgent care center where he was brought by the local emergency squad after collapsing at a local shopping mall. Mr. James is well-known to the staff because of his brittle diabetes and repeated problems over many years in maintaining tight control. You are completing his discharge papers so he can return home. As he is getting ready to leave, you say to him: "Mr. James, we are really concerned about your family health."

Take some time to carefully think about what you might have meant when you said this. Discuss the possibilities with some colleagues and identify ways they might interpret family health in this situation. After you have considered this, then think about how Mr. James might have understood what you said. How are the ideas similar? Different? What are the potential implications?

Developing Nursing Knowledge

The field of nursing has used borrowed theories in practice without thoughtfully considering their derivation, intent, or application. Although borrowed theories were once used without question, their appropriateness to nursing is sometimes questioned. How do we know that we know? *Knowing* is a dynamic process of experiencing and comprehending the self and the world and has both creative and expressive dimensions (Chinn & Kramer, 1991). Several years ago, Carper (1978) reviewed current nursing literature and described the four patterns of knowing as (1) ethics, or the moral knowledge of nursing; (2) esthetics, or the art of nursing; (3) personal knowledge, or intuitiveness; and (4) empirics, or the science of nursing. We might generally conclude that knowledge (e.g., values, ideas, facts, beliefs, ideas, information) is developed in many ways and is what persons possess within and are able to express, share, or communicate to others. Scientific methods or empiricism provides a foundation of knowledge firmly grounded in reality and provides the most objective knowledge because it has been tested and is supported by evidence.

 ### Cooperative Learning

Form a group of three or four persons. Discuss your individual worldviews or paradigms about what family health means. Identify where you agree and where you differ. Based on the group sharing, see if you can reach a consensus. In three to five sentences, explain the group's family health paradigm. Make a separate list of the areas where you did not agree or could not reach a consensus.

▓ The Family Health Construct

Notice the term *construct* as it is associated with family health. Constructs are invented for special scientific purposes and have intrinsic theoretical meaning, but they only possess empirical meaning when observational terms have been identified (Chinn & Kramer, 1991; Fawcett & Downs, 1992). Constructs are the result of thought and are not "immediately accessible to direct sensory observation" (Fawcett & Downs, p. 22). A construct implies that the combining or arranging of parts or elements forms something. Use of a construct provides a way to initiate discussions about relationships of complex ideas in a systematic way. Polit and Hungler (1999) define *construct* as "an abstraction or concept that is deliberately invented (constructed) by researchers for a scientific purpose" (p. 698). According to Kerlinger (1986), a construct is a concept with additional meaning and has been "deliberately and consciously invented or adopted for a special scientific purpose" (p. 27). Family health includes complex variables and is viewed as a construct.

Where does one begin to explain the term *family health?* If one is a linear thinker, then the logical thing would be to start at the beginning. But where does family health begin? Family health has individual, multimember, extended, and intergenerational perspectives that include individual and family variables. In other words, individuals have a set of characteristics, but being part of a family means that every individual is dynamically influenced by and influencing others. Family health is influenced by the state of the individuals that comprise the family, but it also has systemic processes that take place within a multimember group.

For instance, a mother may be home alone and feeling stress free. Three children arrive home from school clamoring loudly for snacks and are at odds with one another. At the same time, the family dog rushes into the kitchen with its muddy paws on the newly mopped floor. In a matter of moments, the mother has gone from peaceful well-being to major stress! Her equilibrium is unbalanced! She might begin screaming and threatening. What happens as the children encounter her wrath? The dimensions of the multimember group are not always predictable, just as the family health equation has many unknowns that are affected by time and developmental perspectives.

Family health becomes increasingly complex when the impact of extended family and kin relationships is considered. Even when members do not live in the same household and have infrequent contact, these members often continue to play roles in family health. In some families, the thought of the in-laws visiting or of a brother and his family spending an extended weekend have the potential to add to or subtract from family health. Intergenerational relationships often mean that support is available, but they also mean obligations and additional stresses may be implied. Extended family and generational relationships remind family members about responsibilities to maintain traditions, attend celebrations, and revere honored family relationships. The complex variables associated with family health are almost countless.

▓ Summary

Nurses require some foundational understandings about the frameworks that have been used to build nursing knowledge in order to more fully understand family health. This chapter provides background relative to knowledge development. It describes some troublesome aspects related to the meaning of language, and it discusses some problems that may occur when terms are not made explicit. Attempts are made to clarify what is implied by the term *family health* and make it accessible to readers.

Test Your Knowledge

1. Briefly explain what is meant by the term *concept*.
2. Describe what it means to operationalize a term.
3. Identify what is meant by the term *conceptual model*.
4. Define the term *theory*.
5. What is meant by the term *family health*?
6. Identify ways your personal beliefs about family health may differ from what has been described in the chapter.
7. Explain two or three reasons why nurses need to consider family health from broad perspectives.

Chapter

Family Concepts

3

CHAPTER OBJECTIVES *At the end of this chapter, the reader will be able to:*

- Identify the different ways *family* may be defined.
- Describe ways family diversity affects nursing practice.
- Identify a variety of ways to describe family health.
- Explain relationships between family health and ecological models.

Defining Family

> *Never doubt that a small group of thoughtful committed citizens can change the world; indeed, it's the only thing that ever has.*
> Margaret Mead

Confusion about concepts closely associated with family, family nursing, and family health makes discussions difficult. Much of the field of nursing's body of knowledge about family is in formative stages, and great opportunities still exist to clarify meanings, operationalize concepts, and formulate care models. Comprehensive and coherent models to guide family practice continue to be illusive. Stronger evidence about what defines family-focused care is still needed. Some attempts to describe family health have focused on dimensions such as functionality, psychosocial aspects, or the ability of members to successfully complete tasks. According to Anderson and Tomlinson (1992), family health is complex, lacks consensus, includes too many borrowed constructs, and is deficient in theoretical constructs that tie its multiple interacting systemic factors together. "The lack of specific paradigmatic emphasis that recognizes the family system, and the confusion of differing definitions of family

health leaves the direction of nursing practice and nursing research unclear"
(p. 57).

Families are viewed as systems, with the whole being greater than the sum of the
parts. Use of the term *family* seems to imply that others have similar assumptions and
meanings, but with the failure to make meanings explicit, the family will too often be
interpreted as white, middle class, heterosexual, two parents, and of Euro-American
ancestry. Many myths about families come from white, middle-class people's projecting
their experiences as national trends or uncontested facts (Coontz, 1992). Dominant
cultures have ways of swaying what characterizes a traditional family and what is
universally desirable and standard. The failure to define the term *family* explicitly means
that unintended ideas become standards for judgments, comparisons, and biases, and
that powerful groups distinguish others as "they" or "them." Newman (1997), speaking
about the nursing discipline and its paradigm, stated: "We are moving from attention on
the other as object to attention to the we in relationship, from fixing things to attending
to the meaning of the whole, from hierarchical one-way intervention to mutual process
partnering" (p. 37). In single published works, speeches, or conversations, authors,
policymakers, educators, and health-care providers often slide from one definition to
another without noting differences. What does it mean when religious activists speak
of family values? When legislators speak about family health? When physicians speak
of family practice? When nurses talk about family care? Ideas are too often oblique and
unclear.

Coontz (1992) has concluded that "there is no one family form that has ever pro-
tected people from poverty or social disruption, and no traditional arrangement that
provides a workable model for how we might organize family relations in the modern
world" (p. 5). The Western family seems to be in flux, and it is common to encounter
reconstituted, blended, single-parent, homosexual, foster, interracial, immigrant, and
homeless families. *MSN Encarta*, the online encyclopedia, defines *family* as a basic social group united through bonds of kinship or marriage that provides its members with
protection, companionship, security, and socialization. Legal definitions of *family* before the 1960s mostly described the nuclear family. Some laws have been contested, but
most state laws and local ordinances continue to support this view even though society
presents contrary evidence. In the United States, federal guidelines provide one way to
understand family. The U.S. Census Bureau defines *family* as a group of two people
or more (one of whom is the householder) related by birth, marriage, or adoption and
residing together; all such people (including related subfamily members) are considered
members of one family. A household may be composed of one such group, more than
one, or none at all. A family household is a household maintained by a householder
and includes any unrelated people who may be residing there.

A useful definition of family is "a group of people, connected emotionally and/or by
blood, who have lived together long enough to have developed patterns of interaction
and stories that justify and explain these patterns of interaction" (Minuchin, Lee, &
Simon, 1996, p. 29). A definition of *family* used in studying alcoholic families is "a
set of interconnected individuals acting together to produce a unique social unit that
changes in a predictable fashion over time" (Steinglass, Bennett, Wolin, & Reiss, 1987,
p. 13). A family "is characterized by two or more persons related by birth, marriage,
adoption, or choice," and possess "socio-emotional ties and enduring responsibilities,
particularly in terms of one or more member's dependence on others for support and
nurturance" (Allen, Fine, & Demo, 2000, p. 1). Stuart (1991) suggested critical family

attributes are:

- A family is a system or a unit.
- Members may or may not be related or live together.
- A family may or may not have children.
- Members have commitments and attachments to one another that imply present and future obligations.
- A family functions to protect, nourish, and socialize its members.

Focusing on member ages and family life stage (e.g., engagement, marriage, parent-hood, families with various aged children, retirement), subgroups (e.g., single parents, adolescent parents, families with chronically ill children, stepfamilies), context (e.g., cultural, social, political, historical, and temporal settings), and diversity (e.g., race, ethnicity, homosexual, interracial) are important issues when considering family def-initions. If family is examined as a collective unit composed of individuals, then four properties might be considered:

1. Absolute qualities that describe the individual
2. Relational qualities that explain member interactions
3. Comparative qualities that describe members' similarities and differences
4. Contextual qualities that describe features relevant to the whole (Lazarsfeld & Menzel, 1969)

A crucial aspect for describing the term *family* rests in knowing how individuals vary their conceptions across stages of family development and how and when a family of origin is transformed to a family of procreation (Brennan & Wamboldt, 1990). It appears that interpersonal communication and social transactions are germane to the development of family conception. Some agreement about family definitions may rest in seeing them as basic social groups, spousal units, cohabitational units, or parent-child units (Trost, 1988). Although some families stress consanguinity, conjugality, or sharing a domicile, others have few restrictions and accept a wide variety of social groupings as family (Trost, 1990). Perhaps an appropriate definition is "the family is who they say they are," a description that "is based on the family's beliefs about their conception of family rather than who lives in the household" (Wright & Leahey, 2000, p. 70).

Family definitions emphasize biological ties or structural relationships, functional and emotional relationship aspects (Amato, 2000), and members with long-term com-mitted relationships (Tomm, 1994). In her textbook on the family, Friedeman (1998a) defines family as "two or more persons who are joined together by bonds of sharing and emotional closeness and who identify themselves as being part of the family" (p. 9). In Hanson's (2001a) text on the family, she defines family as "two or more individuals who depend on one another for emotional, physical, and economic support. The members of a family are self-defined" (p. 6). A family is a group of individuals bound by strong emotional ties, a sense of belonging, and fervor for involvement in the lives of one another (Wright, Watson, & Bell, 1996). Friedemann (1995) says family is a structured organized unit that is composed of subsystems defined by emotional bonds and respon-sibilities that interact with its environment. Individuals comprising the family unit have relationships with the members, family, and environment. Ganong (1996) said families have an ethic of privacy, are value laden, are influenced by the sociocultural context, and multigenerationally continue over time. The term *family paradigm* refers to "the family's shared view of its environment [a view that] may be partly a product—directly or indirectly—of the perceptual and cognitive response dispositions of its members and the influence of these dispositions on one another" (Reiss & Elstein, 1971, p. 121).

Critical Thinking Activity

Use three pieces of paper for this assignment. On the first sheet of paper, write two different definitions of *family*, one from the perspective of what you know about families in the United States and one that captures a world or global perspective of the term.

When finished, pass your definitions to a classmate who can then suggest ways to modify or expand the definitions. Consider your classmate's suggestions and then rewrite your definition on the second sheet of paper reflecting his or her suggestions.

Next share your revised definition with a different student and repeat the process. Rewrite your final version of the definition on the third sheet of paper.

Compare the definition within your group and select the preferred definition. Have a group discussion about the process of defining families from different perspectives. What ideas did you learn from the critique of others? Did continued work on the definitions make them better?

Share your first and last definitions with some of your classmates. Identify if there are differences between definitions of families from U.S. perspectives and more global perspectives. What might be the implications for nursing practice and research?

Family Diversity

Tensions between those who view families from various perspectives lead to questions about whether an ideal family form exists or if a particular process has an inherent rightness that supercedes others. Debate about the superiority and rightness of a particular family type often persists as if members had some innate ability to independently choose among parents, ancestral heritage, and contextual background. The plurality in the modern world family differs greatly from past views of the ideal family, and myths about the "normal" family must be examined. Educators, practitioners, and researchers must grapple with ideas that "alternative" family forms are less "normal." McAdoo (1993) suggested that emphasis placed on family strengths and positive modes of adaptation provides positive approaches for addressing family diversity.

Teaching nurses and students about responsible interactions with families from diverse backgrounds must be undergirded with a strong commitment to fuller understandings about notions of cultural care, family diversity, and faithful allegiance to ensuring that culturally appropriate health care is provided (American Academy of Nursing Expert Panel on Culturally Competent Health Care, 1992). A general consensus exists within the field of nursing that culturally competent, sensitive care is necessary for meeting diverse client needs; however, ways to ensure effective modes to teach and fully learn principles are still conundrums. According to Friedman (1998), areas of family diversity that nurses need to consider include:

- Race, ethnicity, and religion
- The immigration experience
- Generational differences
- Language
- Class and poverty
- Residence and regional differences
- Family forms

Content about culture and family diversity need to be integrated as conceptual threads throughout curricula at the undergraduate, graduate, and doctoral levels.

Classroom lectures provide information and a theoretical basis for practice, but experiential opportunities are needed to fully understand caring responses to human diversity. Knowledge alone does not impart competence or proficiency. Rather, encounters with differences in ethnicity, race, gender, class, and sexual orientation through clinical experiences, practicum, and internships are needed so bias, prejudice, and other feelings can be personally engaged. Learning strategies that can be used to address family diversity include:

- Creating emotional climates that foster open contexts, respect for difference, and nonjudgmental attitudes
- Using assignments that expose divergent viewpoints and contradictory ideas
- Encouraging active student dialogue and engagement
- Using small groups to involve opinion-sharing conversations about multiple realities in diverse families
- Including reflexity or self-reflection as a teaching strategy to critically examine knowledge, experiences, and perspectives
- Discussing the realities of diverse families
- Selecting clinical sites that promote opportunities for learning experiences about diversity and culturally competent care
- Using writing assignments that include both interviews and library reviews (Friedman, 1998)

Respect for differences, tolerance of ambiguity, and discussions about diversity can be part of classroom and clinical experiences, but nurses must personalize them in terms of their own biases and prejudices. Oppression and discrimination are rooted in stereotyping, ethnocentrism, homophobia, and other "isms." Cultural competence means using opportunities to face the discriminatory actions and attitudes one often sees in others but ignores in oneself.

Allen et al. (2000) suggest some questions to consider and answer for embracing the diversity in families in the United States and the rest of the world:

- Should we focus on similarities or differences?
- What is the best way to characterize family diversity?
- Can and should families be compared against a benchmark?
- Can research on white, middle-class, heterosexual families be generalized to other families?
- Can outsiders understand insiders?
- Are existing family theories relevant for inquiries about family diversity?
- What criteria should we use to evaluate families?
- Should oppression and privilege be described subjectively or objectively?
- Why do different methodological approaches often generate different findings?
- Should we make our values about family diversity explicit?

Diversity is a critical issue that must be anticipated and addressed if nursing is going to attend to the schisms between the therapeutics needed to address health.

 ## *Reflective Thinking*

What is your cultural background? Although many Americans have great knowledge about their race, many have far less knowledge about their family ethnicity and any associated cultural traditions. If you do not know your cultural background, then you may want to gather some of this information from close and extended family members. After you have identified your cultural background, list 8 to 10 things from your family experience that seem pertinent to family health. How many of these items are culturally influenced? Discuss your findings and conclusions with other students and compare and contrast lived cultural experiences that affect family health.

Families within the Community Context

The preponderance of the evidence about family is compounded when families are viewed from household or contextual perspectives. Interactions with friends, neighbors, peers, coworkers, professionals, and others and relationships encountered at school, work, and play environments all have the potential to affect health. For example, a low-income single mother lives in a small apartment with two elementary-school aged children. The playground in the apartment complex is a thoroughfare for unemployed persons who have been known to misuse alcohol and abuse drugs. The children want to go outside and play. Their mother thinks the fresh air and activity would be good for them, but she keeps them inside because she has housework that has to be done and is afraid to leave them unsupervised. Does this neighborhood environment affect family health? If you were the nurse seeing this mother on her clinic visit, what information would you still need in order to suggest interventions to promote family health? What kinds of questions would you need to ask?

Laws, policies, social institutions, culture, traditions, and the media also affect families. Do these aspects have the potential to impact family health? If so, in what ways does this occur? Let us return to thinking about our low-income mother. She has just learned that the state laws governing her family income have changed. The new law states that she can no longer stay home with her children and receive welfare support. The law now demands that she go to school, work, or receive some form of training in order to retain her eligibility for welfare. Although she is willing to obey the law and appreciates the opportunity to improve her economic situation, she has concerns about the safety and care of her two children. Who is going to get them off to school, see that they are on the school bus, and provide after-school care until she arrives home in the evenings? The law provides financial coverage for transportation for her, but not enough for the many places she needs to go to ensure her children's care and safety until she returns home. Although the law provides some financial assistance, the places where the care is available entail leaving her children with strangers. Although this mother is concerned about the well-being of her children, she does not believe that taking her children to a stranger's home via public transportation in all kinds of weather increases their health. How does social policy and national law potentially affect family health? How does a nurse providing family-focused care respond to the larger systems that impact family health? What kinds of knowledge do family nurses need about health policy and advocacy?

Although family health is characterized by the complex ways household members interact within their context to obtain, sustain, and regain maximum health for all, this definition excludes the complex interactions with larger systems and nurse roles. Merely agreeing that family-focused care is needed to promote family health provides little direction for addressing complex care needs or evaluating outcomes. If family health is to be viewed as an achievable outcome related to family-focused care, then it seems logical that relevant family models and theories are needed. According to Gilliss

(1991a), in order to develop a science of family nursing, it is vital that "we are more attentive to the development of paradigms and theories that adequately address the nurse and family together" (p. 21).

 Critical Thinking Activity

Ms. Jones has called the health department for assistance, and you are the nurse who answers the phone call. She is quite distressed and is having some difficulty talking to you. It seems that she may be having a flight of ideas and is not thinking logically. She tells you that one of her children, a 2-year-old boy, is ill. He has been running a fever for several days and has vomited throughout the night. She also tells you that she has a 4-month-old infant and she has run out of baby formula. She explains to you that she is a single parent, has no transportation of her own, and has no insurance benefits.

What should you do to assist her? Prioritize the needs you have identified. What are the outcomes you want to achieve? List all the possible alternatives for helping her that you can identify. Which interventions will you select? What kinds of follow-up care do you think might be needed? How will you evaluate the outcomes? What does family health look like in this situation?

Family Care from Global Perspectives

Few models are inclusive enough to take broad ecological perspectives into considera-tion when thinking about the many variables associated with family health. Compelling evidence to substantiate that health is inextricably linked to the places where we live and the health of others now exists. Increased worldwide travel, growing rates of im-migration, and internationally linked economies provide proof that events that occur on one side of the globe quickly disperse. Infectious diseases and epidemics can spread swiftly with profound impact on families and communities throughout many continents (i.e., HIV, AIDS, mad cow disease).

The objective of the World Health Organization (WHO) is the attainment by all peoples of the highest possible level of health. Health, as defined by the WHO is "a state of complete physical, mental and social well-being, not merely the absence of disease or infirmity" (World Health Organization, 1944, p. 29). This ideal health state was later redefined as "the ability to identify and to realize aspirations, to satisfy needs, and to change or cope with the environment. Health is therefore a resource for everyday life, not the objective of living. Health is a positive concept emphasizing social and personal resources, as well as physical capacities" (World Health Organization, 1986, p. 426).

Health is characterized as a holistic phenomena and an ecological relationship of per-sons in relationship to their environment. In 1977, the World Health Assembly decided that the WHO's major social goal should be that all people attained a level of health that permits them to lead socially and economically productive lives. The purpose is not an end to disease and disability, but rather an assurance that medical services are available for everyone's needs and that targets are available to verify that health resources are evenly distributed and essential health care is accessible to everyone. The WHO's goal is to see that families are free from avoidable burden of disease so that they can shape their lives.

The WHO in Europe originated the idea of Healthy Cities in about 1985 and envisioned health as the result of more than medical care. The Healthy Cities movement spread to Canada and the United States and now includes projects in well over 1000 cities worldwide, with more starting all the time. People are viewed as healthy when they live in nurturing environments and are involved in community life. The Healthy Cities concept took into consideration the important influences of context or the places, surroundings, relationships, and opportunities related to individuals. The projects highlighted the interconnections among diverse elements and societal problems and suggested that the solutions to both community and quality-of-life problems were interwoven. Community strengthening and empowering are approaches used to solve problems, provide support, and increase health.

Family Systems

The term *family system* is often used to describe medical- and health-related professionals and resources that impact health and illness concerns of individuals who belong to families. The nature of family nursing has been argued from several perspectives over the years. Family as a system must be explained in terms of its complex interactions among the characteristics of its individuals and its unitary whole. Von Bertalanffy (1950) is usually credited as one of the first people to describe general systems theory. Family as a system has been viewed as foundation for nursing practice, and several have described this perspective (Friedemann, 1995; Friedman, 1998a; Hanson & Boyd, 1996; Hanson & Mischke, 1996; Neuman, 1989; Wright & Leahey, 2000). Tomlinson and Anderson (1996) suggest a family health system model that builds on the Neuman Systems Model (1989) "where family health embraces more than the health of individuals as a part of a family and recognizes the family health system as a central phenomenon of nursing practice" (p. 137) would be helpful. Steinglass (1992) stated that systems theory provides a meaningful way to integrate biology and family dynamics and was the best available framework to tackle issues related to primary care practice, clinical course of illness, and organization of service delivery. Friedemann (1995) describes the systemic organization of family in terms of environment, person, family, health, and family health with dynamic targets of control, growth, stability, and spirituality used by the system to find congruence. "The process dimensions of system maintenance, system change, coherence, and individuation encompass the concrete behaviors necessary to strive toward the abstract targets" (p. 10). Friedman (1998a) stated that the three grand theories needed to assess families are systems theory, structural-functional theory, and developmental theory. However, Doherty (1992) points out that there is no central family theory; rather, a variety of theories in the family science field focus on "how families create shared meanings, how families change over time, how families handle stress and resolve conflicts, and how families develop habitual patterns of interaction" (p. 31).

Family Nursing

One definition of family nursing is "the provision of care involving the nursing process, to families and family members in health and illness situations" (Friedman, 1998a, p. 34). Friedman states that family nursing is a specialty area that cuts across nursing specialties and depends on how *family* is conceptualized (i.e., family as context, family as the sum of its members, family subsystem as client, family as client). Names used for family nurses (e.g., family health nurse, family nurse practitioner, family nurse clinical specialist) add to the confusion about practice roles (Bomar & McNeely, 1996). Roles seem to differ based on practice settings, types of clients, beliefs and assumptions about families, and nurses' education levels. Family nurses have long focused on the provision of services and problem resolution rather than what promotes "the discovery and enhancement of family capacity" or the ability to promote their own health and healing (Hartrick, 1997, p. 65).

A difference in the way nursing care is delivered has to do with whether *family* is described as client or as context (Tomlinson & Anderson, 1996). Approaches to family nursing might be from four different perspectives and include family as context, family as client, family as system, and family as component of society (Hanson, 2001). Friedman (1995) differentiates between nursing of an individual within a family and nursing of the family system. She explains that a focus on the member within a family implies a need to consider the individual's systemic interchange with the family and the environment and nursing actions need to be congruent with clients' goals. Nursing of the family system is based on the family's judgment of what constitutes normality or congruence and is aimed at process dimensions and system maintenance.

Summary

Understandings about the term *family* are slowly moving in new directions, but for the most part, nurses mainly attend to the care of individuals with few concerns about family health. Many definitions of *family* exist, and nurses must make meanings explicit. Issues related to diversity are especially important when the focus is on family. Family health needs are closely aligned with household context—an area still needing to be more fully investigated. Nurses need additional education about family and the forms of practice needed to optimize health for all members.

Test Your Knowledge

1. Define the term *family* and explain three ways care might be different from merely providing care for individuals.
2. Explain why it is appropriate for addressing family related to individual health-care concerns and give an example of when it would be especially important.
3. Give three examples of family diversity and explain how these aspects may affect nursing care.
4. Provide a definition of *family health* and describe how your definition might influence the ways nursing is practiced.
5. Give an example of an individual health issue and explain how a nurse might target the family system to improve the outcome.
6. Give an example of an individual health issue and explain how a nurse might target a contextual system to improve the outcome.
7. Identify four things that nursing educators should be concerned about if they are going to teach student nurses about family care.
8. Describe what is meant by the idea of "think family."
9. Discuss three things that are important for students to learn about family nursing.
10. Explain whether an ecological or a systems model would be the better approach to meeting health needs.

Health and Family Health Concepts

CHAPTER OBJECTIVES *At the end of this chapter, the reader will be able to:*

- Differentiate between the concepts of health and family health.
- Identify several different ways the term *family health* is defined.

No one can whistle a symphony; it takes an orchestra to play it!
—Anonymous

Health is a concept that has wide recognition and many associated meanings. The term family health is widely used by health-care practitioners, including nurses, but the concept is seldom defined or operationalized. Although the phrase is broadly used in literature, authors often use the concept loosely within single works and fail to provide precise or clear definitions. The purpose of this chapter is to provide readers with a discussion about variables and factors related to health and family health concepts. Findings from the author's research about health and family health are provided.

Being Unhealthy

In the author's research about family health, composite definitions of *unhealthy, health*, and *family health* were derived. Being unhealthy was viewed as more than the presence of disease, illness, or disability (Table 4–1). The term was described as a condition experienced when pain or biophysical or emotional symptoms prevented the self-efficacy needed to perform usual tasks, created the inability to fulfill normative roles and social obligations, and created a sense of powerlessness in accomplishing previously desired activities. Subjects saw themselves as unhealthy when pain, biophysical symptoms, or emotional conditions interfered with their ability to fulfill desired activities. A key indicator of being unhealthy was the inability to perform the usual expected family roles and fulfill obligations related to duties and responsibilities. In other words, as

Table 4–1	Factors Viewed as Unhealthy

- Presence of pain or biophysical or mental health symptoms
- Disruption of usual roles
- Unfulfilled obligations
- Limited self-care
- Disparity between desired and actual behaviors

long as persons continued to perform some semblance of what members viewed as normative, they were considered healthy. This meant that members' chronic illnesses, disabilities, and even terminal illnesses were not necessarily interpreted as impediments to daily health activities and the suffering individuals were not always viewed as unhealthy. Self-care limitations were frequently described as unhealthy, especially when the limitations interfered with desired tasks and activities. Self-efficacy appeared to be an important measure for circumscribing the bounds of who was healthy or unhealthy.

Defining Health

In the author's dissertation research, health was associated with not being sick, but it extended beyond disease and illness. Participants described health as the absence of illness or disease and the ability to actively engage in daily life activities (Denham, 1997). Family members in the dissertation study described health in four ways:

1. The absence of illness or disease
2. The ability to actively engage in life
3. A balance among multiple family life dimensions
4. A holistic phenomenon with physical, emotional, social, spiritual, and ecological dimensions

Health was also viewed as a balance of multiple life dimensions such as members' needs, developmental characteristics, gender differences, and factors related to chronic conditions. Participants described physical, emotional, social, spiritual, and ecological relationships to health.

Participants in the study of family health during bereavement provided similar ideas about health, but they also added some factors (Denham, 1999b). For this subject group, health meant not being so sick that one could not work or be physically active. One participant said good health was being "fit enough to do what you want to do" and bad health "means you can't." As the subjects described what it meant to be healthy individuals, they described things such as the ability to perform usual daily activities, fulfill family roles, and be their own persons. Other things identified by most participants were the ability to maintain control over their lives, mental well-being, and faith or feelings of spiritual connectedness. Members with terminal illnesses were viewed as healthy as long as they could maintain some independence, complete some self-care needs, and participate in some activities of daily living.

In the third research study (Denham, 1999c) in which the participants were viewed as more vulnerable families, health was described as not being physically sick, having the ability to take care of basic needs, and feeling good about yourself and others. These family members discussed biophysical, emotional, psychosocial, environmental, and spiritual spheres of health. Many participants also described health in terms of routine patterns related to "healthy living." For example, they viewed eating right, exercising, performing self-care tasks, doing meaningful things, and having support systems as important factors for being healthy.

Findings from the research corroborate much of what is found in the literature and support the view that health is more than the absence of illness and disease. Participants described holistic aspects of health that included—but extended beyond—biophysical indicators. In all three studies, health extended beyond disease and illness and was often associated with:

- The ability to work or be physically active
- Not being sick
- The ability to take care of basic needs
- Having active participation in family roles
- The ability to have some control
- The ability to complete usual daily activities
- Having emotional well-being
- Having spiritual connectedness
- Having personal individuation

Even when suffering from an illness or coping with a terminal illness, others tended to view members as mostly healthy when they are able to maintain independence, complete at least some self-care needs, and participate in some activities of daily living. Health included the ability to have some control over self-care, participate in usual roles and daily life activities, and achieve meaningful accomplishments. Mental and spiritual aspects were repeatedly described.

Defining Family Health

Definitions should provide clear representations of ideas. Family health is frequently discussed, but few attempts have been made to provide a broad, overarching definition of the term. Although the literature reflects wide use of the term, it remains ambiguous and lacks conceptual clarity. References to family health often reflect the opinions, knowledge, and experiences of professionals, but family health research often lacks operationally defined concepts. Many nurses and others frequently refer to family health by describing functional, psychological, and biological aspects of individuals and families. Family health is often described as a goal of nursing, but clear, decipherable outcomes related to that goal are usually nonexistent. The current literature is even less consistent in providing clear definitions of family health than the health concept. Although families are often described as potential support systems for health, few family-focused investigations about family health have been completed (Backett, 1992; Duffy, 1988; Gilliss, 1991a; Ransom, 1986; Thomas, 1990).

Table 4–2 provides the findings from the three family health studies about the things the participants reported as family health influences. In the dissertation study (Denham, 1997), family health was described as a dynamic and complex concept more greatly influenced by multidimensional household variables, member interactions, and the cultural context than by individual members' occasional medical encounters. It appeared that the participants viewed family health as the dynamic ways members holistically cared for one another using communication, cooperation, and caregiving to develop and sustain health routines within the contextually embedded household. Subjects mostly viewed their families as healthy, but they reported that they occasionally experienced less healthy or unhealthy times. Individual members often identified themselves as "healthy families" even when a member was experiencing illnesses, living with a chronic condition or disability, caring for a dying member, or grieving a loss of a family member. The term *healthy family* was mostly used to explain a family state in which functional and relational aspects of life were viewed as manageable. For example, one family with three children described rather serious health concerns for two of them and extensive

Table 4-2	Family Health Influences

Study No.1

- Family context (e.g., family membership, extended family, spaces within the home, neighborhood location, peer and social relationships, biological heritage, cultural traditions, community resources, the larger environment, social policies, state laws, access to medical care)
- Family relationships (e.g., communication, coordination, caregiving)
- Participation in health-related routines

Study No. 2

- Family context (e.g., member resources, household factors, member assets or deficits)
- Family relationships (e.g., family togetherness, closeness, and fun; shared values among members; mutual respect, support, and care; shared sense of humor)
- Individual and family health behaviors

Study No. 3

- Family context (e.g., household resources or deficits, social capital, household and neighborhood factors, public policy, political milieu)
- Family relationships (e.g., processes of communication, cooperation, and caregiving influenced over time; family development; unique member needs and values; household boundaries)
- Member and family health routines (e.g., self-care, diet, mental health, family care, preventive care, illness care)

Source: Denham, SA: The definition and practice of family health. Journal of Family Health 5(2):133–159, 1999a; Denham, SA: Family health: During and after death of a family member. Journal of Family Nursing 5(2):160–183, 1999b; Denham, SA: Family health in an economically disadvantaged population. Journal of Family Nursing 5(2):184–213, 1999c.

disabilities for the third, but the family members still viewed themselves as a "healthy family" because they were able to provide for one another's needs, could manage the stress levels, and loved one another.

In the study (Denham, 1996b) that included bereaved family members who had used hospice services, *family health* was described as members caring for one another's well-being (i.e., mental, emotional, spiritual, and biophysical needs). Participants described family health as a collective experience influenced by values and goals in which members enabled one another to fulfill roles, accommodate changes, use household assets and resources, provide support, and address unique health needs. Families sought to find symmetry between solidarity and individual needs in order to balance the unpredictable competing demands. Although dying and death were viewed as unhealthy for that individual and stressful for the family, participants viewed members' shared time together during the experience as health promoting.

Economically disadvantaged families seemed more idealistic in their views of family health than the other family groups. They vacillated between hope and despair as they frequently faced erratic household changes and threatening systems that were beyond their control. Family health was described as a complex and dynamic balance of individual and family variables influenced by member interactions, household resources, personal and family routines, neighborhood threats and supports, conflicting values of the larger society, and institutional policies.

Family context, member relationships, and health routines were identified in all the studies as important family health influences. In the Family Health Model, family health is viewed as a process of multimember interactions and health-related behaviors that evolve over time that members use to attain, maintain, sustain, or regain the health of individual members and the family as a whole. Complex contextual factors that may or may not be under the family's control shape family health differently for diverse families. For instance, the Appalachian families in the studies viewed extended family, kin, and friends as more important family health determinants than specific health-care services or access to medical professionals. Although traditional medicine and health-care providers were viewed as important contributors to overall health, participants viewed household contexts, processes, and behaviors as more important family health indicators. It is surmised that other families with different cultural contexts have some different ideas and meanings associated with family health. All families have functional processes and routine behaviors that affect individual health practices and the family's definition of family health; these processes and behaviors are inextricably linked to the family context.

Family health is a dialectic challenged by the family health literature and research to integrate the interacting family development, family functioning, and health systems (Anderson & Tomlinson, 1992; Neuman, 1995). A *dialectic* is as a discourse or conversation in which methods of reasoning and intellectual investigation are used to engage beliefs, elicit truths, wrestle with opposing ideas, and examine the tensions among interacting forces. Unfortunately, the nursing discipline has mostly targeted care and services toward individuals and not wrestled as fervently as needed with the implications of the complex family systems. This neglect has resulted in continual slippage among ideas such as family as a system, family health systems, family nursing practice, health and illness cycles, family health, and family health promotion. Discussion of these concepts often results in confusion, with levels of meaning neither clearly differentiated nor easily discerned.

Family health is more than the sum of the health of individuals and is not clearly discernible through individual assessments (Loveland-Cherry, 1996). Friedemann (1995) describes family health as congruence, a dynamic process that occurs as a result of balancing stability, growth, control, and spirituality in response to a changing family environment. "'Family health' is a concept that is often referred to in the literature and is identified as a goal of nursing intervention; however, it is seldom defined." (Loveland-Cherry, 1996, p. 23). Mauksch (1974) emphasizes that a *family health estate* includes the interdependent relationships of health of the individual and of the family and that its exploration should be in terms of individual and family health–related roles, tasks, knowledge, attitudes, values, and beliefs. Tomlinson and Anderson (1996) have argued that "family health should link family structure, function, and health variables; incorporate the biopsychosocial and contextual system aspects of nursing; specify the paradigm view; and address the levels of family interaction with the nurse" (p. 137). Five realms of system level phenomena related to the family's experience of family health have been described in terms of processes in the areas of interaction, integrity, coping, development, and health (Anderson & Tomlinson, 1992). Family health care can also be described as the process of providing families with health-care services within the scope of nursing practice.

Family Health and Illness

The family health and illness cycle was originally developed by Doherty and McCubbin (1985) for a special issue of *Family Relations* as an attempt to organize the health and illness literature and provide a way to sequence family experiences. The cycle is best viewed as categories of family responses to illness and health as members interact with health-care systems through the phases of health promotion and risk reduction, vulnerability and disease onset or relapse, illness appraisal, acute response, and adaptation to illness and recovery. Viewing the family patterns might be helpful to family nurses as they provide care at specific time points and provide assistance when exploring previous illness-related experiences. However, "this framework does not capture the complex dynamics involved in multiple illnesses in family members," and the model does not "show all the important interactions between the family and other social groups" (Doherty & Campbell, 1988, p. 27). Additionally, the model makes the events appear as if they are separate occurrences rather than simultaneous ones.

Most attempts at health promotion have been viewed from individual perspectives, with less attention aimed at how to include and empower the family. *Health promotion* refers to activities aimed at maintaining or enhancing clients' well-being through the appropriate use of resources (Pender, Barkauskas, Hayman, Rice, & Anderson, 1992). Pender (1996) differentiated between health promotion (i.e., strategies related to potentiating individual lifestyle and personal choices in a social context) and health protection (i.e., strategies with environmental or regulatory measures that safeguard populations and thwart health insults). When family health is discussed, most would probably agree that health promotion and protection are also included.

Family Health in the United States

Who are the gatekeepers for family health in the United States? In actuality, one might argue that no gatekeepers exist; however, it has been the social role of government to protect the public's health. Goals of public health hinge on the need to protect the community against risks associated with interpersonal contact and communal life (Institute of Medicine, 1988). Public health aims at protecting, promoting, and restoring health by using science, skills, and beliefs to develop and enact social behaviors that change with technology and values. In the United States, many different federal agencies exist to oversee and direct health-related activities. The Department of Health and Human Services houses the Health Care Financing Administration (Medicare and Medicaid), Public Health Services, Department of Agriculture, Department of Defense, and Environmental Protection Agency are some of these agencies. Each federal department has many agencies, and multiple agencies often operate within similar areas of concern. Each state has a public health system that is responsible for the health of the residents within state boundaries. The business of public health is largely handled at the local level by county health departments. A principal responsibility of each county agency is to carry out the national and state mandates and manage a broad spectrum of health services. Agencies vary in their abilities to collect and analyze health data, respond to crises, plan for and evaluate health services, disseminate health information, and influence health policies locally. The events of September 11, 2001 provide evidence of ways federal, state, and local agencies can work effectively to address family health needs. These events also point out the deficiencies in some systems.

The American Association for World Health is the only private national organization in the United States dedicated to funneling a broad spectrum of critical national and international health information to Americans at the grassroots level. The organization's mission is to reach all rural and urban communities and aid local leaders to influence positive health practices by implementing programs that promote wellness and prevent disease. Since 1979, *Healthy People* has been a national health promotion and disease prevention initiative that brings together national, state, and local government agencies; nonprofit, voluntary, and professional organizations; businesses; communities; and individuals to improve the health of all Americans, eliminate health disparities, and improve the years and quality of healthy life (US Department of Health, Education, & Welfare, 1979). Goals of *Healthy People 2000* were to:

1. Increase the years of healthy life for all Americans
2. Decrease health disparities for all Americans
3. Increase the access to preventive health-care services for all Americans through targeting 22 priority areas related to health promotion, health protection, and preventative services (US Department of Health and Human Services, 1990)

These national health objectives have widely impacted the missions, goals, and planning objectives of state and local health departments throughout the nation.

Healthy People 2010 identifies 28 leading health indicators that represent the ideas and expertise of a diverse range of individuals and organizations concerned about the nation's health (US Department of Health and Human Services, 2000). National health objectives provide a road map to identify the most significant preventable health threats, establish national goals, and identify interventions that reduce these threats. The major premise is "the health of the individual is almost inseparable from the health of the larger community and that the health of every community in every State and territory determines the overall health status of the Nation" (US Department of Health and Human Services, 2000, p. 3).

Although annual costs of national health expenditures have steadily risen over the past two decades, the monies spent for public health remain only a small proportion of the total budget. In 1998, a total of $1,149.1 billion was spent on health care, but only 3.2 percent of these dollars were spent to address public health activities (National Center for Health Statistics, 2000). In 1998, 75.4 million persons made outpatient visits for medical care; this is an overall rate of 28 visits per 100 persons (Slusarcick & McCaig, 2000). Black persons had higher rates of visits than whites, and women visited more frequently than men. A total of 829.3 million visits by people seeking medical care in physicians' offices, or 3.1 visits per person, were made in 1998 (Woodwell, 2000). Although women (60.3 percent) made more visits than men (39.7 percent) to seek medical care from physicians, persons age 75 years or older each made an average of 6.6 annual visits. About 89.8 million of the total visits were injury related, with 70 percent of these identified as unintentional injuries. Blood pressure checks and upper respiratory infections were the most common reasons for seeking medical care. In 1996, there were 13,500 home health and hospice agencies that provided services to 2.4 million home health patients and 59,000 hospice patients (National Home and Hospice Care Survey, 2000). Although more than twice as many women received home health services than men, far fewer gender differences were noted when it came to those receiving hospice care. Almost all of these health-care episodes and costs were related to the needs of single individuals, with little, if any, attention aimed at family needs.

Nursing Organizations and Family Health

The International Council of Nurses (ICN) is a federation of national nursing associations that represents nurses in more than 120 countries. Founded in 1899, the ICN is the world's first and widest reaching international organization for health professionals that strives to ensure quality nursing care for all, sound global health policies, the advancement of nursing knowledge, worldwide respect for the nursing profession, and a competent and satisfied nursing workforce. The ICN states that individuals—given opportunities, knowledge, and access to services and resources—have the capacity to produce their own health and the health of their families. The organization focuses on globalization, identifying how health care and nursing practices need to respond and evolve. Health determinants and health promotion are viewed more broadly than by the traditional health sector. Health is viewed as related to many factors, including shelter, food, education, social security, health care, social services, income, respect for human rights, and employment. These determinants shape values, lifestyles choices, coping skills, and health behaviors. The ICN serves as a leader for thinking about nursing and the health of the world's families from international perspectives.

As a result of the ICN's commitment to addressing current health-care needs and concerns about nursing opportunities for practice, they have recently published a monograph entitled "The Family Nurse: Frameworks for Practice" (Schroeder & Affara, 2001). The monograph provides an overview of the author's knowledge about and experiences with family practice models in selected countries based on interviews, observations, and literature review. The monograph describes four different models for describing family nursing: (1) An individual family member is the client and the reason for initiating care, (2) family is client, but an individual family member is the reason for initiating care, (3) family unit is both the client and the reason for initiating care and services for families in specific communities, and (4) a variation of the first model but here the family nurse functions in two different health care areas utilizing case management, collaboration, and has a strong knowledge about individual health priorities. Each model has potential for use in international settings and requires a highly skilled nurse that has education and experience in many advanced areas of nursing. Aspects of the Family Health Model could serve as complementary to all of these family practices.

Sigma Theta Tau International, which was founded in 1922, includes approximately 120,000 nurses residing in more than 90 countries and territories, with 406 chapters located at 503 college and university campuses in the United States and other nations. This professional nursing organization aims to create a global community of nurses who lead in using scholarship, knowledge, and technology to improve the health of the world's people by increasing the scientific base of practice. The society seeks to aid in the development of more inclusive perspectives of professional practice that extend beyond North America.

Health in the Literature

Concerns about health research include the need to better understand the contextual aspects and differentiate between consumer and provider viewpoints. Colantonio (1988) found that laypersons were more concerned about functional messages and positive terminology when discussing health, but professionals were mainly focused on illness. Consumers define health broadly and suggest that practitioners and researchers use multidimensional health models (Kenney, 1992). It is important to view persons contextually when considering health and include "the social, political, and environmental factors affecting the health of differing populations" (Pender, Walker, Sechrist, & Frank-Stromborg, 1990, p. 122). High risk, ethnic diversity, biophysical characteristics, developmental levels, and cultural backgrounds are all contributory health factors (Pender et al., 1992). The literature has clearly shown that health is affected by poverty, culture, socioeconomic factors, and environment (Evans, 1994; Kagawa-Singer, 1993; McLeod & Shanahan, 1993; Nelson, 1994; Weinart & Long, 1987). Although health research includes many variables, factors related to the embedded context, developmental perspectives, and complex multimember interactions are largely ignored. Implications of health attributes, resiliency factors, and confounding antecedents are seldom fully considered. Fragmented and reductionist approaches to the study of health result in inconclusive evidence about the strengths of the competing relationships among the myriad of possible variables. Programmatic studies of health that include well-defined or operationalized family groups, longitudinal designs, interdisciplinary perspectives, and ecological frameworks are often missing when one reviews the body of literature that touts itself as family related. Practice and research that center on isolated variables and ignore the complex dynamic health relationships continue to impede knowledge development pertinent to family-focused care.

Family Health in the Literature

Family health definitions have been mostly given from the professional or expert position rather than from family perspectives, and semantic slippage is often prevalent within single investigative works. Definitions often reflect functional perspectives, less often include contextual points of view, and rarely include biophysical aspects. Family functioning and adaptation have been widely used to conceptualize family health (Barnhill, 1979; Bigbee, 1992; Fisher & Ransom, 1990; Friedmann, 1991; Grey, 1993; McCubbin,

1989). Others have explained family health from developmental perspectives (Blecke, 1990; Duvall & Miller, 1985; Lasky & Eichelberger, 1985; Lau et al., 1990). Family health has also been described as the household production of health, with the home identified as the developmental niche (Berman, Kendall, & Bhattacharyya, 1994; Harkness & Super, 1994; Schuman & Mosley, 1994). Family health has been investigated in relation to societal concerns (Franks, Campbell, & Shields, 1992; McLeod & Shanahan, 1993; Wise & Lowe, 1992; Zlotnick & Cassanego, 1992), in relation to patterned family behaviors (Bennett, Wolin, & Reiss, 1988; Boyce et al., 1977; Campbell, 1991; Fiese, 1993; Keltner, 1990, 1992; Rogers & Holloway, 1991; Steinglass, Bennett, Wolin, & Reiss, 1987, Thomas, 1990); and as a socially constructed phenomena (Backett, 1992; Cox & Davis, 1993). Despite all that has been written, models for understanding the depth, breadth, and scope of family health are lacking.

Anderson and Tomlinson (1992) noted that family health studies are thwarted by conceptual ambiguity, confusion in defining the unit of care, and a failure to include health as the central construct. A prolific body of literature that fails to provide a definitive description of the health phenomena increases the obscurity of the family health construct (Friedman, 1992). The terms *family health* (i.e., more than the absence of disease or dysfunction) and *family health promotion* (i.e., behaviors that increase well-being) are often used interchangeably, but a need continues to describe these ideas as distinct terms or concepts (Bomar & McNeely, 1996). The failure to clearly define the family health construct and the lack of consistency in its operationalization impede the usefulness of the family health concept.

🕴🕴🕴🕴🕴🕴 *Cooperative Learning*

It is amazing how easily things can be glossed over when we read and do not give careful consideration to what we are reading! Form small groups with your class. Each group should identify a specific family or health textbook to decide whether definitions are clearly provided for the terms *health* and *family health*. Groups should identify whether these definitions are consistently used throughout the text. If the terms are used differently, list these meanings and describe how they agree or conflict with the original definitions provided. Share the findings as an in-class discussion and discuss potential implications.

Test Your Knowledge

1. Describe what is meant by the term *health*.
2. Explain how the term *health* is different from *family health*.
3. Identify ways nurses' perceptions of health and family health influence their practice.
4. Do you consider *family health* and *healthy family* as different concepts? Why or why not?
5. Discuss your definition of *health promotion* and describe how it affects your current nursing practice.
6. Identify three ways national agendas or organizations perceive health and could influence family health practices.
7. Describe the work of a nursing organization that impacts family health.

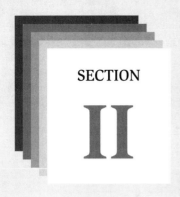

SECTION

II

Contextual Aspects of Family Health

Chapter

5

Family Context: A Dimension of Family Health

CHAPTER OBJECTIVES *At the end of this chapter, the reader will be able to:*

- Differentiate between views and consequences associated with holistic and reductionist thinking.
- Identify phenomenology as a perspective to understand the "messiness" of family health.
- Compare and contrast *family as context of care* with *family as unit of care*.
- Discuss the implications of contextualism.

Family Health from Contextual Perspectives

> *In the middle of difficulty lies opportunity.*
> *The important thing is to not stop questioning.*
> *Imagination is more important than knowledge.*
> —Albert Einstein

Nurses often discuss the term *environment* as an important aspect of individual and family care, but ideas associated with the term often remain vague and not clearly delineated. Most family models place greater importance on the innate qualities of individuals and the personal interactions between them than on the effects of the contextual environment where they live, work, and play. This chapter provides a foundation for deliberating about contextual care and emphasizing the importance of family context to family health. It is important that nurses understand where knowledge derives from and how it impacts practice. Family context affects family roles, member interactions, functional capacities, individual health behaviors, and family health. Nurses must gain greater familiarity with contextual aspects in order to understand the tremendous influence imparted by the embedded environment on family households and daily lives.

It is often suggested that family health should be considered from contextual perspectives, but full discussions about what this means related to practice are generally absent. Most discussions about environment have been about mechanisms relevant to individuals' health rather than family health. A literature review, which was completed to identify the ways nurses focused on the environment, indicated that the greatest focus was on the immediate or institutional environment from the patient's or nurse's perspective. Kleffel (1991) referenced a total of 53 studies, but only four studies focused on the local community, and a single study addressed the social, economic, and political contexts of the environment. Kleffel concluded: "There is a paucity of nursing literature dealing with contemporary environmental issues" (p. 44) and that nursing research seldom addresses the ecological causes of the prevalence, severity, and duration of illnesses. Descriptions of what characterizes family care and ecological perspective are often vague or missing.

Urie Bronfenbrenner, professor emeritus of Human Development and Family Studies and Psychology at Cornell University, has influenced persons from many disciplines through his work as a developmental psychologist, teacher, scholar, and contributor to social policy development. When Bronfenbrenner (1979) formulated his ecological theories of human development, he said the present state of developmental psychology was "the science of the strange behavior of children in strange situations with strange adults for the briefest periods of time" (p. 19). One might question whether nursing is largely a science about ill and diseased individual care, practiced in ill and disease care situations, with other illness and disease care providers for the briefest periods of time. Most nurses do not focus on health promotion, disease prevention, or risk reduction; rather, they focus on individual care for those seeking medical management for episodic illnesses or disease management in agency or institutional settings. Nurses are mostly acquainted with individual care and possess little knowledge and few skills to deal with family-focused care.

 ## Reflective Thinking

Nurses generally learn about family in their early nursing education and believe that because they occasionally talk with or encounter families in some ways that they are providing family care. Take some time and earnestly think about your personal experiences with patients and their families.

How much thought have you given to including the family in the care needs of the patient? How often do you seek to discover the diverse needs of patients and families as they live in their households? What things do you assess about the family? What interventions do you use that include family members in meeting client needs? When are you most likely to include families in your plans? When are you least likely to include families in your assessment, interventions, and evaluations?

> After you carefully consider your own experience, talk to a nurse colleague
> and brainstorm about things you might do to increase your skill of including
> family in your clinical practice. Discuss these ideas with others and identify
> variations in the ways nurses address family in practice.

Views of family from systems perspectives permeate much of the thinking in nursing and certainly help understandings about some health interactions. However, system thinking does not consistently include holistic or contextual perspectives that affect family care needs. Clear articulation of what is meant by holistic care and careful identification of implications could be a mammoth task. Although nurses give lip service to beliefs about holistic care and environmental impact, reviews of nursing assessments, care plans, interventions, and patient outcomes generally fail to produce evidence that supports these beliefs. Comprehensive models that address the holistic and environmental contexts believed important are mostly nonexistent.

Although medical approaches increasingly discuss the need for more holistic perspectives, most practice models continue to emphasize the family as a unit without fully understanding the meanings and effects of the members' family experiences in their day-to-day lives (Hartrick & Lindsey, 1995). Nurses seldom reflect on the impact of member interactions or the interactions with the environments as part of health. Challenges continue to develop knowledge that includes astute awareness of fundamental postulates, abilities to envision alternative viewpoints that perturb the current paradigms, and openness to marginal and current ideas (Hartrick, 1995; Maturana & Varela, 1992; Olds, 1992). In other words, nurses need to become discontent with the status quo experienced in practice settings and ask troubling questions. The development of innovative care models to address broad family needs will occur when nurses allow themselves to think outside present practices prescribed by the systems in which they are employed. Development of knowledge is an evolutionary process that questions previous conjectures and allows ideas to be reformulated when they result in practices that fail to achieve optimal outcomes, meet specified needs, or have meaning. Today's nurses stand on the edge of a practice frontier of family nursing and family-focused care that is yet to be fully engaged.

Cartesian Thinking

Rene Descartes (1565–1650), a mathematician, resolved that the world was dualistic and things could be solved in mechanistic ways. He asserted that the mind and body existed independently of one another, but each could be acted on by science. From a Cartesian perspective, one often arrives at the mistaken view that because the mind and body are separate, a single objective truth is possible, attainable, and desirable. Cartesian thinking has allowed us to dissect persons into distinct parts that detach them from the whole. Cartesian thinking allows us to view persons as objective reality that can be explained and known within their distinct parts. This type of thinking also permits us to think that minds and bodies are unconnected or at least not fully dependent on one another. This form of thinking means that when problems occur, solutions are sought to "fix the problem."

At the beginning of the 20th century, when the major causes of disease and illness were related to infectious and communicable diseases, Cartesian thinking allowed people to solve many dilemmas. Naming the problem, identifying the cause, and devising a cure resolved the solutions to many past scientific enigmas. However, results of Cartesian thinking often disallow potential confounding factors outside the dimension of interest and neatly resolve the "messiness" associated with problems. Cartesian thinking permits one to parcel health problems into parts or compartments. However, research supplies evidence about multiple causation of health risk and illness concern. For instance, psychoneuroimmunology provides evidence about the interconnections among emotions, the immune system, health, illness, and disease. Findings about abuse and violence provide evidence about the interplay of individual, family, environmental, and societal causes. Today's family health concerns focus on complex issues such as living with chronic diseases and disabilities and responding to new knowledge about genetics and diseases. Focusing on single health determinants and solitary cures in one realm seems too simple a solution for complex family health problems. If one aims to use the foundation of knowledge as a way to structure new models for future needs, then holding too tightly to traditions useful in the past may become stumbling blocks. To prepare for future health-care trends, insightful questions relevant to family health and current societal needs are needed.

Unraveling the "Messiness" of Family Health

Current technologies and practices are challenged by the "messiness" found in the complicated needs of today's families. Some needs inherent to family care are:

1. The diverse needs of multiple members
2. Difficulties with understanding the complex variables that potentiate and negate health
3. Interrelated causes of problems
4. Time-related effects of causes and treatments
5. Developmental variations of multiple persons sharing a common household
6. Longitudinal patterns across multiple generations

In order to fully understand the family health concept, it seems that greater attention is needed to the complex interactions over the life course of members' developmental processes within households that are embedded in evolving social contexts. Merely attending to individual medical needs seems shortsighted. Attention to short-term outcomes and costs and narrow consideration of long-term ones could ignore important evidence and preclude the critical thinking necessary to ascertain more beneficial family health outcomes.

Evolving family health paradigms need to be innovative, identify key priorities, and focus on comprehensive measures and interventions to meet the complex needs of today and tomorrow. Science concentrates on the objective—things that can be seen, heard, tasted, felt, or validated in measurable ways. Although the need to accumulate empirical data in scientific ways continues, the data must be expanded. Bronfenbrenner (1979) stated: "It seems to me that American researchers are constantly seeking to explain how the child came to be what he is; we in the USSR are trying to discover not how the child came to be what he is, but how he can become what he not yet is" (p. 40). Greater understanding about the impact of embedded contexts and social changes on present and future development and processes is needed.

The effects of context on functional processes are deeply entangled relationships that are not easily separated. Disentangling this "messiness" requires increased understandings about member-to-member, member-to-context, and family-to-context relationships. Member-to-member relationships occur within the household niche, but they are also influenced by things such as relationships, friendships, and acquaintances outside of the family. For example, peer relationships influence the thinking and actions of pre-adolescent teens, and employers affect the attitudes of parents. *Member-to-context* relationships are those that occur between an individual or family subsystem and settings beyond the boundaries of the household niche. Thus, church attendance and a youth's participation on a high school football team may both affect the family, but the impact on members may be different. *Family-to-context* relationships refers to relationships that occur between a family and embedded contextual settings beyond the boundaries of the household niche. For example, neighborhoods can influence a family's sense of security or risk, job adequacy, educational effectiveness, and accessibility to health-care services. Other contextual factors associated with family health are historical periods, economic conditions, political positions, and the social milieu.

 ### Critical Thinking Activity

Form a group with three or four of your classmates and work together to complete this exercise. Consider Bronfenbrenner's (1979) statement: "It seems to me that American researchers are constantly seeking to explain how the child came to be what he is; we in the USSR are trying to discover not how the child came to be what he is, but how he can become what he not yet is." Each person should first identify what it means to take the perspective of "explain how the child came to be what he is" and then the perspective of "discover not how the child came to be what he is, but how he can become what he not yet is."

After you have worked separately, then your group should share ideas, identify where you agree or disagree, and consider if the group brings new ideas to individual perspectives.

Objective versus Subjective Perspectives

In the past, subjective data were viewed as less verifiable and were often discounted by academics and scientists. Whereas inductive reasoning is the process of coming to conclusions based on evidence, deductive reasoning is viewed as an argument based on logical principles rather than the assessment of evidence. Empirical evidence is compatible with the results of systematic observation and experiments and has served to support or falsify theories, thus either affirming or denying the existence of foundations of knowledge. *Logical positivism* is a term applied to the philosophy that underlies the scientific approach and assumes that there is a fixed, orderly form of reality that can be observed and objectively studied. *Positivism* assumes that nature has a consistent order that is independent of scientific observation. Hacking (1983) described ideas characteristically associated with a logical positivist approach to natural science:

- Emphasis is placed on the difficulties associated with absolutely falsifying or verifying theories.
- Sensory observation is the basis for all genuine knowledge.
- Discussions of causation are really no more than talk about a concurrent confluence of certain types of events in a particular time and space.
- No physical necessity forces things to happen, so what remains are regularities between types of events and the ability to postulate wider ranges of possibilities.
- There is hostility toward things unobservable.
- There is opposition to metaphysics or the fundamental nature of reality and being, which are studies of things outside of objective experiences.

Popper (1959) stated that science seeks theories that are logically consistent and can be falsified. However, although scientific laws go beyond what can be actually experienced, we are left in the dubious position of never being able to absolutely prove truth; instead, we can provide evidence of fallacy. Popper concludes that a scientific theory must be provisionally accepted until it can be falsified, but even then the theories are not discarded based on single refuted incidents. He held that one should accept the theory that is best corroborated by evidence, provides the greatest number of true statements, and is most testable. If it is not possible to ascertain absolute certainty, then one is faced with understanding available truth. Popper argues that science is not subjective, but it is not fully objective, either. Although the inductive process might be viewed as the hard evidence outside the scientist who observes it, most now agree that the act of observation itself influences what is observed. Popper rejects the view that induction is the pinnacle of scientific investigation and substitutes falsifiability in its place. Individuals encounter reality based on perception; the things they choose to see; and the contributions their minds make as they interpret space, time, and causality. Popper's arguments allow us to conclude that although science implies seeking truth, knowledge is always limited in some ways by the ignorance of those pursuing it.

In current practice, nurses consider the subjective reports about pain as valid. In 1999, the American Pain Association (Dumas et al., 1999) stated that pain should be assessed as the fifth vital sign. The subjective report is recognized as a clinical measure that should be assessed with the same degree of respect and regularity as other vital signs. The objectively measured vital signs are not viewed as indicators of pain, but the subjective self-report using a numerical scale is viewed as the gauge of pain intensity. Empirical evidence has shown that individuals' reports about their pain experiences are reliable indicators. The acceptance of a subjective indicator as an optimum pain measure resulted after a body of research provided evidence of its value.

What do we do with self-reports in other areas? In clinical practice, a patient's reported experience is a desired part of the assessment process. At times, medical diagnosis is elusive and difficult to confirm, yet individuals continue to report persistent symptoms (e.g., fibromyalgia, reflex sympathetic dystrophy, phantom limb pain), and abnormal clinical laboratory values are not always easily linked to diagnosed problems. Although evidence about relationships between stress and systemic conditions (e.g., cardiac conditions, gastritis) continues to grow, diagnosis is often difficult when tests fail to identify problems. Assessment data includes symptoms, but it less often includes inquiries into causation related to contextual relationships or social conditions.

For example, a 23-year-old woman with type I diabetes is brought into the emergency department by a friend. The woman has a blood sugar of 626 mg/dL and is lethargic. The assessment results in prompt and appropriate medical attention, but only the immediate circumstances leading to the emergency and presenting symptoms have been appraised. The medical response is appropriate, the patient's blood sugar is lowered, her mental alertness returns, her functional ability returns, and she is discharged home after several hours in the emergency room. Although interventions are aimed at the immediate risks imposed by the emergency, far less is done to identify or intervene in the lifestyle behaviors, personal interactions, contextual factors, or the social structures that impact the individual's condition. After the emergency subsides, time is seldom taken to identify the family, peer, and social issues that support or threaten health. Interventions tend to be generic, and a "one size fits all" response is provided. The "messiness" surrounding complex family concerns often dissuades practitioners from providing more comprehensive approaches. Nursing has predominately aimed to meet the presenting needs without exploring alternative possibilities.

Nurse scientists intent on rigor in design often exclude contextual factors and thus eliminate the possibility of findings that could provide more comprehensive understanding about family health. For example, a researcher might take many approaches in proposing a study seeking to answer the question: "What causes differences in siblings' health-seeking behaviors?" Although discrete individual holistic characteristics of siblings might be investigated and analyzed, important factors might not be included. Variations among siblings' health and health behaviors related to their unique genetic makeup, age, and gender might be considered, and concepts such as motivation and self-efficacy may be included in a study. However, it is less likely that family functional status at different developmental stages of each child, variations in life course, peer relationships, and nonshared environments would be explored. The effects of discrepant peer relationships and nonshared environments may be essential determinants for understanding variations in the health conditions of multiple members. More inclusive models for conceptualizing the "messiness" associated with holistic care and embedded context are needed.

♦♦♦♦♦♦♦ Cooperative Learning

The following task has three components.
1. Identify what the term *holistic care* implies to the student.
2. Identify what things might be considered the "messiness" of holistic care.
3. Analyze how nurses can assess and intervene in the "messiness" of holistic care.

Form groups. Each group should discuss individuals' descriptions of holistic care and come to some consensus about a definition. Then each group should list all the things they perceive as the "messiness" of holistic care. After the list has been completed, prioritize the list twice: (1) based on the importance for nurse assessment and intervention and (2) based on patient and family need.

Compare the two lists and identify where they differ. What implications do these differences have for nursing practice?

When all groups have completed the assignment, groups should share their definitions of holistic care and what they discovered about the "messiness" of holistic care from nursing and patient perspectives. Is there a consensus about specific ways nurses might better intervene in providing holistic care?

The Naturalistic Paradigm

A response to the logical positivism of scientists has been a naturalistic paradigm in which reality is not viewed as a fixed commodity but instead is seen as a construction of the individuals participating (Politt & Hungler, 1999). *Postmodernism* is a term often associated with naturalistic paradigms, and it implies a way to take apart or deconstruct old ideas and structures and rebuild or reconstruct them in new ways (Politt & Hungler, 1999; Ward, 1997). A postmodern perspective is less about unearthing or labeling an objective existing truth and more about placing things into categories or reframing them in particular ways; it is more about bringing ideas forth and less about discovering distinct qualities (Ward). Researchers who use naturalistic perspectives are inclined to view reality as relative and possibilities of different interpretations as observations. Aims are not to falsify or verify the constructions, but merely to observe them.

In the past, findings from qualitative research and naturalistic studies were often viewed as less scientific. Presently, qualitative findings are perceived more positively and considered a way to develop middle-range nursing theories. Qualitative research provides the opportunity to focus on questions related to social experiences, address questions about the ways life experiences are created, and describe things that give meaning to life (Denzin & Lincoln, 1994). Simple discussions about a single reality are difficult, and qualitative research helps explore the multiple realities that coexist. Using naturalistic perspectives seems an appropriate way to understand family health because it is a complex construct with many seemingly unrelated variables. Nurses come into practice with different perceptual realities based on their life experiences, personal values, beliefs, and traditions. These realities create lenses through which knowledge is built and experiences about family health are interpreted.

Phenomenology

In clinical practice, nurses continuously interpret situations and project possibilities. Interpreting requires understanding about what is to be interpreted. The projection of possibilities can only occur after understanding occurs; some might refer to this as circular rather than linear thinking. Nurses who maintain separateness or take aloof positions are at risk for misinterpreting things that others view as meaningful. Prior knowledge and experience can provide frames of reference that may be deterrents to discerning the meanings of others' experiences. The term *bracketing* is often used to imply the need to make visible what one believes and a willingness to set it aside in order to comprehend the phenomenon of interest. Nurses who desire to understand experiences contrary to their own must acknowledge and set aside personal beliefs, values, attitudes, biases, and prejudices and appreciate the perspectives of others.

The family context provides information interpreted through experiences and provides a way to appreciate diverse viewpoints. For example, a recent HBO program called *The Corner* provided an alternative point of view about family, drug use, and health. Although nurses would generally see being high on drugs as unhealthy, drug addicts in this program saw the "daily fix" as the way to "get well." Whereas other family member saw the inability to obtain drugs as health negating, outsiders saw fiendishly seeking drugs as being unhealthy. Another's perspective provides a way to reframe situations. Goals and viewpoints of others are often different from those of professional helpers; unless the "expert" is willing to have a dialogue about the disparate values, it is unlikely that the help given can alter behaviors.

Studying family health from contextual perspectives implies coming to understand developing persons within the ways they interpret essences and through their experiences. Family health is a collective memory experienced by individuals within the embedded context and shared in some respects by others. Van Manen (1990) states that persons have consciousness and act purposively "in and on the world by creating objects of 'meaning' that are 'expressions' of how human beings exist in the world" (p. 4). He emphasizes that the purpose of phenomenology is not to solve problems but to understand meanings. *Phenomenology* is a means of understanding family health within the context of experience (Hartrick & Lindsey, 1995). Phenomenology aims to make phenomena explicit, identify universal meanings, and describe ways that nurses can encounter families in naturalistic or household settings.

Georg Hegel (1770–1831), Edmund Husserl (1858–1938), Martin Heidegger (1889–1976), Jean-Paul Sartre (1905–1980), Hans-Georg Gadamer (1900–), and Paul Ricouer (1913–) have been viewed as the foremost philosophers in the study of phenomena or field of phenomenology. Phenomenology begins with concerns about experience and conscious awareness and "is a rigorous science whose purpose is to bring to language, human experiences" (Streubert & Carpenter, 1999, p. 61). Patton (1990) distinguishes between phenomenology as a philosophic perspective and as a research method and notes that phenomenological inquiry focuses on the question: "What is the structure and essence of experience of this phenomenon for these people?" (p. 69). Phenomenology strips away the particular and objective and encourages views of essences. *Essences* are defined as "elements related to the ideal or true meaning of something, those concepts that give common understanding to the phenomenon under investigation" (Streubert & Carpenter, p. 46). Individual and collective thinking about things, persons, and events identifies the essences of shared experiences, but they may also be a way of speaking them into existence, valuing meanings, and developing a common language to explain experiences. Language helps us name and know things in our experience. Essences are sometimes referred to as viewpoints, perspectives, or paradigms, and they provide opportunities to be present in worlds viewed differently from others. Families encountered in practice are likely to have essences that differ from those of the nurse.

Hermaneutics, or the study of interpretation, is an important aspect of phenomenology and naturalistic inquiry. Heidegger (1962) said understanding begins when language resists meaning and ends when language yields meaning; thus, we can only project possibilities when we have adequate understanding. Heidegger gave hermeneutics an ontological dimension, which he referred to as *dasein,* a term used to describe understanding and interpretation as essential features of being. Understanding and interpretation seem somewhat circular as the past is brought into the future. Gadamer (1994) said understanding starts when language resists meaning and ends when language yields meaning. In order to fully understand family health, projected meanings must be discovered, interpreted, and analyzed. Continual dialogue with a family about their situation results in communication about their particular situation.

Gadamer (1994) described experience as what occurs when we encounter the negative or unexpected and it awakens us to the insights that can be gained from other situations. Insights are realized when statements are seen as responses to questions. The only way to fully grasp a statement is to understand the question to which the statement is an answer. The question directs its own meaning and is realized by the response. According to Gadamer, the search for a question partly involves determinations about the context and community that give rise to the answer. Either the situation or the persons who are subjects of inquiry do not always foresee the conclusions. According to Hartrick and Lindsey (1995), nurses have gathered information but have forfeited understanding of the information; have diagnosed family functioning but have failed to recognize the experiences and meanings of family health; and have focused on diagnosis and treatment but have neglected to address health promotion and healing processes. The field of nursing has not yet clearly delineated what is meant when the context of a family's lived experience is referred to, and this can be a problem for describing the scope of practice.

🕴🕴🕴🕴🕴🕴 *Cooperative Learning*

List the ways quantitative and qualitative research perspectives can provide different understandings about health and family health. Discuss the differences that should be considered in studying individuals versus families. Compare the benefits and the threats to discovering knowledge posed by each perspective.

Examine two different research studies relevant to family health; one should use quantitative methods, and the other should use qualitative ones. List the benefits and threats identified in each study. Discuss ways each study contributes to nurses' knowledge about family health.

Contextualism

Clinical practice lacks appropriate assessment tools, intervention strategies, and evaluation measurements necessary for family as unit of care. Bell (1995) described the isomorphism of nursing as a situation in which the processes in one system influence those in another system, with the result being functionally similar outcomes. Whenever isomorphism occurs, repeated patterns interfere with the production of creative thinking, innovative ideas, and new visions. Isomorphism can occur when teachers encourage students to learn in ways that result in lockstep adoption of predominant attitudes and ideas without critically weighing alternatives. Isomorphism occurs when institutions socialize practitioners and discourage questioning traditions or majority actions. Isomorphism can also occur when patients influence nurses to think about family issues in the same ways they do. Bell stated:

> Isomorphism describes the suction we fight when it is easiest to simply repeat the pattern of the dialogue that maintains more of the same in family nursing. More descriptions of family responses to health and illness at the expense of describing and testing interventions are more of the same. More descriptive studies of questionable rigor that fail to address the research issues that are unique to the study of families are more of the same. More research reports at the risk of undervaluing clinical practice issues, teaching strategies, or discussions of family theory and policy are more of the same. More bland and safe discussions at the risk of raising controversial issues for critical debate and scholarly inquiry are more of the same (p. 6).

Family nursing needs practitioners, educators, administrators, and researchers who are ready to think beyond traditions and dare to be different. Models that conceptualize the multiple threads of the embedded context are needed to supply more succinct understandings about the overt and covert implications of member-family-context relationships. "Contextualism views any events in the context of other events and presupposes a multiplicity of events in which the past, present, and future form a coherent and interconnected totality" (Hartrick, 1995, p. 140). Ecological perspectives support understanding the meanings of past, present, and future phenomena of family experiences.

Family as Context

Family's Multiple Contexts

The family itself is a context for its members, but it is also embedded into multiple contextual systems in ways that all family members may not experience simultaneously, consistently, or congruently. In other words, individual members within families have different experiences, so each member and the member interactions contribute to the exchanges that comprise the family's contextual view. Members' views of their context are fluid, evolve and change over time. They have contrasting views that cumulatively provide insight about family health. The family configuration and membership has myriad possibilities. Assumptions about who comprises the family should be avoided;

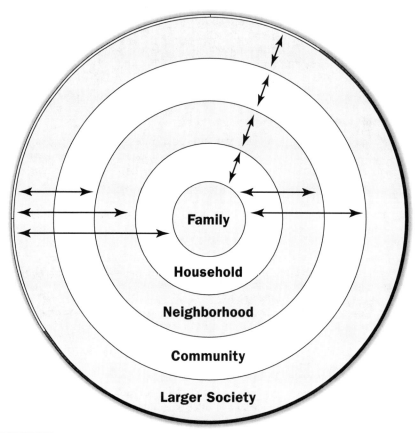

Figure 5-1 Family as context.

instead, the reported information provided by members should be identified. Families are composed of members who may be related through marriage, blood, or numerous situations resulting from choice. The likelihood of meeting Western families of the more traditional type or what we have called *nuclear families* is far less likely than in earlier historical periods. Regardless of the immediate family state, the trajectory of members' lives together over time includes situational changes that may have profound, lasting, distinct, uncommon, and diverse effects on its members.

The family is a context for its developing members, but it is dynamic and evolves over the life course. Members do not always perceive or interpret alterations in similar ways. While the family is evolving, the larger societal environment or the embedded context creates direct and indirect effects that also impact members. The family consists of individual developing members, dyads, and triads embedded in household, neighborhood, community, and greater societal contexts (Fig. 5-1).

Family members affect and are affected by each contextual aspect. Members interact with one another within some shared contexts and react to one another as a result of what is experienced within nonshared contexts. Members encounter similar and dichotomous experiences as they encounter their various contexts throughout the life course; these all have the potential to affect individual and family health. Singular and shared experiences result in both individual and collective meanings that impact the family's identity.

Leaders in the field of family nursing have repeatedly called for the discipline to more concertedly consider the family as the unit of analysis (Feetham, 1990; Gilliss, 1983; Uphold & Strickland, 1989). Although increased focus on the family as the unit of study has occurred, most clinicians still lack the knowledge and skills necessary to differentiate between the family as the unit of care and family as the context of care. *Family as the context of care* implies that individuals are the focus of care, and family is the backdrop. In contrast, *family as the unit of care* implies an understanding that within the family dwell individuals who have unique needs and share some common characteristics, traits, strengths, resources, threats, and liabilities. However, if the family is the unit of care, then it becomes a target of care even when interactions relate to individuals. The focal point of family-focused care is family as the unit of care.

Family as the Unit of Care versus the Context of Care

Whenever family is the context of care, attention is mainly focused on individuals' needs, with less consideration given to the linkages between the individual, family, and family context. Care is generally aimed at meeting the presenting individuals' specific needs, but little attention is directed at the precipitating family history, past or present member relationships, or future goals or expectations. When the family is viewed as context, the care provided usually implies that treatment, education, and counseling have addressed the symptomatic needs of singular persons with minimal input of family members. From this perspective, caring seldom seeks to identify the strengths, resources, needs, relationships, and behaviors of the entire family in relation to the needs of the individual. From a practical sense, nurses who see the family as context often ignore the strength or threats imposed by the family as members impact one another and the effects of interactions on the family as a whole (Table 5–1). When the family is the context of care, clinicians often make assumptions about families based on the needs and perceptions of a single individual. Family as context may include some assessment of family-related information, but interventions are mainly aimed at single individuals. Considerations of alternative care forms that include the entire family, or at least some other members, seldom occur.

When family is viewed as the unit of care, the scope of family takes on a more holistic and inclusive view of the multiple members and their interrelated strengths, unique limitations, and shared resources. Individuals have distinct differences that include biophysical characteristics, perceptions, values, behaviors, and meaning making that may be similar to others in the family but may also differ. Family as the unit of care implies an understanding about potential health impacts that result from member relationships, interactions, and transactions. Family members perceive a family identity and often view members as connected to or separated from this identity. This family

Table 5–1   Family as Context versus Family as Unit of Care

Family as Context	Family as Unit of Care
Individual is focus of care	Individual and family are target of care
Family is in the backdrop	Family is in the forefront
Family is composed of individuals	Family is a unified whole
Individual data reflect family	Family data reflect individuals
Care of individual	Family-focused care includes family group, individual, family subgroups, family contextual systems

identity often has links to multiple members' beliefs about health, wellness, disease, illness, and health-care services. Viewing the family as the unit of care implies that the family includes individual members even when they are not currently dwelling within the household. For example, if a mother gives up a child for adoption or if a member dies, the effects of these relationships continue even years after the occurrence. Likewise, adults retain linkages to their families of origin even when they have relocated, and families of procreation affect members even when they do not live within the same household. Family as the unit of care creates long-lived associations that linger over the life course and are pertinent to individual and family health.

The family context is largely embedded. In other words, although family members have some awareness of the multiple realms that characterize their ecological context, few individuals could fully describe linkages without some prompting through an assessment process. Assessment requires a high level of communication expertise in order to interact with families and their members at individual, relational, and transactional levels. Wright and Leahey (2000) provide an excellent discussion of communication skills and interview techniques for conducting family assessments. Their text is highly recommended as an additional source for learning about family communication, interviewing, and counseling.

Assumptions about Family Context

Assumptions about the family context form are foundational to the Family Health Model. Assumptions are the notions or axioms that are usually taken for granted but assumed to be true. Table 5–2 discusses the underlying assumptions related to family context that were instrumental in conceptualizing the family as context in the model.

These underlying assumptions identify the bias that family health is directly and indirectly influenced by the embedded context in which families dwell. Context begins with the members themselves, but it also includes all aspects of the larger societal systems. The context is the stage for interactive relationships and discourse, the places where functional relationships occur, and the settings for enacting family health routines. The family context is integral to health and provides multiple settings where members are positively and negatively influenced over the life course. The context not only includes family members and the household location but also the politics and the social and public policies of the historical time that impact a given context. As the context is altered over time, family health is influenced by factors related to the multiple life contexts. The length of time in a given context may influence members, and even brief periods can have profound and lasting effects. Older persons have been significantly impacted

---

Table 5–2 **Assumptions Related to Family Context**

- Family context has robust implications for individual and family health.
- The family context is dynamic and interacts with individuals, family systems, and families.
- Individuals are affected by the family context even when they are not present in it.
- Some aspects of family context can be directly observed as well as manipulated, but some aspects are more discreet, less observable, and difficult to manipulate.
- Actions and responses that affect any single-family member or aspect of the family context have the potential to affect the actions and responses of other members.
- The assessment of the family context includes data about individuals, family subsystems, family, and the embedded household context.
- Context contains traits related to persons, places, events, situations, social mores, and time.
- Culture, tradition, religion, and social values are contextual determinants.

by the context of their families of origin, which continues to be an important influence across the life course.

🏃🏃🏃🏃 *Cooperative Learning*

Assumptions provide a foundation for understanding implications of comprehensive assessment of family members and their ecological context. Form a group of three to four students. Each student should read through the list of assumptions related to the contextual aspects of family health and make notes about his or her immediate impressions. After everyone has had time to review the assumptions, the group should spend some time discussing them, sharing their impressions, and identifying where they agree or disagree. Each group should reach a consensus about the two most important assumptions a family nurse should consider and be able to state a rationale for their selections. After the groups have adequately discussed their ideas, they should take turns sharing their ideas with the entire class.

Summary

Nurses often overlook contextual perspectives when they consider health. Assessment that ignores pertinent factors imposed by the embedded context often results in conclusions and interventions that overlook important health determinants. Focusing on pathology while ignoring pertinent contextual factors too often leads to care that treats symptoms but ignores causes. Failure to see the impacting causation as possibly environmental, systemic, and outside the individual results in seeing events as solitary rather than contextually embedded. At times, individuals are blamed for causes of problems, and the impact of community or environment as causative agents is overlooked. Thus, responses are too often made only in terms of the individual, with inadequate responses to community, social, and political events that may be germinating agents. Family-focused care must include the family as the unit of care. Primary care needs to include families and where members live, work, and play. Views of family households as a primary context for health broaden the scope of possibilities for causation and cure. In order to address the health needs of families, nurses must acquire knowledge, skills, and experience that are based on broader understandings about the effects of embedded contextual systems.

Nurses prepared at the generalist level may not be adequately equipped to fully implement care plans appropriate for family as the unit of care. Although diseases and illnesses may be central in individual care, today's concerns involve systemic issues such as violence and abuse, substance abuse, early intimate sexual encounters, peer pressures, caregiving for members with chronic illnesses, lack of resources, and inadequate supports. Health risks are often related to problems such as income disparity, educational inequities, family fragmentation, underemployment, lack of skills, poor housing, and risks imposed by the environment. Nurses require better understandings about the family context in order to be equipped to address family needs. High costs associated with health care compel practitioners and care providers to envision alternative ways to meet demands. Although medical management will always be appropriate, possibilities related to the family as the unit of care need to be more carefully conceptualized.

Test Your Knowledge

1. Thoroughly describe what is implied when nurses speak about providing holistic care.
2. Describe what is meant by the idea of family context. Give three examples.
3. Identify differences between the ideas of empiricism and naturalistic inquiry.
4. Discuss the advantages and disadvantages of objective empirical data.
5. Discuss the advantages and disadvantages of subjective qualitative data.
6. Explain what is meant by the idea of family as the context of care.
7. Operationalize the idea of family as the unit of care and list three ways nurses might intervene if the family member receiving care has asthma.

Chapter

6

The Family Microsystem as the Context of Family Health

CHAPTER OBJECTIVES *At the end of this chapter, the reader will be able to:*

- Identify traits and dimensions pertinent to the family microsystem.
- Explain potential relationships between aspects of the family context and health.
- Compare and contrast the potential effects of the family context on the processes of becoming and well-being.

Ecological Contexts

> *There are many hypotheses in science which are wrong. That's perfectly all right; they're the aperture to finding out what's right. Science is a self-correcting process. To be accepted, new ideas must survive the most rigorous standards of evidence and scrutiny.*
>
> —Carl Sagan

Contextual ideas are similar to invisible threads that link life aspects across time and persons or subliminal themes that impact and influence throughout the life course. The impact or influence of these contexts may not be obvious or immediately evident and may be easily overlooked or thought to be insignificant. This chapter more fully explains the contextual perspectives of family health germane to the family microsystem. Contextual systems are multidimensional, potentially static or dynamic, global in perspective, transactional in nature, and mediated by individuals' actions (Wachs, 1983). Ecology is a science concerned with relationships between living organisms and environments, but the term also refers to experiences that affect organisms. In the Family Health Model, the context refers to the forces, processes, and experiences that shape health over the life course. The ecological context provides a way to appreciate health from diverse cultural, ethnic, racial, religious, historical, political, sociological, and international perspectives. Ecological contexts affect all persons regardless of where they are born or the places where they live. This chapter describes family's contextual factors and explains potential health relationships.

Familiarity with the language of ecological systems is important for understanding the potential impact of embedded context on health. The Family Health Model uses the terms *microsystem, mesosystem, exosystem, macrosystem,* and *chronosystem* to identify the concentric contexts that affect health (Box 6–1). These concepts provide ways to conceptualize relationships and interactions pertinent to the well-being and processes of becoming associated with development and health. It is not possible to discuss all the possible relationships between context and family health that exist, but some examples are provided in this chapter. Better understandings about the contextual systems should offer ways to envision how unique and shared environments affect developing persons and families. Infinite variations exist in the ways families define themselves, exchange information, and interact with larger environmental systems. Family context might be compared to a labyrinth with complex pathways, dead ends, and endless unanswered questions. The context provides a way to view family health from alternative paradigms.

Box 6–1 **Terms Associated with the Embedded Ecological Context**

Microsystem
The microsystem is the immediate and principal environment in which developing persons and significant others share meanings, objects, resources, and information. It includes interactions between individuals, subsystems, the family, the household niche, the neighborhood, and the community.

Mesosystem
The mesosystem is the multiple settings in which individuals actually participate. Although these settings may not be physically connected, they are not independent of one another.

Exosystem
The exosystem is the multiple settings in which developmental processes related to individual and family health occur. Although the individual does not actually participate in them, these systems still directly affect developmental processes, well-being, and health.

Macrosystem
The macrosystem is the complex, interrelated, and shared societal systems (e.g., ideology, political systems, social institutions, laws, morality). It characterizes the culture or subculture and includes things such as ethnicity, socioeconomic factors, religious beliefs, and traditions that have the potential to impact individual and family health.

Chronosystem
The chronosystem refers to passages of time and the altering changes related to individuals, families, and embedded contextual systems. Measurement and influences of change can be measured over time, through the life course, and by historical periods.

Source: Ideas based on Bronfenbrenner, U: The Ecology of Human Development: Experiments by Nature and Design. Harvard University Press, Cambridge, Mass., 1979; Bronfenbrenner, U: Ecology of the family as a context for human development: Research perspectives. Developmental Psychology, 22:723–742, 1986, with permission.

Ecological dimensions contain ideas about factors that contribute to and confound family health. By examining each area separately, one can more clearly distinguish between variables associated with specific contextual spaces and identify places where overlap, intersection, and boundaries occur. Just as a set of Russian dolls has similar and different characteristics, so do family's embedded systems. Greater appreciation for the impact of space, time, and family traits enables one to differentiate between various triggers with potential health effects. Although it is not easy to discriminate contextual spaces or dimension, an ability to identify these spaces as internal or external to the person and family provides additional ways to understand health.

Impact of the Ecological Context

The pervasive impact of ecological contextual systems begins in early life—perhaps even in utero—and retains the potential for causal relationships throughout the life course. The technical languages used by various disciplines are often divisive and interfere with communication. It is purported that considering prospective causes embedded in family context can increase understandings about health. Buying into the idea that the context (e.g., family culture, community resources, social milieu, political ambience) is a key determinant that affects health refutes assumptions that health problems are mostly inherited or lifestyle traits. Views that context and health are correlated implies things such as:

- Health risks are influenced by social and political policies.
- Accountability for sustaining the environment is a global responsibility.
- Population-based care may hold greater promise for family health than continued focus primarily on individuals.

The Family Health Model assumes that the family is affected by:

- Members' inherited and acquired traits
- Relational interactions among individuals, subsystems, and families as they are impacted by and impact context over the life course
- Relational interactions with others beyond the boundaries of the family of origin and procreation
- The cultural, social, economic, and political influences of the embedded household niche
- Health information, knowledge, skills, and experiences of family members and others with whom the family interacts
- The beliefs, values, traditions, behaviors, and routines of family members and related others
- Threats, risks, and the availability of resources

As stated earlier, the contextual domain has an internal and an external environment. The ecological context includes traits of family members, such as values, beliefs, attitudes, abilities, intelligences, personalities, behaviors, and biological attributes. Family members may have biophysical, emotional, psychological, and genetic similarities or differences. Traits may retain their original essences throughout the lifespan, but they may also be altered. It is probable that within single households, related and nonrelated family members share some traits but also have some differences. Learning and behaviors initiated within the family of origin and those established in a family of procreation influence family members. The shared contexts provide a collective experience with great potential to affect at least some health determinants of multiple members in similar ways. Member traits are affected by the unique characteristics of the household niche, community factors, historical time period, and political milieu.

Box 6–2 **Assumptions about Contextual Relationships and Health**

- Health is affected by member participation in a variety of contexts.
- Health is influenced by dynamic interactions among multiple family members within the household niche and various contextual influences.
- Family members' shared and distinct contextual influences affect health.
- Interactions that occur within a specific context or as a result of a context can enhance or threaten individual and family health.
- Contextual pressures encourage individuals to learn, seek, and value some health knowledge and behaviors and ignore other health knowledge and behaviors.
- Contexts can create resistance to individual and family health behaviors and potentiate negative responses.
- Larger contextual systems provide moral ideologies; resources and threats; and patterns of rights, responsibilities, and obligations that cause resistance, acceptance, or challenge to health.
- Embedded contexts provide an almost infinite number of possibilities for considering health-related interventions in a variety of contexts and at different developmental stages over the life course.
- The embedded context is in the forefront of individual and family health rather than in the background.

Bronfenbrenner (1979, 1986) described the ecological context in terms of nested sectors of society that overlap as family members have face-to-face interactions. Although a triangular notion is sometimes useful to consider distinct interactions and competition between family members and the larger society, a concentric configuration provides a better way to understand interactions among the contextual sectors. Some assumptions can be made about potential associations between the family, context, and health (Box 6–2).

Lewin's (1936, 1951) work greatly influenced Bronfenbrenner's thinking about the ways boundaries separate spaces from one another while increasing and decreasing their permeability. The firmness or permeability of boundaries of various contextual sectors determines the ease of access and openness to change. In the Family Health Model, contextual spaces have as great a potential to affect health as functional processes. Transitional or interactional processes are viewed as functional aspects of family health. Individuals often use functional processes to choose contexts for interaction, but some contexts are imposed and not chosen, and others encroach on members without their conscious awareness.

Literature Examples of Ecological Context

Although the literature about the family context and variables relevant to health are not major forces in thinking about health, substantial evidence about relationships between context and health exist. "Society exists as a shifting structure of groups and of positions to be occupied, a structure to be differentiated along a number of dimensions: socioeconomic, ethnic, age level, gender, and lifestyle" (Goodnow, 1995, p. 367). For example, an ecological framework was used to study adherence to treatment and health status of children with diabetes (Auslander, Thompson, Dreitzer, & Santiago, 1997). Sociodemographic, family, and community predictors of mothers' satisfaction with their children's medical care and medical outcomes were identified. Mothers' level of satisfaction was related to their adherence to the medical regimen and did not account for differences in child health status. Mothers who described greater concern with racism and family stress were less satisfied with medical care than mothers reporting less stressful environments. Using the Family Health Model to understand variables in this study, family stress corresponds to functional processes of family health, but the environmental causes and racism are viewed as contextual aspects. Family-focused care would target the child's medical needs but would also consider interventions aimed at racism and environment important for improving family health.

A study (Black, Dubowitz, & Starr, 1999) that examined relationships between paternal roles, residence, and the well-being of 3-year-old children from low-income African-American families found no differences in children's cognition, receptive language, behavior, or home environment related to the father's presence. Although relationships were identified between paternal roles and children's well-being based on father differences, the biological relationship of the father and parental marital status were not significant. When fathers lived in the home and were satisfied with parenting roles, played with children, and made financial contributions to the family, the homes were more child centered and children had better cognitive and language competence. Children also had fewer behavioral problems when fathers were employed and satisfied with their parenting roles. All variables were not affected by the presence of the father in the home. Based on the Family Health Model, functional processes here include parenting roles and child outcomes, and context includes the presence of the father, employment, and other community factors. Family-focused care would aim to promote positive father involvement in the lives of children but would also ascertain which contextual influences most affected the fathers' participation and satisfaction with parenting roles.

Greater emphasis on gender differences and social inequalities as health determinants is needed. Analysis of data from the 1994 Canadian National Population Health Survey identified that health effects were caused by gender, social, structural (i.e., age, family structure, education, occupation, income, social support), and behavioral determinants (i.e., smoking, drinking, weight, physical activity) (Denton & Walters, 1999). Findings indicated that social inequality was the most important health determinant, but men and women differed in health predicting factors. Social structural factors (i.e., high-income category, working full time, caring for a family, social support available) were more important for women than men. Smoking or alcohol consumption was a key health determinant for men, but weight and physical activity were more important for women. A study (Allison, Adlaf, Ialomiteanu, & Rehm, 1999) that focused on young adults' risk behaviors concluded that social context influenced behaviors and should be included in health promotion interventions. A study of Australian adolescents and parents investigated relationships among family capital, children's attributes, family settings, and adolescents' aspirations (Marjoribanks, 1998). Findings indicated that:

1. Family contexts are moderately to largely associated with children's academic performances and adolescents' aspirations.
2. Relationships between family contexts, children's attributes, and adolescents' aspirations are mediated by adolescents' perceptions of their parents' support.
3. Gender-related differences exist between associations among family capital, attributes, family settings, and adolescents' aspirations.

This study implies the possibility that complex relationships between individual attributes or contextual variables, as well as functional processes, contribute to health. Using the Family Health Model, these studies suggest that the context is an important indicator and predictor relevant to health. Family-focused care would not only consider biological factors or behavioral processes, but would also determine which interventions related to the larger contextual systems would enhance health outcomes.

The literature provides many examples about the effects of contextual variables on health, but context is often only viewed in terms of sociodemographic factors. Although education, employment status, income, and other factors are important, they are not the only relevant contextual factors. A problem with only looking at these variables is that they tend to make individuals more accountable but ignore potentials related to the effects of larger societal systems, politics, morals and values of powerful populations, and time. For example, although we may hold individuals accountable for smoking behaviors, their choices are also influenced by contextual factors over time (Denham, 1997). Although health outcomes are often linked to lifestyle behaviors, a growing body of research affords evidence of the importance of environmental relationships.

𝕥𝕥𝕥𝕥𝕥𝕥𝕥 *Cooperative Learning*

Identify a current social problem. Spend some time independently reflecting and making some notes about your ideas before sharing them with others.

For example, consider the use of alcohol. Who is to blame if an individual chooses to abuse alcohol? Although the first response might be to blame the individual, thinking that he or she decided to participate in abusive drinking, be temperate in use, or refrain from imbibing. Is it possible that other influences exist? What are those influences over the life course? Take a few minutes and list some family factors that might contribute to the drinking behaviors individuals choose. Then think about other factors (e.g., school, work, friends, the community, the media, the law) that may contribute to individual choice.

After time for reflection and completion of lists of factors, three to four students exploring the same issue should join together in small groups and compare ideas. What has been overlooked? What are the contextual factors that potentially alter the choices made and resultant behaviors? What are the implications for nursing? Describe ways that nurses can intervene to provide care for the individual with the problem if family is the unit of care.

Family Microsystems and Their Parts

The family microsystem is neither a small nor a solitary system. As individuals live together over the life course within household niches, each member experiences similarities and differences in the contexts encountered. Within the household niche, family members engage in roles, activities, processes, and relationships that are referred to in the Family Health Model as *functional processes*. Member functions are not only affected by the family household but also by larger contextual systems (i.e., exosystem, mesosystem, macrosystem). Members and family subsystems interact with larger contextual systems to construct unique family health paradigms (Fig. 6–1).

Even when individuals share a household, differences in birth order, residence in different geographical locations, impacts by diverse historical periods, and exposure to dissimilar contextual systems mean that members do not all have the same life experiences (Box 6–3). Although some characteristics may be common to families, others may be different.

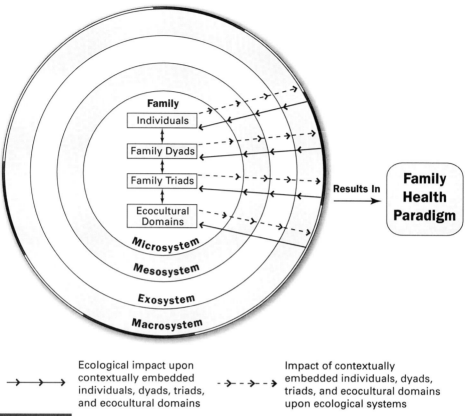

Ecological impact upon contextually embedded individuals, dyads, triads, and ecocultural domains

Impact of contextually embedded individuals, dyads, triads, and ecocultural domains upon ecological systems

Figure 6–1 Ecological framework of family health. Member functions are not only affected by the family household, or microsystem, but also by larger contextual systems such as exosystem, mesosystem, and macrosystem.

Box 6–3 **Aspects of the Family Microsystem**

- Characteristic traits of all members viewed as family (e.g., genetics, gender, age, race, ethnicity, culture, education, spirituality)
- Dyad and triad relationships internal to the family
- Dyad and triad relationships external to the family
- Intergenerational relationships (e.g., kin traditions, rituals, religion, valuing, collective memory, social class)
- Household niche (e.g., physical structure, material goods, immediate surroundings, tangible and intangible family resources)
- Immediate neighborhood (e.g., proximal relationships and processes)
- Larger community (e.g., institutions; federal, state, and local agencies; employment opportunities; support systems; health-related resources)

Changing Family Contexts over Time

Findings indicate that major changes in the composition of American families have occurred over the past quarter century (McCubbin, McCubbin, Skolnick, & Skolnick, 1999; Thompson & Han, 1999). Although many still value traditional views of nuclear families, others think and live differently. The U.S. Census Bureau informs us that the percentage of children living with two parents has been declining among all racial and ethnic groups. In 1997, 32 percent of all U.S. births were to unmarried women (National Center for Health Statistics, 2000). There are 11.9 million single parents in the United States, with 28 percent (20 million) of all children in the United States younger than age 18 years living with one parent (U.S. Census Bureau, 1998). Children who live in one-parent households are substantially more likely to have family incomes below the poverty line than those with two parents. Most children who live with single parents live with a single mother. In 1998, 68 percent of American children lived with two parents, down from 77 percent in 1980. In 1998, 76 percent of white, non-Hispanic children lived with two parents compared with 36 percent of black children and 64 percent of children of Hispanic origin (America's Children, 1999a). Some children live with a single parent who has a cohabiting partner; 16 percent of children living with single fathers and 9 percent of children living with single mothers also lived with the parent's partner (America's Children, 2000). Although parenting is a functional process related to health, the absence or presence of parents, race, and economics are contextual factors that are equally important.

In the past, intermarriage was rare, and social mores encouraged unions within race, ethnicity, religion, and even community. Although 3 to 4 decades ago, it was unusual to see interracial couples in large cities, now they are seen in rural communities, magazine advertisements, and daytime soap operas. On June 12, 1967, the Supreme Court decision in *Loving v. Virginia* struck down a miscegenation law that forbade mixing of the races. Laws against miscegenation in America appeared as early as 1661 and remained unchanged for hundreds of years. In some states, interracial marriages were not legal and were viewed as criminal, punishable by large fines and long prison sentences. Interracial marriages have increased more than 400 percent in the past 30 years. According to the 1990 U.S. census, there were 1.5 million interracial couples with 2 million children. Just as Americans are forming relational alliances different from some accepted in the past, families in other parts of the world are also finding that honored ancestral traditions are crumbling and new patterns are being developed. Contextual perspectives create questions about genetic futures and health and illness patterns when races are less distinct and health implications when traditional practices are altered.

Traditional views of families with single heterosexual marriages in which children are conceived and cared for seem tenuous today. Today's families are melded (e.g., previously married parents with biological children or stepchildren); single-parent, formerly married families; never-married families (e.g., single parent with biological children); unmarried families (e.g., never married to one another but living together for extended periods of time with biological children, stepchildren, or both); homosexual families with biological, adopted, or stepchildren; grandparent families (e.g., with biological relationships to children for whom they assist and support financially); adopted families (e.g., married partners with foster, adopted, or biological children); and others.

Reproductive technologies redefine family, and questions about genetics, cloning, implantation, adoption, surrogacy, and choice impose ethical and contextual concerns. A family may include children conceived through *in vitro* fertilization using donors who may or may not be biologically related or families with children conceived through surrogate births who may or may not be biologically related. In the Family Health Model, contextual concerns may relate to health implications of serial contexts in which individuals reside across a lifetime, whether family types promote member health, or whether health routines retain resiliency when the family context is altered.

The family of procreation is usually understood as the place where a man and a woman join economic, emotional, and supportive resources in order to give birth and have a place to rear children. Some parental roles and responsibilities are formally established by a nuptial agreement sanctioned by laws of the land and society, but family diversity is widely visible even when not sanctioned. Marriage provides a mechanism to care for offspring from birth to maturity, but birth rates for unmarried women show significant variations since 1980 (Ventura, Martin, Curtin, & Mathews, 1999). Some patterns of procreation have changed dramatically in the United States over the past two decades. Contextual perspectives cause nurses to ask questions about the effects of these changes on the health of mothers, children, and families and identify appropriate interventions. For example, some health needs and concerns of a first-time parent who is a teen mother could be very different from those of a mother in her late 30s. Family-focused care would encourage the nurse to consider potential health risks and resiliency factors in terms of family context and not merely consider whether the mother can care for the infant's biological needs. Family-focused care causes nurses to consider health potentials related to past, present, and future contextual factors and spaces.

Exploration of all family types would take more pages than allowed in this text, but it is suggested that variations alter family contexts. For example, older families without children during their years of generativity may differ from others with adult children, those raising grandchildren, or ones that acquired children from other relationships. Families with preschool children may be contextually different from those in which a child has a physical incapacity, mental disability, or chronic illness. Families in their middle adult years (e.g., age 40 to 60 years) raising preschool children may be very different from those who are seeing children off to college or those with children in prison or socially conflicted roles. Older families with higher gradients of social capital, economic prosperity, and health may look different from those with ill members, fewer material goods, or less support. The Family Health Model encourages nurses to consider the potentials related to changing contexts and factors over the life course that might influence health that are different from functional processes and interactions.

Reflective Thinking

Adults often hold fast to beliefs, values, and attitudes deeply rooted in their early life experiences. Valued ideologies are often closely adhered to, and time is seldom spent intensely examining what is believed or the reasons for the beliefs. Implications of beliefs are often ignored unless a need arises to defend them. In fact, many seek information that confirms or supports their beliefs rather than engage ideas that contradict them.

Nurses are often involved with families that are different from their own. How do you cope with these differences? How well do you cope? How do you respond professionally to persons with cultures or ideas that you view as negative? What happens when your work environment presents situations that manifest biases or prejudice? How do you respond when you personally feel one way but professional practice calls for actions contrary to your deep-seated ideas? Can you identify some particular examples of how you have responded?

Consider an issue related to family context that does not feel comfortable. For example, how do you feel about cohabiting adults who choose to raise children outside of wedlock? What about gay or lesbian partner alliances and issues of adoption? How do you feel about white families raising black children? What do you think about fathers being the custodial parents of preschool children?

Choose one issue related to family that causes ambivalence and identify your values and beliefs. Can you identify some positive aspects? What are the negatives? Can you identify why do you believe as you do? Given your personal values, beliefs, and attitudes, could you act professionally and competently? What are the biggest challenges? Are there things you need to alter or change?

Individual and Family Development

In the Family Health Model, individual and family development is viewed as a functional process influenced by embedded contextual systems. Development is altered by personal, social, and environmental factors. The focus has mostly been on individual development, with less concentration on what is implied by *family development*. Development is viewed as integration of race, class, gender, and culture (McGoldrick & Carter, 1999).

> Gender, class, culture, and race form a basic structure within which individuals learn what behaviors, beliefs, values, and ways of expressing emotion and relating to others will be expected to demonstrate throughout life. It is this context that carries every child from birth and childhood through adulthood to death and defines his or her legacy for the next generation. The gender, class, and cultural structure of any society profoundly influences the parameters of a child's evolving ability to empathize, share, negotiate, and communicate. It prescribes the child's way of thinking for his- or herself and of being emotionally connected to others (McGoldrick & Carter, p. 28).

For example, an analysis (Arber, 1997) of more than 20,000 women and men age 20 to 59 years identified the importance of analyzing gender data for educational qualifications, occupational class, and employment status. Although educational indicators were good predictors of women's self-assessed health, chronic illnesses were more closely linked to work and household conditions. Findings indicated that husbands' unemployment had adverse consequences on wives' health. Arber concluded that health measurement in women should consider changes in marital status, employment, and household circumstances. In the Family Health Model, these factors would be viewed as contextual, with the potential to influence individual and family development.

In talking about human development, Luscher (1995) stated that systems originate in broad sociocultural and institutional structures to create belief systems that are transmitted to immediate family settings, affect proximal processes or interactions, and ultimately create belief systems in developing persons. In other words, individual and family development are affected by the larger contextual systems in which they are embedded even when awareness of the influence is lacking. In this model, individual traits are viewed as contextual (i.e., genetic traits, gender, age, race, ethnicity, culture, education, spirituality). Although some traits (e.g., genetics, race, ethnicity, gender, intelligence) seem absolute and unchangeable, others (e.g., cultural traditions, education, health) are expected to change over time. However, even traits viewed as absolute might be subject to change. For example, a person who believes he or she has been wrongly sexually identified may undergo hormone treatments and surgical intervention to physiologically change his or her sexual orientation to align him- or herself with psychological perceptions rather than gender assignment by a physician, parents, or society. In this case, the context would be shifted dramatically as the individual takes on a persona different from the one previously held. Are nurses prepared to address the needs and concerns of transgendered individuals or provide care to support the developmental conflicts related to the contextual change? Family-focused care would not only target needs associated with hormonal or surgical treatments but would also include issues and relationships with larger contextual needs.

A young man graduates from college and goes overseas as a member of the Peace Corps. Although a separate household has been established in a distant place, the members of the family of origin still view this adult son as a family member. How does the move or change of context alter the young man's development? How does the separation affect family development? If the family has a home computer and regularly interacts using e-mail, this new form of interaction that entails sharing ideas, information, and feelings in different ways may be a way to overcome the physical separation and promote developmental processes. However, if the young man goes to a remote place where communication is impossible, would the developmental effects be different? Family-focused care would ask questions about relationships between context and development that occur across the life course.

 ## Critical Thinking Activity

Suppose your practice as family nurse in a neighborhood urgent-care clinic entails regular interactions with the Green family. The staff at the clinic is well acquainted with this family because of the chronic asthma of their 10-year-old son, Tom. Mr. Green, a local businessman, has served several years on the city council, and his wife is an elementary school teacher. Financially, they are comfortable and have adequate health insurance for needed services. They have two other children, Alice, a 14-year-old daughter, and James, a 16-year-old son. You know all of the family members from their frequent visits.

On this particular visit, Tom has had a flare-up of his asthma, and his mother has brought him in for a breathing treatment. Although the physician and the respiratory therapist are providing Tom with care, Mrs. Green pulls you aside and says that she needs to talk with you confidentially. You locate an empty conference room and sit down to talk. By this time, Mrs. Green is visibly distressed. You anticipate that she will discuss Tom's asthmatic condition because it has been a continual cause of family concern. As she begins to talk, you immediately recognize that her concern is not about Tom, but James.

Mrs. Green tells you that the family has been going through a great amount of stress because of James and that this stress caused Tom's present asthmatic episode. The Greens relocated to this community from a neighboring state after James' birth. It seems that when James was born, the obstetrician was uncertain about the gender of the child, and the Greens were told that he had a sexual anomaly. The child had what appeared to be a partially formed penis, through which he urinated, but he also had what might be a small vaginal opening. James had no testicles but had what appeared to be a single, poorly formed ovary and a single fallopian tube. The family was faced with the crisis of gender. The obstetrician and others encouraged the Greens to identify the child as male, and a surgical procedure closed the vaginal opening.

The present crisis has been developing for some time. During puberty, James became especially withdrawn and somewhat depressed. His smaller size and lack of interest in athletics has often been the cause of ridicule from peers and occasionally from his father. Over the past few months, James has repeatedly expressed to his family that he is not a boy, but a girl, and wants to be treated as such. He has taken to wearing female clothing when at home and wants to change his name. Lately he has been asking about the possibilities of surgery that would change his gender to what it should be. This situation has created a rather tense home environment, with continual arguments among family members.

As the family nurse, how should you address this family health issue? What are the contextual concerns? What developmental factors might be impacted by the family's context? What will you say to Mrs. Green? What suggestions would you give for follow-up care? If family is the unit of care, what interventions might be needed?

Race, Ethnicity, and Culture

Most U.S. families have an immigrant heritage, but many have no memory or valuing associated with these roots. In fact, many of the United States' families see immigrants as people other than themselves. Some families are of different racial, ethnic, or cultural backgrounds and continue to live near extended family members, but others have inter-mingled, intermarried, and reside in communities where diversity is common. Ethnicity may be important to some, but many Americans neither know about nor value their heritage. Although some focus on stereotypes, others are blinded to differences. Within some families, it is possible to identify a great deal of intergenerational conflict based on race and ethnicity (Carter & McGoldrick, 1999a). Although whites are the majority in America, predictions suggest that by 2050, their numbers will be matched by populations of Hispanic, blacks, and Asians. The racial, ethnic, and cultural patterns of earlier generations have dramatically changed and continue to be altered. Diversity is not only a factor that affects Americans but also one that concerns other nations. Migration, media influences, ease of travel, and rapid change all affect families in ways never imagined a few generations ago. Family-focused care suggests that nurses consider these contextual factors when they complete assessments, create care plans, consider appropriate interventions, and evaluate outcomes.

The identification and meaning of race becomes increasingly complex as children with mixed racial and ethnic heritage are born. How useful is race as a variable associated with health when ancestries are mixed? Although a biracial person may be raised in one cultural context, he or she might perceive closer alignment with the other. In what ways do race and ethnicity affect nurses' practice with families? How do persons of the same race or ethnicity differ intergenerationally? In what ways do these factors related to race, ethnicity, and culture affect individual and family development? What are the potential influences on health? For example, immigrant parents may have beliefs and practices that are different from those of their children and grandchildren. A nurse interested in treating family as the unit of care may need information about cultural differences pertaining to these generations in order to fully address individual health needs.

Culture is certainly associated with race and ethnicity; however, all persons have culture even when they are oblivious, indifferent, or unaware. Cultures may have cor-related symbols, traditions, celebrations, rituals, and practices that are not consciously thought about by members but are observable by others. Members within the same family may have generational differences in the ways they value and practice cultural behaviors. Culture includes factors that give rise to beliefs, values, attitudes, and behaviors. Marginalization of some individuals and families based on racial, ethnic, cultural, and even gender divisions continues to be problematic worldwide. Some might argue that more variation exists within a group than between groups. The context of race, ethnicity, and culture have meanings beyond their labels and have the potential to affect the processes of becoming, development, well-being, and health of individuals and families. Family-focused care targets understanding the implications of these contextual factors and their relevance to health needs.

👫👫👫👫 *Cooperative Learning*

The class is divided into five groups. Each group is assigned a different family type (e.g., African-American, Asian-American, European-American, Hispanic-American, Native American, middle-class white). Your group should complete its assignment independently and prepare a handout to share with all class members. Your instructor will set a date for completion and schedule an in-class discussion to compare and contrast findings.

Each group should answer the following questions:

1. Which various ethnicities and cultures does each family type have?
2. What are the number and percentage of Americans that fall into this group?
3. Where in the United States do most families of this type live?
4. What is the median family income for your group? What kinds of work are done by most wage earners in this group?
5. What is the educational preparation for most family members in this group? Are there variations of education based on generations? If so, what are they?
6. What are the major health risks for family members in this group?
7. What cultural practices of families in this group might be strengths for health?
8. What cultural practices of families in this group might be threats to health?
9. What kinds of housing do most families in this group live in?

After group members have answered these questions, decide what it might mean for nurses concerned with family as the unit of care. Discuss the implications for individual and family health. Prepare a handout that synthesizes what your group has learned and its potential implications for health and nurses.

Age of Members

The ages of family members are viewed as part of the family context in the Family Health Model, and they affect developmental expectations. A family household with a 14-year-old mother; her newborn infant; the teen mother's siblings, who are 10 and 12 years old; and a 30-year-old, unmarried mother may present different concerns than a household in which the teenage mother and newborn live alone or one in which a young woman lives with the 18-year-old father of her child. How might the context affect this young mother differently if she lived with siblings who were 10 and 12 years old, but the home had two parents who were 34 and 36 years old? What might it be like if the teen mother gave the child up for adoption but continued to live with her family of origin?

Age is a factor in each setting, but the context of each one presents potentially different outcomes for the newborn, mother, and others. Age neither indicates maturity nor the ability to provide child care, but the family members' ages provide some developmental information about the members that could be pertinent to health outcomes. How might a nurse intervene differently based on these different family contexts?

Intelligence, Education, and Employment

Intelligence, education, and employment are also contextual factors that have the potential to influence health. A person without a formal education may not lack intelligence, and having a college degree does not necessarily identify intelligence. Formal education is important, but questions about the values and ability to learn about particular life tasks or health needs may be of greater concern to nurses. Questions about the value of education relative to a situation may be as important as the need for education. What education is needed? What is the purpose of the education? Why does it matter? Answers to specific questions may produce more helpful information than merely knowing whether a person completed high school or has a degree in chemical engineering. Contextual concern focuses on whether persons have developmentally appropriate knowledge and skills needed to complete life tasks and address health concerns. The world's families do not have equal opportunities to obtain formal education, but many people are eager and able to learn what is necessary for good lives and health. Reasons why persons have less formal education may rest more in larger contextual systems than in the abilities of individuals.

According to Marmot, Fuhrer, Ettner, Marks, Bumpass, and Ryff (1998), findings from the National Survey of Mid-life Developments, a study about socioeconomic gradients in mortality during midlife, show that higher education predicted better health and mediating variables (e.g., household income, parents' education, smoking behavior, and social relationships). Kohn (1995) suggests that education and work are part of the same process rather than competing factors and that education determines job conditions, work complexity, and individual personality. Persons with higher education often acquire jobs with greater financial security, fewer risks, better health-care coverage, and a larger stream of social networks. Higher education may increase job opportunities and employment choices, but work conditions and value orientations may have as much to do with contextual systems as intelligence or abilities.

Another concern related to education has to do with the organizational structure of the educational system and the ways it affects individual learners. Although we might view an individual as self-directed and motivated to learn, one must inquire about the contextual factors that support individual behaviors. Which success factors in an educational structure are products of individual personality? Which ones are related to teacher excellence, a budget for teaching aides, or a system that ensures quality and opportunity for all learners? After years of researching relationships between personality, education, and occupation, Kohn (1995) concludes:

> People learn from their experiences, and learn most of all from having to cope with complex and demanding experiences. There is more to education than attuning people to the printed page, important though that is (p. 151).

Biogenetic factors with the potential to influence intelligence can also be viewed as contextual (e.g., learning potential, developmental disability, exceptionalness). For example, a child with genetic or developmental disabilities may still have the ability to learn, but the child may proceed at a different pace from those without disabilities. Abilities to learn differ based on contextual and individual traits. A study of children's verbal IQ scores and relationships to their parents' education, genetics, and environment found greater variability for environment than genetic heritage, but parents' education, genet- ics, and environmental factors also affected the children's scores (Rowe, Jacobsen, & Van den Oord, 1999).

Old ways of measuring educational impact may be less effective because of current trends such as magnet schools, charter schools, homeschooling, continuing education, second life careers, and Internet asynchronous learning modes. Many children start preschool earlier, and higher numbers of children attend day care with some educa- tional component. In 1997, 48 percent of children were enrolled in preschool compared with 45 percent in 1996. Preschool enrollment increased among black, non-Hispanic children (from 45 to 55 percent) and among children living in poverty (from 34 percent to 40 percent) (America's Children, 1999b). However, in 1998, about 8 percent of the Nation's 16- to 19-year-old young adults were neither enrolled in school nor working, a significant decrease from the 9 percent found in 1997 (America's Children). Merely as- sessing grade level or possession of a degree of formal education only provides a partial picture of the broad contextual relationships between health, intelligence, education, and employment. Family-focused care implies a need to consider factors that enhance learning, capabilities, and resources relevant to health outcomes.

Spiritual Context

In the Family Health Model, *spirituality* is viewed as an important contextual aspect and is defined as an innate trait of all persons that concerns connectedness to self, others, and a higher power; transcendence to places and energies beyond one's own being; and an essence of meaningfulness. Spirituality often includes religion, faith systems, sacred principles, worship, symbolic meanings, and ritual practices. Friedemann (1995) suggests that spirituality is a family target that leads to congruence, hence family health. She describes spirituality in terms of togetherness, individuation, and commitment but also explains it as a means of reducing isolation and finding connections and comfort. Fish and Shelly (1978) describe spirituality in terms of love and relatedness, forgiveness, and a search for meaning. Although most persons have some sense of spirituality, it may wax and wane over a lifetime and be expressed outside of formal religion.

Religion is defined as an acknowledgement of an ultimate reality or deity and usually refers to inward and outward expressions of belief guided by doctrine. Religion of- ten demands adherence to specified beliefs and symbolic practices. Religion may have a classification such as Christianity, Hinduism, Islam, or Judaism; be discussed as denom- inations such as Catholic, Protestant, Baptist, Mormon, Lutheran, Jehovah's Witnesses; or be referred to in terms such as fundamentalist, reformed, or orthodox. Religions usu- ally have authority, guide values and beliefs, define what is right and wrong, identify the expectations of followers, and unify members. Religion and spirituality provide a life context and are often associated with health and illness. Dying persons may not have attended church or followed religious practices for decades, but when faced with an uncertainty, they may return to beliefs they learned in their families of origin.

Some persons fulfill spiritual needs through religion, but others use things such as poetry, arts, nature, music, exercise, and other things. Spirituality is often evoked when the human spirit is distressed (e.g., during grief or suffering or when searching for a reason to be, seeking answers to life's questions, or facing eternity). Spiritual needs occur when persons feel isolated from others, lack a sense of purpose, and experience a need for relationships to fill life voids (Carson, 1989). Although the scientific academy often undervalues the strength, influence, and power of religion and spirituality, it is viewed as an intrinsic contextual aspect of individuals that has meaning for family identity, values, and behaviors related to health. Family-focused care includes considerations about spirituality and religion as immediate rather than afterthoughts.

Genetics and Family Health

Biogenetics is another contextual aspect of individuals and families. The Human Genome Project presents evidence with a tremendous potential to impact health. Although important relationships exist between genetics and disease, nurses and others may be ill-prepared to address basic genetic principles, genetic testing processes, and implications of testing (Jacobs & Deatrick, 1999). Counseling about risks requires specialized knowledge that presently extends beyond the expertise of many nurses. Gene testing for rare hereditary syndromes and family diseases will offer new options and challenges. In the near future, some oncology nurses will assess hereditary risks; offer susceptibility testing to those who may benefit; and provide follow-up counseling, support, and referral (Biesecker, 1997). Many ethical, legal, social, and practice issues will be re-evaluated in light of knowledge derived from the human genome. Nurses working with families experiencing chronic illnesses, developmental disabilities, hereditary conditions, and issues related to conception and birth will be especially challenged by genetics.

Developmental behavioral genetics is the study of genetic and environmental influences on individual differences in the development of behavior (Plomin, 1983). Genetic research may have its greatest impact for clinicians in terms of understanding the environment and how the environment relates to development (Plomin, 1995). In behavioral-genetic studies, the environment is either estimated or indirectly measured, but questions center around the ways the genotype or person and the environment interact to influence development (Wachs, 1983). Arguments about nature and nurture are being challenged by research that indicates development involves a substantial contribution from genetic factors and relationships to family environment measures. A rapidly growing body of evidence indicates that relationships exist between genetics, health, disease, and behavior linked to individual differences, environment, and the interactions among them rather than either nature or nurture processes (McClearn, Vogler, & Plomin, 1996).

According to Plomin (1994), genetics rarely accounts for more than half of the variance in any research; thus, nonshared environmental influences may help explain nongenetic factors related to behavioral differences for children within the same family. Genetically similar siblings raised within the same family differ in personality and psychopathy in ways that are not explained by genetics and appear to be related to within-family processes or nonshared environments (Dunn & Plomin, 1991). Conventional strategies of matching children on a family-by-family basis are often inadequate for understanding why siblings are so different. In a literature review about adolescent psychopathology, children's behavioral genetics and nonshared environments were considered factors related to depression (Pike & Plomin, 1996). Findings indicated that environment and genetics are important for understanding childhood psychiatric disorders and that nonshared sibling environments are especially salient. The proposed health model suggests that family genetics and contextual systems have health implications. Family-focused care entails assessment, interventions, and outcome measurement in both areas.

Family Household

The U.S. Census Bureau states that a household includes all people who occupy a housing unit. A household consists of a single family, one person living alone, two or more families living together, or any group of related or unrelated people who share living arrangements. The Census Bureau designates one person as the householder, usually the person who owns the home or is responsible for paying the rent or mortgage. A housing unit is described as a house, apartment, mobile home, group of rooms, or single room that is occupied as separate living quarters. Separate living quarters are those in which the occupants live and eat separately from other people in the building and which have direct access from the outside of the building or through a common hall. The Census Bureau definition of a household is appropriate for use in the Family Health Model.

In the Family Health Model, households are identified as niches or embedded settings in which (1) family members dwell; (2) family members share values, beliefs, information, and resources related to health; and (3) behaviors related to health are performed. Households are the places where individuals learn health information, develop health values, and participate in health-related behaviors. Family culture guides values, traditions, and rituals relevant to the health practices of members. The household is the institution in which "production, consumption, and social reproduction are organized" and other dimensions of social order manifest themselves through the dyad and triad interrelationships (Berman, Kendall, & Bhattacharyya, 1994, p. 207). The family household is the place where families use their available resources to produce health (Schumann & Mosley, 1994). Individuals are likely to live in several geographic locations and residences over the life course, but others may live in a single location and the same or a similar residence for an entire lifetime. Household factors affect health outcomes and could assist in the development of effective interventions (Harkness & Super, 1994).

The household niche provides a way to understand the contextual setting in which members spend time caring for themselves and one another. The Family Health Model views the interactions among individuals, family subsystems, families, and larger contextual systems mostly occurring from the household perspective. The household is "a mediator of both environmental risks and programmatic interventions to promote better health" (Harkness & Super, p. 217). The household is the place where individuals develop and members interact related to their health and illness needs. The household has implications for the health of individuals and the family, as well as implications for intergenerational transmission of health patterns. Family-focused care would not only consider characteristics of individual members but also those of the household niche that might be relevant to a specific health concern or individual and family well-being.

Immediate Neighborhood or Community

Households are situated in neighborhoods and are associated with communities and larger contextual systems. Definitions of neighborhood might be different depending on the cultural context of the family (e.g., housing development, low-income projects, gated community, apartment complex, farming community, dormitory, prison block). Community is often defined in terms of its geographic area and agencies, institutions, businesses, services, law enforcement, and others. Children usually attend school in the community; adults have jobs there; and members may vote, shop, attend to religious practices, and pay taxes there.

A family may be congruent with societal expectations or present a gross contrast to neighborhood norms. Neighborhoods and communities may have values that support or threaten family lifestyle and individual health. The races, religions, ethnicities, and cultures of residents may be barriers or strengths to accessing resources related to health and well-being. If residents are viewed as marginal or less acceptable, then they may be viewed as threats to the welfare of the community and may not have access to the same resources afforded to others. The geographic location of the family household may facilitate access to services or resources, but it may also be inhibiting. Neighborhoods can:

- Influence the ways family boundaries are established
- Influence the activities that individuals participate in when they are at home
- Influence who members regularly interact with outside the family network

---

Box 6–4 **Propositions about Relationships Between the Context and Family Health**

- Health learning and behaviors that are reinforced across multiple contexts are more likely to be consistently adhered to by family members.
- Health learning and behaviors adopted by family triads are more consistently adhered to than health learning and behaviors of single individuals or dyads.
- Families with more open boundaries have members more accepting of information and behaviors to improve health.
- Health is increased when genetic potentials are increased and environments are stable and advantaged.
- Health potentials are greatest when environments are disadvantaged and disorganized.
- Consistently sustained interventions aimed at contextual systems over extended periods increase the degree of health actualized in given environments.

Playmates and friends are often established based on neighborhood proximity. Macintyre (1994) suggested that the production of health is a consequence of variations of social mechanisms over the life course as material resources and psychosocial and biological factors interact. Neighborhoods and communities may offer different resources pertinent to health-care services and the availability of professionals to meet health needs, but they may also be the perpetrators of environmental threats that cause increased risks for illness and disease. Health inequalities are related to (1) physical or social environments; (2) the availability of information, resources, and experts; and (3) the accessibility, affordability, and availability of services. The Family Health Model suggests that health is not a unique individual quality; rather, it is one that is enhanced and placed at risk by larger contextual systems. Family-focused care targets not only individuals and families but also the advantages and disadvantages, threats and assets, and strengths and limitations imposed by neighborhoods and communities.

Summary

The concept of a *microsystem* is an embedded context that includes concrete and abstract ideas related to family life and health (Box 6–4). Although nurses have some knowledge about environments, concerns seldom include the ways contextual systems integrate all developmental aspects to influence health and illness. The Family Health Model emphasizes the powerful ways contextual systems shape family processes and health outcomes. The microsystem is only one aspect of the embedded context, but it is the one with which family members are the most aware and familiar. The microsystem not only includes family members and their unique traits but also the household niche, neighborhood, and community. Family-focused care proposes that nurses complete individual assessment related to specific illness or health needs but also include family dyads and triads, household, neighborhood, and community context influences. Plans of care for individuals would also include interventions for issues related to the family context.

Test Your Knowledge

1. Describe what is meant by the terms *ecological context* and *family microsystem*.
2. Explain what is implied by contextual influences on the health of a developing person.
3. Identify three ways the ecological context can potentially affect health.
4. Choose three contextual aspects of the family microsystem and describe each.

5. Compare and contrast the potential effects of residing in multiple family contexts over the life course.

6. Discuss differences the nurse might anticipate related to an individual's educational attainment and health.

7. Identify two cultures with which you have some familiarity and compare the potential effects of that culture on individual health and family health.

8. Do you think that health risks differ for families living in rural or urban settings? Support your answer using contextual perspectives.

9. Discuss three health implications imposed by employment.

Chapter

7

Broader Aspects of the Family's Embedded Contextual System

CHAPTER OBJECTIVES *At the end of this chapter, the reader will be able to:*

- Identify aspects of the microsystem, mesosystem, exosystem, macrosystem, and chronosystem that are relevant to health.
- Describe the potential interactions that occur between individuals, family subsystems, and families and the broad contextual systems in which they are embedded.
- Describe potential relationships between the embedded context, development, health, and well-being.

> *Verily all things move within your being in constant half embrace, the desired and the dreaded, the repugnant and the cherished, the pursued and that which you would escape.*
> —Kahlil Gibran, The Prophet

Although understandings about the family microsystem are important, nurses who desire to provide family-focused care must also possess knowledge and skills that pertain to the larger contextual systems that affect the lives of individuals and families. This chapter provides a description of the dimensions that influence the lives of individuals, family subsystems, and families: the exosystem, mesosystem, macrosystem, and chronosystem. The complex processes that transpire among embedded systems are not insulated events; rather, they initiate, sustain, mediate, and terminate dynamic processes that pertain to development, health, and well-being.

The Chronosystem and Its Pervasive Effects

In 1988, the Institute of Medicine gave the nation a wake-up call when it declared that the public health system was in disarray and was characterized by poor organization, inadequate capacities to fulfill the public's needs, and the inability to make or act on decisions to meet the public's needs. The report suggested meeting population needs, strengthening the nation's public health capacities, and focusing on prevention and health promotion. According to the Institute of Medicine (2000), the "health of all people is profoundly affected by scientific, technical, economic, social, educational, and behavioral factors that are changing at an unprecedented rate as the world economy becomes increasingly interconnected" (p. 85). Boundaries between public health and medicine are being redefined as more agree that health care must focus on individual treatment as well as the health of populations. "We now recognize that each person's health and well-being are shaped by the interaction of genetic endowment, environmental exposures, lifestyle and food choices, income, and medical care" (Institute of Medicine, 2000, pp. 59–60).

The 21st century brings changes in structures that affect societal changes, class, cultural contexts, politics, economics, communication, and international ideologies. These structures have the potential to affect individuals, families, and communities throughout the world. This chapter provides a way to understand the effects of contextual systems on families, communities, and populations.

Characteristics of the Chronosystem

The *chronosystem* provides ways to comprehend differences in time experienced by individuals and families. Lives are linked and families are constituted by social interdependence (Elder, 1995), but personal choice, chance, and context affect members differently over time. For example, siblings live together in the family of origin and share many things, but as they reach maturity and become more independent, some things change and some remain fairly constant over time. Individuals also experience imprinted moments of time that seem like anchors for ordering and giving meaning to some life aspects. For example, the assassination of President John F. Kennedy is a time recalled by many as a historical point for ordering other life events. Time shared with others at college, on a baseball team, or as a comrade in battle may unite individuals in unique ways that give special meanings and identities. Birth and death are times when family and friends are drawn together to celebrate traditions and mark the lives of others in memorable ways and give them distinctive importance. Normal growth and development, lifecycle transitions, and movement from place to place are events shared by most individuals, but the distinctiveness of these phenomena is experienced differently. Box 7–1 provides a list of chronosystem concepts that people commonly use to mark time. Chronosystems have to do with the timing of events, number of events in a given time, the length of time of events, and perceptions of time over time.

Box 7-1   **Concepts Related to the Chronosystem**

- Actual passage of time
- Special moments in time
- Age differences
- Intergenerational transmission
- Historical past
- Experienced and unexperienced present
- Desired futures

Chronosystems include normative and non-normative events (Bronfenbrenner, 1986). Normative events are times that developing persons and families anticipate and relate to things such as birth, marriage, school entrance, puberty, graduation from secondary school, joining the workforce, military service, retirement, episodic illness, and death in old age. Normative events are culturally bound within specific social contexts at given points in time. This means that those who are born in different generations; live in diverse social settings; or are members of different religions, races, ethnicities, or cultures identify what is normative in different ways. Normative events often embrace shared meanings relevant to family identity and entail traditions or rituals. The timing of normative events is often a unifying one, and although events sometimes include challenges, they are generally viewed positively. Families usually spend time preparing for normative events and have expectations about roles, responsibilities, and duties relevant to their timing.

Non-normative events appear unexpectedly and are times for which families are unprepared; they are sometimes viewed as crises such as the birth of a child with a genetic anomaly, getting a divorce, getting suspended from school, being fired, relocating, winning the lottery, receiving traumatic injuries, dying prematurely, or dealing with chronic illness. Non-normative or unpredictable life course events occur within historical contexts (e.g., wars, famines, natural disasters, the rise and fall of political regimes, economic instability) and are often interpreted based on the type and duration of the experience. Individuals and families tend to be less prepared for these times; usually lack traditions, rituals, or support to help cope with them; and view them as threats. Whether events are normative or non-normative, time has meaning related to development, health, and wellness.

The Chronosystem as a Life Course

The Family Health Model suggests that the embedded context is the genesis, or starting point, at which social processes that affect the lives, values, behaviors, and behaviors of individuals, family subsystems, and families occur. This model focuses on a social life course, lives in time and place, human agency, the timing of lives, and linked lives. Box 7–2 provides some terminology and definitions related to chronosystems, development, health, and well-being. Elder (1995) described the life course as an emerging paradigm that enables one to understand the social forces that shape and develop people's lives and the multiple contexts that affect life consequences. Age-graded trajectories, historical influences, self-regulation, interdependent relationships, and perceptions all influence the life course.

When considering the chronosystem, one must ask questions related to the timing of events and health. Do events that occur within a close time frame infer causation? Are similar events happening to different people, or is the same event happening to

---

Box 7–2 **Effects of the Chronosystems on Development, Health, and Well-being**

Social Life Course

Interwoven age-graded trajectories are subject to change, future options, and short-term transitions from birth to death. Each trajectory has a series of linked states; thus a change in state results in a transition embedded in the trajectory. Change has the potential to create a complex interplay between context and health.

Time and Place

Developmental processes are shaped by sociocultural trajectories. Historical time and place present restraints, opportunities, priorities, and values reflected in life course behaviors. Historical change is never uniform across communities, so variations in context have the potential to enhance or threaten development, health, and well-being.

Human Agency

Individual choices among situational and perceptual options form foundations for outcomes. Persons are agents who can contribute to their health, but contexts outside their agency enhance or restrain their actions.

Timing of Lives

Age is not the only measure of time; sequence, pace, incident types, duration of situations, the availability of options, and the presence of constraints also mediate choices.

Interdependent Lives

Lives are linked to one another, specific contexts, the timing of historical events, and choices based on situational and perceptual options. Actions have domino-like effects on the lives of others presently and over time. Linked lives such as family subsystems, family, kin networks, friendships, and colleagues provide opportunities and threats to development, health, and well-being.

Source: Ideas based on Elder, GH: The life course paradigm. In Moen, PG, Elder, H, and Luscher, K (eds.): Examining Lives in Context. American Psychological Association, Washington, DC, 1995, pp 101–139.

---

different individuals correlated with one another? What effects does the timing of a specific event have on development? Health? Well-being? How do we know the effects of time in relation to the duration of experiences? In what ways is the timing of societal events related to health? Why do persons who share experiences over time interpret them and respond to them in dramatically opposed ways? Meaningful questions about the timing of events and the effects on linked lives need to be asked to gather evidence to guide practice. The implications of the chronosystem on contextual systems provide unique ways to ascertain and evaluate functional processes and interactions.

 Reflective Thinking

In this exercise, you will draw a healthgram. First draw a line to represent your life, with the beginning point identifying your birth and the end representing your death. Should the line be straight, circular, or angular? Mark a place to designate where you presently see yourself and think about the age you might be when you eventually die.

On the top of the line, indicate important events, diseases, illnesses, exposure to risks, and times of support experienced thus far in your life course. Under the line, indicate your age, where you lived, whom you lived with, close friends, and associates.

You can make this very detailed. You may want to include employment, stresses, peak moments, and so on. The exercise asks you to recall things in many realms of your past. After you have completed your healthgram, see if you can identify any trends that evolved over time. If you have completed this exercise independently, ask yourself whether your data could be more complete. You may want to discuss it with some family members or others who might provide different perspectives.

Finally, based on your personal history and present health patterns, consider what you know about your family health history and genetics. What do you see in your health future? At what points in the past have changes occurred? What do you see for the future? What can you do now or in the future to enhance your health? After adequate time is available to complete the activity, discuss with other students the way that time in relationship to development, health, and well-being could enhance learning about chronosystems.

Aspects of the Mesosystem

Individuals do not develop alone or within vacuums; rather, they develop in the context of others, and the social environment of individuals exerts both negative and positive potentials on the life course. The *mesosystem* is the multiple influences experienced by developing individuals as they interact with family subsystems and family within the household niche (Box 7–3). A family may have several members, but each one encounters a somewhat different life experience, depending on things such as age, maturity, abilities, choice, and chance. Extended kin relationships, peers, school, play, work, and special interests are all factors that influence member interactions and functional processes that impact development, health, and well-being. Although the household is usually the principal context for interactions, as the members get older, mature, and establish more extra-household linkages, these interactions expand. Members may spend more time away from the household, increase their time with outsiders, and expand their social networks.

Peer Relationships

Whenever a person moves into a new setting, the potential for forming new peer relationships exists. Peer relationships may occur between a family member and a person outside of the family circle or may occur between members within the family circle. For instance, a toddler who usually stays at home may make new friends through caregiving arrangements if the mother returns to work, or cousins who regularly interact might

---

Box 7-3 **Aspects of the Mesosystem**

- Peer relationships (e.g., dyads, triads, close kin, friendships)
- Preschool, school, and child-care processes
- Work (e.g., unemployment, underemployment)
- Play: Adult and child (e.g., sports, social activities, personal hobbies, vacations)
- Health-care systems (e.g., services used, relationships with providers)
- Social support systems (e.g., club memberships, church affiliations, support groups)

Box 7–4   **Interactions Relevant to Development, Health, and Well-being**

Perception

The world extends beyond the immediate situation and includes other settings, activities that occur in those settings, relationships among the settings, influences of contexts where face-to-face contact does not occur, patterned beliefs, lifestyles, cultural traditions, and spirituality. Perception has to do with the ways individuals, family subsystems, and families view, interpret, value, and give meaning to contextual events.

Action

Individual capacities to accurately interpret interactions that occur in diverse systems and settings, use the systems and settings available, and reconstitute systems and settings.

Development-in-context

Development-in-context is a dynamic feedback system that includes multiple systems and contexts. Development, health, and well-being of individuals, family systems, and families are impacted differently, which affects other interactions across the life course.

Ecological Validity

Ecological validity includes practice and research perspectives pertaining to developmental, health, and well-being of individuals, family subsystems, and families in multiple contextual settings over time. The goal is not the testing of hypotheses but discovery of whether changes have been produced in perceptions and behaviors in diverse contexts at different points in time.

Source: Ideas modified from Bronfenbrenner, U: The Ecology of Human Development: Experiments by Nature and Design. Harvard University Press, Cambridge, Mass., 1979.

---

form a peer relationship that extend beyond usual familial ones. Bronfenbrenner (1979) suggested that:

> Growing persons acquire a more extended, differentiated, and valid conception of the ecological environment, and become motivated and able to engage in activities that reveal the properties of, sustain, or restructure the environment at levels of similar or greater complexity in form and context (p. 27).

Peer relationships assist individuals in reorganizing some personal characteristics, but they also support steadfastness to others. Box 7–4 depicts four levels of interaction of developing persons and their ecological environments (i.e., perception, action, development-in-context, ecological validity) (Bronfenbrenner, 1986).

Preschool, School, and Child Care

In 1999, 54 percent of children from birth through third grade received some form of child care on a regular basis from persons other than their parents, up from 51 percent in 1995 (America's Children, 2000). The number of children living with parents where at least one parent was working full time increased slightly, from 76 percent in 1997 to 77 percent in 1998 (America's Children). When child outcomes are considered, questions sometimes center on whether it is good for mothers to work. Less discussion surrounds issues such as the type of employment; wages earned; ways income is spent; caregiver issues; quality of mother–child interaction; or impact on the child's development, health, or well-being. This Family Health Model forces nurses to cross a variety of sectors related to individual health and examine variations in the impact, outcomes, and effects of systemic processes. Although much is known about how parenting affects children, less is known about the ways children affect parents or how school and child care affect household niches. Family-focused care implies a need to ask questions that have not usually been asked and consider relationships in broader ways.

Work, Employment, and Underemployment

When health and mortality are considered, it is common to see reports that include relationships to parent education and socioeconomic background. Most accept that if education and socioeconomics are improved, then health improves and mortality is reduced. Unfortunately, knowing these facts could result in a failure to acknowledge other risks that may be even more significant. For example, a nationally representative sample of adult women and men participated in a longitudinal study to investigate the degree to which four risk factors—cigarette smoking, alcohol drinking, sedentary lifestyle, and relative body weight—explained relationships between socioeconomic conditions and mortality (Lantz, House, Lepkowski, Williams, Mero, & Chen, 1999). The survey investigated the impact of education, income, and health behaviors on the risk of dying. Although education and income were identified as indicators of mortality and significantly influenced the risks of dying for the lowest-income group, the investigators concluded that mortality was actually caused by a wide array of factors and would persist even with improved health behaviors. It appears that both early and current circumstances cumulatively contribute to explain why people of lower socioeconomic status have worse health and lower psychological well-being (Marmot, Fuhrer, Ettner, Marks, Bumpass, & Ryff, 1998).

The processes related to work and development, health, and well-being are too frequently overlooked. "Work is a big problem waiting to be solved: too much of it for some, not enough for others, and the need to provide good-quality childcare for all of the children on whom the future rests" (Carter & McGoldrick, 1999b, p. 15). Some people work long hours in high-stress environments for fat paychecks, fringe benefits, and prospects of a promising career. Others work equally as hard in equally stressful atmospheres for far less pay, fewer benefits, and uncertain futures. Still others work at trying to find work that pays adequately to meet family needs but are continuously underemployed in service sector jobs that offer minimum wages, no benefits, and little promise of any future. There are those who are unable to find work because of a chronic condition, disability, or lack of skills. Of course, there are also some who just plain do not want to work.

Discussions of employment often discuss the abilities of individuals while ignoring the facts that some businesses use people, love profits, and sacrifice many for the good of a few. Costs of production often center on the skills of laborers and expenditures for health benefits, but issues related to organizational inability to adopt technology, costs related to administrative tasks, or salaries paid to upper management are ignored. Inclusion of the concept of the mesosystem in the Family Health Model implores us to look beyond worker skills, paychecks, and family incomes and question how workplaces affect development, health, and well-being. What are the interactions between employment context and the health of individuals, family subsystems, and families? Family-focused care should cause nurses to ask questions about these interactions.

Sometimes assumptions about relationships inappropriately guide thinking. For example, many might think that a life of farming would be healthier than working in an urban environment. However, a Finnish study (Rahkonen & Takala, 1998) that investigated differences in the health and social patterns of older adults found that farm workers reported more functional disability and poorer health than did white collar workers, with even greater differences observed in men than women. What about relationships between present health and the effects of prior living conditions? An ambitious attempt (Rahkonen, Lahelma, & Huuhka, 1997) to compare childhood living conditions with past and present socioeconomic status with adult health status found that childhood economic problems were significantly related to adult health, and past childhood social problems were weakly related. Unless the context and processes associated with work are closely examined, one might erroneously conclude a situation far more deleterious or optimal than it actually is.

Family-focused care must target contextual factors that appear as more obscure assessment and intervention areas. Nurses must ask questions that address the needs related to populations of workers in single industries rather than merely address the needs of single individuals disassociated from the workplace. For example, occupational health nurses who emphasize family rather than individual care may find contextual systems a way to burrow deeper into safety issues, risk reduction, rehabilitative issues, and health promotion for a family for whom an employer may also provide health benefits. Questions about the long-term effects associated with employment are concerns for the world's people, yet they are not usually taken into account.

Play: Adult and Child

Play, hobbies, and family fun are contextual areas that are pertinent to family health. Although the types of activities may be limited based on finances, skills, availability, interest, and social opportunity, most persons, including adults and children, participate in play, either with others or with family members. As a child, one might recall the horror of being the last one selected to play on a team. What effects does this have when it is repeated often over time? Suppose one enjoys golf, but the fees at the country club or local green are beyond what can be afforded. What if a college student desires to join a sorority that her roommates are considering, but she realizes her family cannot afford the membership costs? Weekend play might consist of yard work, an afternoon of watching football and eating snacks, or a shopping trip to the mall. What do other families do for play? What happens when teenagers no longer want to participate in family activities? What does it mean when children always want to include friends in family activities? These are the kinds of questions that the Family Health Model might cause a nurse to consider when thinking about the mesosystem and planning family-focused care.

Health-Care Systems

When health-care systems are considered, great concerns are often voiced about the adequacy and availability of professionals to meet care needs. Although family members often seek services from the same providers, it is not unusual for some members to have different ones from other members. Although most families may only see physicians infrequently and only for annual physical examinations, well-child care, or emergencies, families that have members with disabilities, chronic illnesses, or a child born prematurely may need multiple providers to address their needs more frequently and over longer time periods. What effects do brief medical encounters have, and how do they differ from extended interactions with multiple care providers? How does care needed by a single member affect other family members?

As family members age, the likelihood of chronic illnesses and the need for extensive services increase. Relationships with health-care providers may have the potential to alter family processes. What happens when a member is faced with hospitalization? How does a short stay for an acute episode differ from long, repeated stays for a chronic situation? What happens to a family when one member needs health resources that the family cannot provide? How do family members support one another when a member acquires a chronic illness such as cancer or diabetes or suffers from a cerebrovascular incident? Family-focused care implies asking assessment questions and planning interventions related to the contextual concerns and functional processes related to health and illness.

Nursing practices related to what is viewed as "good care" continue to evolve, and topics such as the utility of family hospital visitation continue to occur. Not long ago, it was usual practice for families to be excluded from patient care activities, restricted in visiting times, and asked to leave the room whenever interactions occurred between nurses and patients. Some thought it was necessary to reduce interactions in order to allow the patient to heal, and many hospitals imposed policies that isolated patients from their families. Patient records were viewed as belonging to the institution, basic information such as vital signs was kept from patients, and decisions about treatments were made without patient discussion or informed consent. Times have changed; interactions once viewed as detrimental are now seen as protective. More facilities have adopted policies of unrestricted visitation and involve patients' family members in care, discussions, and decisions. The Family Health Model encourages clinicians to not only consider individuals' needs but to also reflect on the consequences that systemic processes may have on individual health and family needs.

🏃🏃🏃🏃 *Cooperative Learning*

In pairs, take 5 to 10 minutes to brainstorm and compose a list of benefits and risks associated with family involvement during the hospital care of individuals. Make sure the list compares things from the family perspective with the nurse's viewpoint. When you have finished, a member from each pair should place his or her items on a blackboard or some other place where the class can view them. Identify items that appear on more than one list. When all items are visible, have a class discussion about the various ideas. In what ways have ideas changed over time? Are changes still occurring? Are there better ways to involve families in patient care than the ones currently in use? What changes are needed?

Social Support Systems

The Family Health Model supports the idea that nurses should act as advocates and consider interactions between family and the social support systems available within the mesosystem. In other words, when a family requires assistance, what sources of assistance are available? What other supports are needed? According to Garbarino and Abramowitz (1992), a social support is "a social arrangement that provides nurturance and feedback to individuals" (p. 65) and "serve as resources in times of physical and emotional need" (Garbarino, Galambos, Plantz, & Kostelny, 1992, p. 203). Caplan (1974) defined support systems as:

> Continuing social aggregates that provide individuals with opportunities for feedback about themselves and for validations for their expectations about others, which may offset deficiencies in these communications within the larger community context. They tell the individual what is expected of him and guide him in what to do. They watch what he does and judge his performance (pp. 4–6).

Support systems can be formal (e.g., social service agencies, community centers, churches, volunteer organizations) or informal (e.g., neighbors, friends, extended family, coworkers). Support usually transpires within the community or a geographic place where families live and interact. Social support can have powerful direct and indirect influences on the lives of families in social, economic, and health components. Community support to provide work-related activities; create mutually satisfactory relationships between teachers, parents, students, and school officials; provide safe and adequate child care; and reduce neighborhood risks are all forms of social support (Garbarino et al., 1992).

Needs and interactions with social support systems vary based on things such as age, maturity, geographic location, knowledge about the availability of services, and abilities to maneuver through bureaucracy. Infants and toddlers usually have few direct interactions with social support systems even though many services are targeted to meet their needs. Rather than support agencies using case finding techniques to locate eligible recipients, systems rely on the skills of parents to navigate the barriers to locating services. Understanding the concept of mesosystem helps one to see that the obstacles to obtaining needed help may be on the side of the provider or the recipient. Although you can lead a horse to water, but you cannot make it drink; it is also true that there is no possibility that the horse can drink if it cannot locate the watering hole! Agencies and institutions deemed to be support systems are often obstructed from those they intend to serve by policies, geographic locations, inept workers, or complex paperwork and procedures. For example, a single parent finds herself unable to work and care for her child, so she seeks help from a local government agency. The immediate tone of the encounter set by the first person contacted could suggest the tone of further interactions. Mothers who feel supported by the agency may take the steps needed to obtain services and have positive feelings about the actions. Mothers with less supportive encounters may still pursue the services because of need, but they may have their sense of self-worth compromised as a result of the experience. How do social supports affect development, health, and well-being? Family-focused care might not only aim at support system referrals but also at assisting families negotiate the organizational systems and cope with the stresses involved.

Focusing on the mesosystem also pertains to seeing that even available social supports can have both positive and negative effects. For example, a working parent might need child-care services. Although extended family members may provide some assistance, services may need to be hired. What happens in the 8-to-10-hour day when others care for the child in an environment outside the household niche? Interactions in that social environment may affect the child's behavior, personality, development, safety, and health. The parent may have some sense of what is occurring in the child-care environment, but clues may not tell the entire story about everything that occurs during the course of the day. How do parents respond to the child at the end of the day? Are their interactions different on nonwork days?

As children grow and mature, they reach out to others in ever-widening circles. Children may be introduced to wider social networks through the church or cultural traditions. Early interactions may serve to reinforce family values, ideas, and attitudes, but as children get involved in activities such as scouts, 4-H groups, or sports, they may meet people who are different from themselves. In what ways do these interactions enhance or threaten what is being taught at home? Do interactions support family values or contradict them? Do support systems strengthen the family's identity? Social networks can instill new values, reinforce them, or bring them into question. For example, a child attends summer Bible school. Parents may notice the child singing new songs, playing pretend games that reflect religious content, or insisting on prayers at meals and bedtime. If the family values what the child is learning, then the actions become more prized. However, if the family does not usually attend church or holds other views, the child might be ridiculed for these activities. Congruency or discord between family values and identity and the larger societal support systems can produce growth or provide conflict for children. Family-focused care questions the results of long-term or repeated conflicts or the compatibility of supports.

Parents participate in social functions that affect the family. Mothers may have hobbies, professional groups, or regular conversations with friends. Fathers may fish, hunt, golf, view spectator sports, belong to civic groups, or stop regularly at a local bar.

Parents may share activities or go separate ways. How do these activities—or lack of activities—affect family processes?

The mesosystem has far-reaching effects on the family. The Family Health Model encourages clinicians and researchers to investigate implications of mesosystem relationships on development and health outcomes. Over time, evaluations may enable nurses to better identify ways to intervene and assist members to balance the inconsistencies between family needs and the impact of larger contextual systems.

Reflective Thinking

Recall your present nursing practice. Think about your day-to-day activities. Have you noticed things about family health that you believe might be related to something outside the family? For example, in caring for a child diagnosed with attention deficit disorder, have you ever considered what other factors might have contributed to the problem behaviors? Or in the case of a sexual abuse or rape case, do you consider what contextual factors might have contributed to the episode (or episodes)? A man with a myocardial infarction is rushed into the emergency department. What possible contextual relationships might have contributed to his condition? An elderly woman is getting her annual mammogram and describes personal happiness, health, and a good life. What contextual factors might have contributed to her good health?

Consider some clients with whom you have recently interacted as you completed their health histories. What questions did you not ask that might provide greater insight into their present conditions? Can you be certain about the contributing factors related to genetics, personal traits, or the household niche? What contextual variables might have also contributed to health risks?

Aspects of the Exosystem

The *exosystem* is one or more settings that do not directly involve individuals as active participants, but these events still affect the family (Box 7–5). The exosystem implores one to consider the dynamic exchanges between families and larger contextual systems where no direct interaction occurs. The exosystem is a reminder that health is not merely confined to family characteristics and processes or interactions of family members with outsiders. The exosystem informs us that although families may seem insulated from external forces, they are not. In fact, health is deeply affected by places where individual members are connected, even when they are not present or not involved in decisions or actions happening there.

Box 7–5 **Aspects of the Exosystem**

- Peer relationships
- Preschool or school
- Work
- Play
- Health-care systems
- Social support systems

Peer Relationships

Peer relationships are frequently discussed in terms of negative and positive benefits, with less consideration given to the broader scope of these associations. Although individuals are certainly accountable for many of their actions, underlying factors may greatly contribute to choices and behaviors. For example, a boy grows up in an urban area where gangs are prevalent. The boy's parents warn him about the risks of involvement with gangs and encourage avoidance. The child wants to heed his parents, but the gang's bullying, threats, and victimization create feelings of social isolation and fear that seem of greater consequence than adherence to parental guidance. The desire for acceptance and the need to belong to larger peer groups has tremendous potential to impact choice in children, youth, and adults. Peer factors impact the psychological, emotional, social, and even spiritual needs of individuals. A geographically isolated mother may want to participate in parenting classes but may lack the transportation to get to the meetings. A community may have a wonderful senior group that welcomes new members, but an inability to drive excludes them from taking part in a potentially enjoyable peer experience. Family-focused care means understanding that decisions made by groups separate from individuals have potential impact on lives of those who do not participate in the decision making. Care might imply facilitating individual actions, but it may also entail collaboration with organizations or larger social systems to change policies or alter practices for the good of the community.

Educational Systems

Decisions at the federal, state, and local levels affect local school districts. Decisions about the inclusion of children with disabilities, rules about universal precautions, and policies for distributing students' medications are often made outside local districts, but these decisions affect local families. The individuals residing within a local area create a potential pool of teachers from which to draw, but teacher abilities, the quality of instruction materials, school levies, and the values of the local school board are factors that affect child learning. Contextual factors beyond the personal capacity to learn may affect grades and academic success. Families are affected by what happens in the classroom. Family-focused care could imply new roles for school nurses and community health nurses as they take more active roles in ascertaining what happens to the health of children as a result of their children's 12 to 13 years spent in a classroom. Questions about the impact of educational systems on individual health and ways to potentiate family health are rarely asked. How can nurses better serve the health of families and communities through access to school-age children? The Family Health Model would encourage nurses to ask questions and seek answers.

Work and Play

Beginning in the 1970s and continuing to the present, communities have been affected by market changes as the United States transforms itself from an industrial nation to one more focused on technology and information. Past opportunities for manufacturing jobs with good pay for those with a high school education or less seem to have disappeared as industries have closed or relocated. For example, one economically solid southern Ohio community faced foreign competition in the mid-1970s as shoe factories relocated and jobs in the steel industry were lost because of shutdowns. Some employees had the option to relocate, but many of them faced unemployment, struggled with retraining, faced relocating to other areas, or took jobs that offered greatly reduced family incomes. Foreign trade and competition created similar scenarios across the nation. Decisions made in boardrooms far removed from household niches, neighborhoods, and communities affected local families. The effects that resulted from lost employment affected aspects of family lives of many people across the nation.

Play is often tied to community economics. As communities prosper, they develop common areas where people congregate to share activities or information. A ball field, city park, community garden area, shopping mall, or local playgrounds are areas that affect opportunities for interaction with others. Many feel great pride when they wear a sweatshirt with a team logo, purchase a ring to symbolize their association with a school or group, or participate in an activity that contributes to a local organization that meets community needs. Persons beyond the individual govern rules about who can join or participate in some play, but these decisions still affect those who do not have a say. For example, decisions about how a community spends its money to support a youth center or library and a decision by the deacons of a local church to open its doors for after-school activities are made outside the family, but they have the potential to affect the family's development, health, and well-being. The Family Health Model encourages family-focused care that looks at community needs and population-based concerns that have the potential to affect the health of individuals and families. Creative and innovative practices that see beyond immediate circumstances and visualize the possibilities that exist between community life and family health are needed.

Health-Care Systems

Whenever health care is mentioned, most people think of physicians, medical care, high costs, health insurance, and illness treatment. Health-care systems are based on Western views of allopathic medicine as the optimal care mode. Employers mostly pay for insurance and health-care costs, but until the past decade, most care was based on a fee-for-service mechanism that directly paid physicians and other providers. In the old system, employers paid for insurance costs, insurance companies paid providers for services rendered, and service users paid little or nothing. By the late 1980s, employers, strapped by continually rising health-care costs, turned to managed care organizations, and the nation experienced a transition aimed at controlling rising costs. In 1999, 91 percent of the nation's employees with health insurance were enrolled in managed care plans, a major change from the 27 percent in 1988 (Institute of Medicine, 2000). The new system instituted capitation; co-pays; and pre-approvals for specialists, surgeries, and expensive treatments, and it emphasized the appropriate use of emergency services. As Americans faced these changes, lobbyists who represented specialized medical interests, media messages from consumer groups, and local and national politics created fears and anxieties about the changes. Managed care organizations encouraged medical providers and health-care agencies to be more businesslike in their operations. They restricted specialist care but encouraged some preventive care. Some physicians, medical organizations, and others raised questions about ethics and the inadequacies of the new systems. Largely uninformed employee groups were unprepared to advocate for their own best interests. As a result of political and economic decisions, the health-care system has had some radical changes, with shifts bringing opportunities and problems for providers and consumers.

A recent report about changes in primary care physicians' and specialists' scope of care identified that 30 percent of primary care physicians and 50 percent of specialists believed that the level of care they were expected to provide under managed care was more than it should be (St. Peter, Reed, Kemper, & Blumenthal, 1999). The investigators concluded that reports that the scope of care was greater than it should be aroused concerns about the impact of changes provided through managed care. Bodenheimer, Lo, and Casalino (1999) suggest that although physicians, as primary gatekeepers, may not provide an optimal care environment, the system should not return to the pre-managed care model of open access to specialists. The authors advised that primary care physicians should devise financial incentives for physicians who coordinate care that manages complex cases, discourages over- or under-referral to specialists, and improves the quality of care.

Although nurses play important roles in the health-care system, forms of reimbursement for nursing care have rarely been separated from other medical costs. The present scarcity of nurses could be a time for rethinking the kinds of services that individuals and families really need to increase their years of healthy life and reduce the health disparities for some population groups. Nurses mostly work in hospitals or other health agencies, with fewer employed in community or public health settings. The Family Health Model encourages rethinking health delivery and envisioning what is needed to meet society's wellness and illness needs. Family-focused care related to the exosystem and the health-care system suggests that becoming consumer advocates involved in health policy development is as pertinent as clinical practice.

Social Support Systems

Being disconnected from the larger society is related to mortality risk and almost every cause of death. "Social connectedness is loosely defined as the amount and quality of interaction an individual has with family, community, school, and workplace, as well as individual perceptions of how much support they have and how much influence they have over their environment" (Larkin, 2000, p. 3). Social isolation has been associated with many diseases and illnesses as well as mortality.

> A big challenge in combating isolation is the scope and complexity of the problem. The causes, characteristics, and outcomes of isolation vary widely from group to group and from individual to individual. For a young mother, the isolation brought on by a lack of transportation and childcare may result in depression and child neglect. For an adolescent, a lack of a nurturing school and positive after-school environment may lead to delinquency, substance abuse, and early sexual activity (Larkin, p. 3).

A study about women with breast cancer and arthritis found that women with more positive social systems and more extensive social networks had higher levels of psychological well-being, regardless of their physical health problems (Heidrich, 1996).

> We now know that a number of pathways link social networks to health outcomes. One is health behaviors: People who are isolated tend to smoke more, be more overweight, and be less physically active. It now appears that social isolation—the feeling of disconnection, of not belonging—is a chronically stressful experience that has a direct biological effect on the body (Berkman, 2000, p. 4).

Studies of health inequalities based on a life history approach should include biological and social beginnings (Wadsworth, 1997). Social support comes from many different directions, persons, systems, agencies, and institutions over the life course. Products of social support can be things such as a sense of community, attachment, connectedness, hardiness, resilience, cohesiveness, tolerance, and civility.

In many ways, it seems as if social support is the opposite of isolation. We often lack consensus about the meaning of social isolation, but most agree that it is clearly an important construct that impacts many aspects of youth and families (Coohey, 1996). What forms does isolation take? The types of isolation are many; social, emotional, physical, geographical, cultural, economic, and technological forms exist. Isolation may result in loneliness; inadequate supports; lack of attachment outside the household niche; marginalization; a sense of being unacceptable; and feelings of alienation, apathy, and abandonment. Consequences of isolation may be an inability to express feelings, secrecy that increases levels of differences, and disassociation from the larger community. Things such as learned helplessness, somatization, substance abuse problems, mental health issues, intergenerational transmission of disease, and social disability may characterize the lives of people affected by isolation.

Society often purposely isolates some groups. For example, criminals and sociopathic individuals are often isolated for the good of society. Although they are not institutionalized, society also isolates other groups such as physically or terminally ill, disabled, and elderly individuals; special education students; and immigrants. In fact, societies frequently isolate persons by gender, social class, economics, economic status, education, religion, color, and sexuality. Chronically ill persons, caregivers, emotionally disabled individuals, single parents, lesbian and gay youths, abused persons, and homeless people also experience isolation. What are the causes of isolation? Reasons might include fear, lack of self-confidence, or anxieties, but societal groups may isolate others because of morality, ethics, laws, traditions, behaviors, environmental pressures, greed or selfishness, or lack of understanding.

The literature widely discusses social isolation related to a variety of issues. Social isolation has been noted to have implications related to abuse and violence (Gelles & Straus, 1979; Maden & Wrench, 1977), a factor in the development of sexual abuse of youth (Fleming, Mullen, & Bammer, 1997), sexually abused women (Gibson & Hartshorne, 1996), battered women (Fiene, 1995; Forte, Franks, Forte, & Rigsby, 1996), school violence (Dupper, 1995), grandparents' caretaking of their grandchildren (Kelley, Yorker, & Whitley, 1997), women in migrant farm families (Rodriquez, 1993), poor Puerto Rican children who migrated with their families (Fontes, 1993), and mothers with low-birth-weight children (Sachs, Hall, Lutenbacher, & Rayens, 1999). Findings indicate that social isolation is a primary characteristic of victims of youthful abuse connected to an increased likelihood of performing life-threatening acts (Hazler, Carney, Green, Powell, & Jolly, 1997).

The early work of Garbarino (1978) described the roles of schools in causing, preventing, and treating child maltreatment based on whether the environment encourages an individualistic ethos and isolation from potent family or individual support systems. Students who are isolated and without best friends are much more likely to become victims than those who do have best friends (Boulton, Trueman, Chau, Whithand, & Amatya, 1999).

The Family Health Model suggests that when social support is considered from exosystem perspectives, issues should not only be examined from the positive perspectives of availability but should also consider what happens when social support is not available. Many of today's risks associated with morbidity and mortality are closely correlated with social and environmental hazards. Whereas Americans value self-reliance and independence, some other cultures value shared responsibility for the care of one another. Family-focused care aimed at reducing social isolation might focus on strategies to strengthen social competence, facilitate connections among family and others, build on individual and family strengths, and increase the sense of community.

𝅘𝅥𝅮𝅘𝅥𝅮𝅘𝅥𝅮 *Cooperative Learning*

Choose a particular community on which to focus. Half of the students should focus on family violence, and the other half should focus on families with children who have physical disabilities. Each group should identify the agencies in the community that provide services applicable to the problems.

Student groups should gather specific information about who the programs serve, the types of services provided, the costs of services, and the ability of the services to meet needs. What are the strengths of the services? What are the gaps in services? Where do services overlap? What needs to change, and what needs to stay the same to enhance the quality of support? Do the available services increase development, health, and well-being? Describe the contributions in each area.

Groups should also investigate the roles nurses have in providing care to these families. Do the community programs employ nurses? If so, what services do they provide? What knowledge and skills are needed to address the needs? How do nurses' salaries equate with those of other nursing jobs in the community? Each group should identify ways nurses might be included in agency programs to enhance care.

Groups should prepare a written summary to share with others. Student groups may want to compare and contrast the findings about the support services and family-focused care for the two family groups.

Aspects of the Macrosystem

The *macrosystem* is the overarching embedded systems that affect development, health, and well-being over the life course. The macrosystem includes ideologies, social expectations, legal and moral perspectives, and cultural or subcultural traditions that affect the reciprocal ways individuals treat and are treated by others (Box 7–6). For example, embedded views about race, ethnicity, religion, gender, class, and age may alter the ways individuals and families view themselves and others. The macrosystem provides a social paradigm that has subliminal effects on values, attitudes, and behaviors. For example, in the early frontier days of American history, it was usual for women to marry in their teens, bear six to twelve children or more, lose several children in either the birth process or to disease, and die before age 50 years. Although these facts may seem appalling today, they represent an accepted way of life in an earlier period. Extrapolating information without exploring its historical significance sometimes allows things to appear as if they were independent choices rather than imposed by the time and context. Although judgment of the rightness or wrongness of behaviors may have moral implications, the appraisal seems fairer if it is underscored with related facts that initially seem less obvious. Most of us are oblivious to the insidious influences of the macrosystem and the ways it compels us to believe and act. We often have the tendency to ignore what is less visible and overlook the covert or subtle ways that we are influenced. The Family Health Model encourages conceptualizations related to health to include the power and pressures of larger embedded contextual systems across the life course.

Box 7–6   Aspects of the Macrosystem
■ Social policy
■ Health policy
■ Public policy
■ Larger environments

Critical Thinking Activity

Nurses often give lip service to the importance of cultural competence in clinical practice, but they may remain naive about cultural differences. For example, we may group all blacks, Hispanics, or Asians together as if they were single homogenous groups. In the United States, all three of these groups are increasing in numbers. Some say that by 2010, one third of the U.S. population will be ethnic and racial minorities and by the year 2030, the minority population will reach 140 million, or 40 percent of the population (Institute of Medicine, 2000).

Choose blacks, Hispanics, or Asians. If you identify with one of these groups, then choose a different one. You are going to make two lists. The first list should identify everything you know for sure about this group. The second list should identify items you are less certain about but often hear about the group. The list can include things such as traditions, diet, health behaviors, personal characteristics, and so on. See how comprehensive you can make your list.

After you complete your lists, go on the Internet and choose a good search engine to investigate the group you have selected. Spend 30 to 45 minutes searching. As you search, make a third list that contains new information or things to support or dispute the items you previously listed. Bring the lists to class on the assigned date. In class, meet with others who reflected about the same group you did. Discuss what you have learned from the experience.

What do you know for sure? What do you need more information about? Where can you find the information you need? What would happen if you moved to a community where your daily work involved interactions with persons from this ethnic group? Are you prepared to address the individual and family needs? What do you need to do to enhance your knowledge and skills to better meet the needs of this group?

Social Policy

Many deaths and disabilities in the United States have behavioral linkages. For example, behaviors directly linked to choice such as smoking, alcohol use, diet, and lifestyle have linkages to morbidity and mortality. The detrimental effects of poverty and threats associated with environmental conditions have also been identified. Although risks associated with behavior and environment are amenable to change, they take large investments of human and social capital. Approximately $1 trillion is spent annually on health care nationwide, but less than 5 percent of the total is used to address the behavioral and social causes of disease, disabilities, morbidity, and mortality (Institute of Medicine, 2000). Discussions about differences in illness and life expectancy have largely focused on individual differences such as economic status and behavior. Less discussion about the effects of social or public policy on disease prevention, influences of the socioeconomic environment on health, or directions of budget allocations has transpired. A recent report by the Institute of Medicine (2000) titled *Promoting Health: Intervention Strategies from Social and Behavioral Research* acknowledges that health, disease and well-being are complex states that develop and change over the life course. Mounting evidence indicates that inequalities are likely to have adverse effects on health and that no single intervention or set of interventions will affect all implicated factors. Although social inequalities associated with mortality are largely caused by a high prevalence of risk behaviors among those with less education and income, a random national sample indicated that socioeconomic differences in mortality are actually caused by a wider array of factors that would persist even if disadvantaged individuals had improved health behaviors (Lantz, House, Lepkowski, Williams, Mero, & Chen, 1998). The cumulative effect of a life course perspective that considers relationships among biological factors, socioeconomic status, and psychosocial conditions that impact health is needed (Hertzman, 1998).

Models that include relationships between the socioeconomic and psychosocial conditions of a society identify much about health determinants germane to persons and populations. Bartley, Blane, and Montgomery (1997) argue that a life course approach is needed to understand social variations in health and the ways policies contribute to high health standards. An English study of a 1958 birth cohort concluded that lifetime socioeconomic circumstances accounted for inequalities in self-reported health at age 33 years (Power, Matthews, & Manor, 1996). A study of ill health among British women compared patterns of social advantage with disadvantage and found that persons with psychological symptoms showed the greatest health variations, and single mothers with dependent children were largely represented in this group (Macran, Clarke, & Joshi, 1996).

However, Kohn (1995) suggested a question of how we can "be certain that what we believe to be social structural regularities are not merely particularities, the product of some limited set of historical, cultural, or political circumstances" (p. 153). Multiple approaches that include broad sectors of society are needed to address complex factors associated with behavioral and environmental risks. The Family Health Model suggests that factors related to biology, development, psychology, economics, environment, policy, and cumulative life events must all be included. Although some determinants imply that appropriately timed interventions are needed, cumulative effects require focusing on prevention and risk reduction. Federal, state, and local revenue streams must support the financial appropriations needed for broad contextual interventions. Philanthropic groups, corporate businesses, private and public sectors, institutions, professional practitioners, policymakers, and others need to merge resources if the nation is to address risks from these broad perspectives and create models of care that touch individuals where they live, work, and play. The macrosystem is a reminder that health is more than individual behaviors and that family health is affected by social and environmental factors. Family-focused care to address macrosystem issues must include team approaches that address multilevel health needs, coordinate care across time and settings, include intersectorial collaboration, and foster policy development.

Health and Public Policy

Citizens in a community are affected by the availability and quality of services in the area. Although some communities may have many available choices, others may have limited or no services. Although federal or state funding for services and programs may exist, the lack of experts or professional providers may limit their availability. Legislators may vote to increase spending to meet specific needs, but wide disparities may still exist in the way these funds are actually used. For example, in the early 1980s, federal legislation was passed to enhance the care of dying persons during the terminal stage. The Hospice Medicare Benefit provides a more optimal way to meet care needs for terminally ill persons during the last 6 months of their lives. In the early 1980s, a grassroots movement embraced the hospice philosophy, and a variety of programs sprung up across the nation. Ideas from St. Christopher's Hospital in London, England, and palliative care practices used in Canada were blended with American ideas to create a unique form of hospice care acceptable to reimbursement systems, professional providers, and families.

Although the funding for programs existed, the locations of households affected whether a program to provide care was actually available. Although persons in urban areas were likely to have access, programs in rural areas were less accessible. Limited leadership; the availability of health-care professionals, start-up funds, or community or physician support; or misunderstandings about reimbursement mechanisms thwarted some efforts. An unwillingness of some physicians to identify a patient as terminal, an uncertainty about the best time to refer a patient for care, a distrust of a system not fully proven, concerns about pain and symptom management, and uncertainties about relinquishing care management to a team were other reasons for the slowness of hospice development in some communities. Also, Medicare provided payment for services for the elderly, but hospice care was not covered in many younger persons' insurance plans. A legislative decision provided a mechanism to fund hospice care, but many hurdles had to be overcome to actually make the services available across the nation.

Health policy is an area where ideas about health behaviors and biological development are likely to become an even more important focus on the interplay between social status and specific diseases (Higgs & Jones, 1999). Future challenges include the identification of the ways revered ideas actually mesh with health promotion needs, whether current health policy addresses these needs, and if health inequalities mainly result from an unequal distribution of societal income or are simply natural phenomena. Although the national concern about chronic disease is growing, health policies and reimbursement systems continue to focus on episodic needs of individuals. Prevention of chronic illness, caregiving needs of a growing elderly population, and the likelihood that most Americans will live with one or two chronic illnesses during their final decades of life are largely ignored by current health-care systems. A life course approach to understand the complex ways biological risk interacts with economic, social, and psychological factors in the development of chronic disease is needed (Bartley et al., 1997). What is the responsibility of government in the health of its people? What is needed to improve the years of healthy life for all people? A large disconnect between health-care needs and market outcomes seems to exist. Are the American people willing to pay higher taxes to cover the costs associated with chronic illnesses, or is the need merely for redistribution of present funds to cover health-care needs differently? What roles should nurses play in policy development? The Family Health Model implores one to not merely evaluate health services as they appear but instead to identify the contextual ideologies that are driving forces in policy development. Family-focused care emphasizes the necessity to compare relationships between current health policy, systemic programs, and economic funnels for current services with trends related to future needs. Nurses' practice roles could involve partnering with consumer or family groups to identify population-based health needs and then collaborating with other health-care professionals, lobbyists, and policymakers to create legislation that more appropriately addresses needs. Roles might also involve model projects to test the effectiveness of comprehensive forms of family practice that tackle a broad scope of family needs.

ᛗᛗᛗᛗᛗᛗ *Cooperative Learning*

Take 5 minutes to pair off with another student. Create lists of the ways the media and societal messages influence alcohol use. How are individuals encouraged to drink or refrain from alcohol use? Get together with another pair of students and choose a note taker. Spend 5 to 10 minutes talking together about ways these messages might affect school-age children. Then spend another 5 minutes discussing the ways media and societal messages affect parents. Finally, spend the last 5 minutes identifying ways a family nurse might use this information in clinical practice. Each group should provide the class with a summary of their ideas.

Larger Environments

The macrosystem context introduces, affirms, and negates health beliefs, knowledge, and behaviors that represent perspectives and paradigms of the larger society. The larger environment begins in the family of origin as the daily events that occur within the household niche among family members and significant closely related others. As time goes by and individuals mature, the larger environment expands to include interactions between the family, mesosystem, exosystem, and macrosystem. Carter and McGoldrick (1999b) described the larger society in peacetime as "as a whole with its laws, norms, traditions, and way of life" and in wartime or in terms of global markets as larger than a single nation or as "spaceship earth" (p. 12).

For centuries, isolated societies were able to maintain primitive ways, distinct languages, and cultural traditions. Technological advances, information-sharing capacities, and globalization have created an avalanche of change that cannot be reversed. Although humans were once limited to hand-transcribed books, the printing press revolutionized the way knowledge could be shared. Before the 1960s, the human race was constrained to the Earth, but Neil Armstrong's walk on the moon forever changed the face of space. When Marshall McLuhan said the "media was the message," he spoke of television's ability to alter individual lives in private homes. Although the larger environment may have once been the neighborhood or community, today it is the world and its interspatial attributes. In the past decade or so, computers and information technologies have revolutionized communication and have extended the horizons of understanding worldwide. Changes that took centuries to evolve can now occur in brief periods and are bringing alterations that will forever remodel contextual perspectives.

The larger environment where we live affects the whole of life and health. When individuals' lives are considered, they must be viewed as embedded in larger contextual systems. Development, health, and well-being are not only affected by genetics, education, and family income but also by larger environments that affect life processes, resilience, cohesiveness, and self-individuation. Health is not just a series of isolated events merely related to individual members; rather, it includes family members' interactive responses as they engage their contexts from a household niche perspective. The Family Health Model encourages nurses to identify ways that the larger environment supports the continuance of present patterns or mediates change. Family-focused care entails practices that must respond to causes and effects related to larger environments and their interactions with individual and family health processes.

Box 7-7 **Challenges That Confront Clinical Practice and Research**

- Identify ways to obtain information about individuals in context rather than merely obtain information about the individual and the context.
- Determine which contexts affect individuals, family subsystems, and family at specific time points versus enduring influences of contexts over the life course.
- Decide which factors across contexts and time are most amenable to interventions and result in the most optimal health outcomes.
- Differentiate the dose (e.g., timing, amount, length of time) of the interventions targeted at specific contextual targets.
- Evaluate differences of the individual as the source of health or disease versus the embedded household niche as the source of health or disease.

Summary

This chapter has provided an overview of the wide-ranging and complex variables related to the embedded context and health. Focus is too often on the immediacy of the case at hand while the impact imposed by the macrosystem context is ignored. Snapshots of the present appear more important than landscape perspectives over the life course. From a macrosystem perspective, the Family Health Model entreats practitioners to understand the implications of embedded individuals, family subsystems, and family household niches over the life course. Many challenges confront researchers and practitioners in clinical practice (Box 7–7).

Health research has focused on controlling for extraneous variables for more rigorous investigative processes. It may be possible that some contextual variables cannot be controlled but can be taken into account. The Family Health Model provides many propositions related to the embedded context that still need to be investigated and tested (Box 7–8). A body of knowledge that furthers understandings about the embedded context and health is needed.

Box 7-8 **Propositions Related to the Family Context**

- Positive interactions that occur within the family microsystem and between the family subsystem, household niche, and diverse external contexts have the potential to enhance individual and family health over the life course.
- Negative interactions that occur within the family microsystem and between the family subsystems, household niche, and diverse external contexts have the potential to threaten individual and family health over the life course.
- Interventions aimed to potentiate individual and family health produce more meaningful family outcomes when contextual perspectives are included.
- Outcomes relevant to individuals are enhanced when interventions also include family subsystems and the household niche.
- Interventions aimed at individual and family health are enhanced when the dyadic and triadic processes and interactions are the targets rather than merely targeting individuals.
- Interventions aimed at individual and family health have more positive outcomes when they affect multiple aspects of the family context and continue over time rather than being single, unrelated, episodic events.
- Interventions aimed at person-process-context will produce more effective health outcomes than interventions aimed solely at singular targets.

Test Your Knowledge

1. Define the term *chronosystem*.
2. Explain and give an example of how the chronosystem affects family health.
3. Define the term *mesosystem*.
4. Explain and give an example of how the mesosystem affects family health.
5. Define the term *exosystem*.
6. Explain and give an example of how the exosystem affects family health.
7. Define the term *macrosystem*.
8. Explain and give an example of how the macrosystem affects family health.
9. Describe a way that a family nurse might use the conceptual ideas about the chronosystem in clinical practice to assess, plan, and evaluate some form of care targeted at family health.
10. Compare and contrast the different ways a family nurse might consider the mesosystem and exosystem when addressing family health.

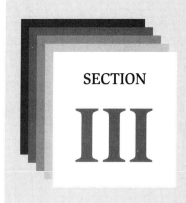

SECTION

III Functional Aspects of Family Health

Chapter

8

Functional Aspects
of Family Health

CHAPTER OBJECTIVES   *At the end of this chapter, the reader will be able to:*

- Discuss ways development and health are products of genetics and environment.
- Differentiate between individual and family development.
- Describe the potential relationships between functional processes and health.
- Identify the importance of dyadic and triadic member relationships to family health.

> *When you are joyous, look deep into your heart and you shall find it is only that which has given you sorrow that is giving you joy. When you are sorrowful look again in your heart, and you shall see that in truth you are weeping for that which has been your delight.*
> —Kahlil Gibran, The Prophet

Achieving a Healthy Family

The term *functional* is often used to describe behavior and interactions within, between, and among persons. Systems function to obtain, store, process, interpret, and use information applicable to health. Family systems have cognitive, utilitarian, and behavioral capacities. For example, one might discuss members' mental aptitudes for learning, abilities to solve problems effectively, or success in achieving personal or family goals. Functionality can be discussed in terms of relationships in which individuals, family subsystems, and families live, work, play, and interact with embedded contextual systems. "Family function is the purpose that the family serves in relation to the individual, other social systems, and society," and these processes are influenced by health of individual members and the family as a whole (Ballard, 2001, p. 84). Family function affects members' development, health, and well-being, but these are also affected by and affect interactions with larger contextual systems. Family members mediate values, beliefs, knowledge, and behaviors that alter many of life's dimensions and can negate or potentiate health. Functionality provides a way to describe obvious and obscure linkages between persons, processes, and settings. This chapter identifies issues related to functionality pertinent to family health.

As previously mentioned, the terms *family health* and *healthy family* are often used interchangeably in the literature. In the Family Health Model, the term *healthy family* refers to the functional abilities of individuals, family subsystems, and families as they develop and live, work, and play to optimize development, processes of becoming, well-being, and health. Satir (1972) said healthy families:

- Are untroubled and nurturing
- Demonstrate patterns of high individual self-worth
- Use direct, clear, specific, and honest forms of communication
- Have flexible, human, and appropriate rules
- Practice open and hopeful links with society

Curran (1983, 1985) said that healthy families communicate well with one another when they listen; share power; use nonverbal messages to express feelings, care, and love; develop patterns of reconciliation; and cooperate to solve problems. Pearsall (1990) suggested strategies to achieve a healthy family through strengthening, comforting, and healing processes.

Healthy family is a process that occurs as members value one another and act in nurturing ways at specific time points and over the life course. It is possible to have a healthy family at one time but a less healthy one at other times. Some aspects of family interactions may be healthy, but others may not be. It might be helpful to think about families on a continuum, with the potential to have more and less healthy times and members. Because families have unique capacities to achieve their goals, it may be more meaningful to consider them in terms of the abilities to accomplish goals they set for themselves rather than compare them with other families. A family might say they are healthy if the members are attaining their objectives and their relationships with each other were satisfactory. Families may see themselves in terms of being healthy without ever considering things such as health, illness, or disease. Even so, nurses can still play roles in assisting individuals and families to achieve functional aspects of a healthy status when they assist them to identify their self-worth or empower them to solve problems.

Family health is an abstract construct with gradients of scale, significance, and flexibility. It is possible to be a healthy family, one with nurturing members who value and effectively interact in a caring way for one another, but still not achieve family health. For example, if a family resides in a poverty-stricken area where food is unavailable, if they live in a war-torn region where life is in constant danger, or if they have recently suffered the perils of a natural disaster that destroyed their community, one might question whether they have family health. In these instances, context can be a greater predictor of family health than the innate family qualities. Although healthy family might imply that family members' functional capacities to achieve family health are available, family health is a more complex process that embraces the interactions of multiple members and contextual systems as members individually and collectively seek a biophysical, emotional, social, and spiritual equilibrium and well-being and maximize processes of becoming. An expanded perspective of family health not only includes cure-oriented medical practices; it is a perspective that also addresses the roles of economics and social policy in optimizing population-based mortality and morbidity, preventing disease and illness, and generating health outcomes. Nurses should be prepared to attend to the multifaceted aspects of family health.

The Nature-versus-Nurture Debate

For more than a century, arguments have persisted about whether the greatest factors that affect human development are genetic or environmental. Some suggest that personality and behaviors are derived from innate traits that are linked to genetics, but others attribute personality and behaviors to environmental influences. Both viewpoints seem useful in understanding development, but neither seems to offer an adequate basis for fully understanding (Bateson, 1998). Bateson suggests that a connectionist model is needed to consider the idea of imprinting as a highly regulated learning process that occurs as individuals physically grow, mature, and interact with the environment. Imprinting entails indelibly impressing formative ideas about behaviors on the memory at early ages. Thus, developing persons become closely linked to the nature and nurture experiences that occur early in life. One could say that the health experiences that occur in the family of origin and the household niche are imprinted as children develop and serve as a foundation for all further learning and practice. It seems most likely that genetic and environmental factors have additive effects on developing persons over time. A connectionist model provides ways to move away from the reductionist and interactionist ideas that characterize the nature versus nurture debate.

Explanations about behavior are often presented in terms of the exclusive importance of genetic or environmental factors. For example, research about social behaviors has attempted to investigate whether the potential for aggressive behavior is mainly genetic or environmental. Research on mice completed in the 1960s used selective breeding to study aggressive behaviors (Lagerspetz, 1964), and later research investigated the interactional and developmental controls of aggression (Cairns, 1972, 1976). Research on mice has found:

1. Within one to five generations, selective breeding can produce aggressive behaviors.
2. The robust effects of rearing, interactional effects, learning, and social organization exist regardless of the animal's genetic background.
3. Social behaviors that can be manipulated through development can also be manipulated by genetic selection across generations (Cairns & Cairns, 1995).

Although humans are certainly not mice, research in mice is frequently used to inform us about human behaviors. Findings seem to indicate that internal and external environments compete and that development involves both mediating and accommodating competing factors. Behavior seems to be more fluid than fixed, and a feedback system appears to exist between biology and context within and across generations.

Are the findings in studies of mice relative to human development? Longitudinal studies that measured deviance and aggression were found to be reasonably predictive in within-individual factors. Additionally, when individual and social characteristics were clustered, school dropout, teen parenthood, and other difficulties were predicted (Cairns & Cairns, 1994). Studies about biological effects of early female maturation have shown strong linkages influenced by the social context (Magnusson, 1988; Statin & Magnusson, 1990). Developing persons appear to have highly predictable trajectories that can be identified in early life, but these trajectories more fully emerge as individuals are influenced by the social context over the lifespan (Cairns & Cairns, 1995). It seems that, at least in some ways, nature and nurture are part of the whole rather than purely dichotomous.

Over the past few decades, the field of early intervention has provided evidence about the ways physiology and environment impact learning and behavior. For example, a study (Calderon & Low, 1998) of children with hearing loss identified that when fathers were present in the home, children had significantly better academic and language outcomes than those without a father present. A study (Calderon, 2000) about the impact of school-based, teacher-rated parental involvement found that although parental involvement was a significant positive predictor of early reading skills, mothers' communication skills and the level of the child's hearing loss were also important predictors. In this study, mothers' use of support services was the strongest predictor of social and emotional adjustment. The child's intelligence was not the only predictor of success; social interactions also played a role. A study (Glascoe, 1997) about the implications of discussions between the parents and providers about developmental problems found that parents seeking health care for their children seem to have more developmental concerns than those without providers. Parents were most likely to discuss concerns about expressive language when they thought their child had health problems, and when parents of disabled children discussed them with health-care providers, children were more likely to be enrolled in special education services. Children with disabilities may have innate physiological characteristics that affect learning outcomes, but parental concerns and behaviors are important variables in the types of care children receive.

Nature and nurture seem to interplay in child learning, development, and physiological capabilities, but both nature and nurture have implications for the entire life course. The Family Health Model suggests that early learning about health within the household niche influences health values and behaviors across the life course. Although genetics and family heritage are viewed as important predictors of potentials related to health, the model suggests that embedded contextual systems and social behaviors are equally influential.

👪 *Cooperative Learning*

Everyone seems to have some opinions about the questions of nature and nurture. Find a partner with whom you can discuss your beliefs about these issues. After allowing time for sharing, form four groups and the instructor will assign a topic:

1. Nature is the most positive influence on child development.
2. Nature is the primary influence on child development, but nurture plays an important role.
3. Nurture is the most positive influence on child development.
4. Nurture is the primary influence on child development, but nature plays an important role.

Choose a recorder to report your group's conclusions. Take time to formulate your ideas, to identify arguments that either support or refute the position, and to provide some rationale for your conclusions. Each group will then discuss its ideas with the class.

Human Development

Theories of Human Development

Volumes have been written about developmental processes, and nurses have studied them throughout their nursing education. A brief discussion of a few of the most influential thinkers about developmental processes is provided to suggest the many important insights pertinent to developing persons. For example, Erikson (1968) described individual development in terms of eight stages of development; Bandura (1982) suggested personal experiences and socialization processes are important for understanding competence and mastery; and Vygotsky (1978) explained ways that historical and cultural changes in children's environments influenced cognition. Piaget (1971) considered ways children at different ages approached problems, and he saw thinking as a series of increasingly complex stages during which learning is revised and incorporated into current thought. He described thought in terms of direct learning, social transmission, and maturation and used the ideas of assimilation, accommodation, and adaptation to describe how experiences, ideas, and encounters change as a child develops. Kohlberg (1981) discussed children's moral development in terms of sensitivity to what is right and wrong. Gilligan (1982) later challenged Kohlberg's ideas, which were based on male subjects. She suggested that whereas male identity was primarily identified with separation and autonomy, girls focused on attachment and emotional connectedness. Boys thought in terms of general ethical principles applied to specific situations, but girls developed an ethic of care that integrated principles with the contexts in which decisions were made. Bowers (1995) discussed the abstract reasoning that allows adolescent idealism, limits the ability to appreciate logical points of view different from their own, and permits egocentric behaviors. These theorists and many others have focused on various aspects of developmental processes, seeing them as series of continuous changes over time with distinct stages vital to generativity, productivity, and achievement. Nurses can extract from their previous learning about developmental processes the knowledge and skills needed to meet health needs through family-focused care.

Critical Thinking Activity

The instructor will assign a different developmental theorist (e.g., Erikson, Piaget, Kohlberg, Gilligan) to you or a group. Identify the key premises of the theoretical framework and list reasons why these premises might not be correct or concerns that you may deduce from alternative possibilities or other knowledge areas. You or your group can present these ideas to the class and discuss ways nurses might use developmental theories to meet health needs.

Human Development

Developmental processes have implications for health across the life course. In the Family Health Model, development is defined as a "person's evolving conception of the ecological environment and his relation to it, as well as the person's growing capacity to discover, sustain or alter its properties" (Bronfenbrenner, 1979, p. 9).

> Human development is the process through which the growing person acquires a more extended differentiated, and valid conception of the ecological environment, and becomes motivated and able to engage in activities that reveal the properties of, sustain,

or restructure the environment at levels of similar or greater complexity in form and content (Bronfenbrenner, p. 27).

A healthy child matures and moves from total dependence and interaction only with the family microsystem to greater independence and interaction with larger contextual systems.

> The ecology of human development involves the scientific study of the progressive, mutual accommodation between an active, growing human being and the changing properties of the immediate settings in which the developing person lives, as this process is affected by relations between these settings, and by the larger contexts in which the settings are embedded (p. 21).

Development affects all aspects of individual and family life, and processes once affected at any point in time possess the potential to cause other changes at other times and places. In other words, development is not only influenced by unique traits and characteristics but also by the context in which households are situated.

A concern related to developmental models is that they mainly focus on psychosocial concerns and are less likely to make connections with biophysical changes or health as a developmental process. Research has mainly investigated relationships between family functioning and psychological health, but only limited studies (Campbell, 1986; Van Riper, 2001) about family functioning and the physical health of family members have been done. Although we know much about developmental variables linked with individuals and parenting, less is known about the impact of the embedded household context on these traits. Kohn (1995) said:

> Social structure had consistent effects on all facets of personality that we studied, and the consistent explanation of these consistent effects was that position in the social structure decidedly affected occupational self-direction and that occupational self-direction decidedly affected personality (p. 156).

The Family Health Model suggests the use of developmental theories for not only considering individuals' functional capacities but also for verifying relationships to health behaviors and outcomes.

Family Development

Several authors have described ways to view development from a family perspective. For example, Carter and McGoldrick (1988) provide a six-stage perspective for use in family therapy that describes family stages:

1. Between families (e.g., unattached young adults)
2. Newly married couples
3. Families with young children
4. Families with adolescents
5. Families that are launching children
6. Families in later life

Duvall and Miller (1985a) have identified eight stages of family development:

1. Beginning families
2. Childbearing families
3. Families with preschool children
4. Families with school-age children
5. Families with teenagers
6. Families that are launching young adults
7. Middle-aged parents
8. Families in retirement and old age

Klein and White (1996) described the developmental tasks of families as:

1. Meeting the biological requirements of families
2. Addressing the cultural imperatives of families
3. Accomplishing the aspirations and values of families

The Family Health Model suggests that developmental tasks are more helpful for addressing family health than family stages.

Several problems seem inherent in stage perspectives. First, neither the ideas of Carter and McGoldrick (1988) nor the ones of Duvall and Miller (1985a) are adequate for fully understanding family diversity. For example, blended families often have both infants and adolescents developing at the same time; homosexual families may raise children who are biologically related to only one partner; and some families wait until their late 20s or early 30s to begin childbearing. Family variations or alternative family types could imply different family stages. A second problem is related to a lack of understanding about the development that occurs in middle age through the old age. The U.S. Census Bureau projects that the number of persons who are older than age 65 years (currently 35 million) will increase 5 million by 2010 and double to 70 million by 2030. The number of persons who are older than age 85 years will double by 2030. Attention has centered mainly on development during parenting stages, but much less is known about development before and after retirement age. Persons now have the potential to live far more years in developmental processes after parenting tasks are completed than years spent engaged in those activities. What effects do altered parent–child relationships in mature life have on child, parent, and family development? What developmental changes occur as parents modify their lives as they approach midlife? How do interactions between grandparents and grandchildren affect development? What developmental changes occur in adult children when they become caregivers for their parents?

Carter and McGoldrick (1999a) have identified concerns related to aging and discuss the needs to view developmental progression and interdependence. Although parenting and mother–infant bonding have been described as interdependent processes (Bowlby, 1969), increased thought needs to be directed to the developmental and functional needs that occur across the life course. Inclusion of larger contextual systems and broader health variables push providers to consider alternative relationships germane to development. Learning about complex interacting variables is costly and time consuming, but some work in this area might provide better ways to articulate deep-seated quandaries intrinsic to health processes.

 Reflective Thinking

Think about childhood development in terms of your experiences and those of your siblings. Try to list some differences and similarities between you and your siblings related to individual health. Do you see yourselves as being more alike or more different? Think about the differences as they relate to individual health. Do you think you are more or less healthy than your siblings? What processes do you think might have contributed to the similarities and differences that you identify?

As you consider these qualities, try to think about what might have accounted for them. Then try to identify what various developmental processes that occurred within your household niche might have contributed to these qualities. What were there different contextual factors that might have contributed? Think about different time periods in your life. What stands out in your memory?

If you have the opportunity, discuss these ideas with your siblings and get their perspectives. Do they see things differently? How might these relationships affect family health?

Functional Perspectives and Family Health

Functional Perspectives and Developing Persons

The Family Health Model is concerned with processes that occur in the household niche as developing persons experience a variety of contextual settings across the life course. Hertzman (1998, 1999) described interactions between childhood development, socioeconomic differences in early life experiences, and psychosocial conditions over the life course as contributors to subsequent health status and system defense factors. Evidence derived from intervention studies in early childhood suggests that cognitive, social, and emotional childhood experiences affect health status and vitality and can be modified in ways that improve health, well-being, and competence in the long term (Hertzman & Wiens, 1996). Although early developmental experiences are powerful health determinants, they are mediated over a lifetime through a variety of contextual interactions. Assumptions about the functional processes relevant to the Family Health Model suggest relationships that nurse clinicians and researchers can tackle (Box 8–1).

The functional status of families aids in understanding the processes related to health. However, some family models have not successfully described, explained, or predicted family behaviors (Keltner & Ramey, 1992, 1993). Friedman (1998) describes the structural-functional approach as an organizing framework for understanding the arrangement and organization of the family and a way to describe family purposes for its own development and societal good. She suggests that the five family functions are affective, economic, reproductive, socialization, and health care. The health-care function "entails the provision of physical necessities: food, clothing, shelter, and health care" (Friedman & Morgan, 1998, p. 404). Artinian (2001) said that a structural-functional framework provides nurses with ways to understand how illness affects the family,

---

Box 8–1 **Assumptions about Functional Processes and Family Health**

- Individuals develop over the life course in response to genetic and contextual traits.
- Individual health is a result of genetic, interactional, and contextual potentials.
- Individuals have beliefs, perceptions, and behaviors that affect health outcomes, but these are mediated by genetic dispositions, family interactions, and environmental contexts.
- Processes of becoming and well-being are influenced by family members' interactions with one another and their embedded contextual systems.
- Initial socialization about health occurs within the household niche and evolves over the life course as developing persons, family subsystems, families, and larger contexts interact.
- The quality, meaning, and effectiveness of core family processes affect health.
- Individuals and families use core family processes to attain, maintain, sustain, and regain health as they interact with internal and external contextual influences.
- Perceptions about what comprises health vary as individuals mature, accommodate change, and encounter contextual influences across the life course.

which processes are needed to optimize functioning, and where to provide interventions. Hanson (2001b) notes that this model encourages a view of family as one of the basic units of society with activities, purposes, organization, and relationships to other social systems that enable nurses to assess the system as a whole, as a societal subunit, or as an interactional system. The Family Health Model is not in direct conflict with ideas depicted through a structural-functional model. However, the Family Health Model does make some distinctions between context and function and views many ideas in the structural-functional model as function related to health processes. However, nursing roles viewed with either model related to functional status could include things such as:

- Teaching and counseling
- Securing knowledge, services, and resources
- Organizing and providing for daily health and illness care needs
- Advocating for what is lacking and needed
- Finding supports for change, processes of becoming, and well-being

Family members who live in the same household may have different needs or goals, use different interactional processes, and respond differently to similar embedded contexts. A study (Richards, Adams, & Hunt, 2000) that compared siblings with one obese sibling and the other within a normal weight range found that even when the genetic relationship was close and the environment was shared, differences in the amounts of food consumed and physical exercise were still identified. In observing family dietary patterns, family members in the same household consumed very different diets and had great variances in the foods consumed (Denham, 1997). Nurses must understand needs unique to families and individual members, as well as the interactive functional processes affected by embedded contextual systems that contribute to or limit health outcomes.

👫👫👫👫 *Cooperative Learning*

The instructor will divide the class into five groups and have you each choose a recorder. Consider a family role that might affect family health. You and your group members should then brainstorm and identify 10 interventions that nurses might consider if addressing needs related to this role. For example, a group discussing parental teaching or counseling should identify specific ways that a family nurse could intervene with families to positively influence individual and family health. After about 10 to 15 minutes of small group discussions, each group will then share their lists with the class.

Dyad and Triadic Relationships

Families are composed of multiple subsystems that can be identified as dyads or triads. As developing persons form close relationships with family members, dyads are initially formed. Each member within the household forms dyadic relationships. *Dyadic units* are dynamic interactions between members with diverse characteristics and meanings. Dyadic relationships are initially formed because of the family context, but persons outside the family boundaries may also become dyad members (e.g., boyfriends, friends, colleagues). Some family dyads are tenacious and tend to persevere over the life course, but the strengths of the relationships may vary with time. Intact dyads with shared goals possess an innate potential to mediate factors relevant to health, but less cohesive dyads may threaten health.

After a family forms dyads, these dyads tend toward resilience. Information from the larger contextual systems is often interpreted by dyads in relation to personal meanings, goals, and family identity. Whenever health needs are encountered, intact dyads use core family processes to *adapt* and *accommodate* factors imposed by member interactions and the larger contextual systems. Adaptation is a passive response to interactions that occur within the household and larger contextual systems that contradict, threaten, or compete with accepted family norms. It is a way to understand how actions, behaviors, and even biological responses are modulated. Accommodation is an active response to existing schemes of thinking and action that occur when members are faced with events or situations when old behavioral patterns are ineffective. Although accommodation can result in some fixed patterns, the process is fluid over the life course, with continual feedback responses from the interactions of multiple family members as new information is received and environmental messages are altered.

The character of dyads is altered whenever other family members or persons enter the context. For example, a mother and toddler may be playing in a usual pattern, but when the father returns home from work, the relationship between the mother and toddler is somewhat altered. Although the father has a dyadic relationship with both the mother and the child, his presence forms a triad, and interruptions affect the play that previously occurred between the mother and child. Dyadic characteristics impact the family's functional capacities. For example, if the father comes in angry and demands to know why the mother is playing rather than cooking his dinner, the context changes from a mother–child dyad to a mother–father one. If the father comes home and begins to play with the mother–child dyad, a triad is formed. It is posited that the strength of a triad is greater than that of a dyad. Entrance of a short-term visitor (e.g., extended family member, friend, neighbor, stranger) into the household may alter usual dyadic patterns, but these behaviors tend to resume after the visitor's departure. Family ideas about things such as boundaries, identity, and traditions influence interactions. Families form complex webs of relationship. Some triads are built on dyadic links, so the strengths and weaknesses of the dyads are inherent in the triads. Each individual has unique views about the strength, value, and effectiveness of the various member relationships.

The formation and interruption of dyads and triads creates family interactional patterns through which members adapt and accommodate to create interactional patterns, with potential effects on development, health, and well-being. Although frequently disrupted dyads may result in altered patterns that threaten family cohesiveness, resiliency, hardiness, or health, congruent dyads or triads have great potential for use in family interventions to mediate or potentiate health. Over time, dyadic interactions form a gestalt, or a pattern of beliefs, attitudes, and behaviors that becomes the context for health routines. The cohesiveness and permeability of dyadic or triadic boundaries have the potential to alter members' health beliefs, knowledge, and behaviors.

Member needs may result in forming temporary, semi-permanent, or permanent relationships with nurses or other health-care providers. The extent of the felt need may determine the strength and extent of the relationship. For example, an infant born with cystic fibrosis may require frequent physician visits. The child and mother may form close bonds with the physician or nurse relevant to meeting the child's health-care needs. This mother may form a semi-permanent relationship with a schoolteacher who needs to know about specific medical regimens to which the child adheres. This same mother may also form a dyadic relationship with a scout leader to ensure that her child can participate in activities similar to other children. The mother also wants to be sure that the leader knows what to do in emergency situations. Nurses can use the potential strengths of family dyads and triads to assess needs and intervene in ways that reduce risks and promote health.

It is proposed that interventions that target dyads and triads rather than single individuals have greater strength and the potential to support family accommodations associated with health concerns. For example, nurses often teach individuals about illness and health-care needs. Teaching seldom includes family needs or multiple members in either a systematic or comprehensive way. It is posited that family functional processes targeted at health-care needs are enhanced when interventions include dyads and triads rather than single individuals.

Reflective Thinking

You have had multiple opportunities to form many dyadic and triadic relationships. Depending on your age and contextual status, you may still consider yourself a member of your family of origin household, you may be part of a family of procreation, or you may live in a variety of alternative forms of households. It is possible that you have lived in several different contexts.

Think back over your life course and recall the dyadic and triadic relationships you have formed within your household niche (or niches). How would you characterize these relationships? Have they changed over time, or do they remain unchanged? In what ways did dyadic relationships influence your health beliefs, health knowledge, and health behaviors? Were there positive effects of these dyads or triads on your personal development, health, or well-being?

What about triadic relationships within your family? Ask yourself the same questions about your triadic relationships. Would you say the triadic relationships are different from dyadic ones? If so, in what ways? How might nurses use the idea of family triads to influence health beliefs, health knowledge, and health behaviors?

Relationships of Proximal Processes to Family Functional Processes

Functional processes have direct relationships with other simultaneous processes that occur within the household. Bronfenbrenner and Ceci (1994) proposed some ideas for a model that includes a genetic paradigm, direct environmental measures, and organism–environmental interactions. They suggested that the genotype or genetic constitution of an individual is influenced by the environment to present a phenotype, or an organism with properties attributed to the genotype and environment. They proposed that heritability increases markedly with the magnitude of proximal processes and results in synergistic effects. *Proximal processes* are the mechanisms through which the genetic potentials for developmental processes are actualized or the ways individuals take their genetic inheritance and actualize them as they mature and interact within larger contextual systems over the life course. It is posited that enhancement of proximal processes and environmental quality can increase genetic potentials, developmental competence, and health. Full realization of genetic potential is strongly influenced by interactions with contextual factors.

The Family Health Model suggests that health is related to genetic or inherited factors that are affected by individuals' proximal processes and the diverse environments they encounter. Family-focused care addresses the functional and interactional processes that occur within the family household as members interact with embedded contextual systems to meet their health needs. Family-focused care implies a need for collaborative relationships to assist individuals, family subsystems, and families with their accommodation processes to attain desired goals. Nurses assist individuals and families to:

- Cope with crisis or stress
- Choose between competing knowledge objects
- Make decisions that influence well-being
- Develop satisfying and meaningful relationships
- Select behaviors that are health promoting
- Avoid behaviors that are health negating
- Modify perceptions of self, others, symbols, and environments that are risk producing
- Acquire resources that promote, maintain, or assist to regain health
- Use immediate and remote environments to potentiate individual and family health

Nurses empower as they assist families to actualize their full genetic potentials by actively engaging their dynamic processes and interactions with larger contextual systems.

Summary

Nurses are generally well prepared to address functional processes with individuals, but interacting with families is an area with which they may lack skills. The daily and cumulative effects of behavioral processes and interactions over the life course have potential to mediate, impede, and facilitate development, processes of becoming, well-being, and health. Functional status pertaining to health outcomes is not fixed; rather, it is malleable as genetic and environmental potentials intersect through the life of interacting family members. Dyads and triads hold promise for rethinking the ways interventions are provided to address family health. Internal familial bonds, ties to extended kin networks, and links with others external to the household niche may be keys to addressing health risks and potentials. Nurses can best address functional needs related to family health by interacting with family subsystems, identifying family goals, and collaborating with family members to address needs related to the embedded contextual systems.

Test Your Knowledge

1. Describe what is implied by *developmental processes* and discuss ways nurses might intervene to promote health.
2. Explain two ways that a family's functional processes can enhance family health.
3. Discuss how ineffective functional processes within a family might threaten well-being.
4. Identify how an embedded contextual system might threaten family health even when the family shares optimal functional processes.
5. Compare and contrast the potential effects of dyadic and triadic relationships on family health.
6. What is meant by the idea of *proximal processes*? Give one example to show how they might be a health threat and another example to demonstrate a positive health effect.
7. List three ways a nurse might use the idea of functional processes to intervene with a family that has a child with chronic asthma.

Chapter

9

The Household Production of Health

CHAPTER OBJECTIVES *At the end of this chapter, the reader will be able to:*

- Describe features of the family household that affect health.
- Explain the term the *household production of health.*
- Identify health practices and behaviors as social constructions of families.
- Discuss ways that ecocultural domains influence members' functions relevant to health.
- Discuss the importance of intergeneration and heritability as family health factors.

> *Great spirits have always found violent opposition from mediocre minds.*
> —Anonymous

Most professional encounters occur within institutional settings, and many nurses never encounter those needing health-care services where they live. Given that most people spend a large part of their time interacting with family members within a household niche, it seems important to place greater emphasis on the household as the niche where health is defined and practiced. The household production of health is affected by events of ordinary life, members' functional capacities, unique health states, and the contextual systems in which the niche is embedded. Although initial socialization about health occurs in the family of origin, early ideas are impacted by many factors that may or may not have a recognizable order. Over time, adherence to some beliefs and behaviors occurs, but others are modified, some are obliterated, and new ones are created. Questions about intergenerational transmission and family function relevant to family health across the life course are important for present and future nursing practice. The Family Health Model implies that just as health has many determinants, approaches to the household as the locus of health production have many implications for interventions by nurses and those in other disciplines.

The Household as the Developmental Niche

Characteristics of the Household as a Developmental Niche

Families have members that share some characteristics but possess other distinct traits. Within the household, developing persons interact to decide the usefulness of health information, interpret health-related experiences, infer meanings about contextual perceptions, and develop behavioral patterns related to health processes. In previous chapters, family members were described as part of the context for family health. Fisher and Ransom (1990) suggested that family is more than context and should be viewed as media and operators through which the family members experience health. They discussed the family in terms of its *ontology,* or the unity that exists between individuals and family. Ontology includes the ways individuals and the family embody each other yet can also be individually described, observed, and treated. Parents and others have enduring influences during critical life periods on children's health beliefs, and these behaviors and interactions continue throughout life.

Harkness and Super (1994) introduced a theoretical framework that they called the *developmental niche.* After studying children's behaviors and development in different cultural contexts, they conceptualized three components of the developmental niche:

1. The physical and social settings of the child's everyday life
2. The culturally regulated customs of child care and child rearing
3. The psychology of caretakers

These subsystems mediate individual experience within the larger cultural context and regulate patterns of health and disease. The household or developmental niche can be viewed as a way to understand child survival and development both from national and international perspectives (Harkness & Super, 1994). Ideas about the household may need to include ideas relevant to policymakers such as rules about family formation (e.g., polygamy, divorce, homosexual or heterosexual cohabitation); child care (e.g., adoption, foster care, parentage); responsibilities toward elderly and developmentally disabled dependents; and intrahousehold allocation of resources (Berman, Kendall, & Bhattacharyya, 1994). Many view marriage as the conjugal unit, but maybe the household needs to be characterized differently to address today's citizens. For example, cohabiting couples are usually not given the same health insurance coverage as those who are legally married, and social values influence employers' decisions about benefits. Thus, some might argue that a disparate employee group is created whose children or cohabiting partners might lack health-care benefits.

Children's behavior, development, and health are influenced by the physical and social settings of the everyday life, cultural customs of child care and rearing, and the caretakers. A study (Farrand, 1991) about child's health status found that attitudes about self, health, and well-being were predictors of health behaviors for children regardless of gender. Green, Kreuter, Deeds, and Partridge (1980) categorically classified health behaviors from functional perspectives: predisposing factors (e.g., attitudes, values, outcome expectations), enabling factors (e.g., skills, resources, knowledge), and reinforcing factors (e.g., social rewards or punishments, physical and material benefits or costs, tangible or imagined outcomes). Individual encounters with sick children often overlook the complex household factors that potentially influence present health concerns and future risks. The Family Health Model entails viewing the embedded household as a primary factor related to individuals' health processes and suggests that nursing practice should include these implications as plans for interventions are introduced.

Household Production of Health

A variety of models can be used to understand the ways households function and achieve health-related outcomes. Anthropologists have tried to explain health behaviors in terms of relationships between cultural beliefs and disease and the determinants that affect the household economy (Coreil, 1990; Schumann & Mosley, 1994). Economics provides a way of understanding the household production of health based on a premise that humans are rational beings and behave according to economic principles (Rosenzwig & Schultz, 1982; Schultz, 1984). Households are repositories for accumulated material goods and are the places where members decide how these goods, time, and other resources will be distributed to meet needs. Members and contextual systems influence these choices. Perhaps the term *choice* is inappropriate because households are not equally ascribed wealth, privilege, or resources, and most actually choose among limited possibilities imposed by contextual systems. Health should not be viewed merely as a household production but also a political construction that affects and is affected by the family (Backett, 1992).

The term *household production of health* has not been fully described in the literature, but it has been discussed as a social construction used by family members to promote, maintain, and regain health (Berman et al., 1994; Denham, 1997; Harkness & Super; Schumann & Mosley, 1994). The household production of health is defined as:

> A dynamic behavioral process through which households combine their (internal) knowledge, resources, and behavioral norms and patterns with available (external) technologies, services, information, and skills to restore, maintain, and promote the health of their members (Berman et al., p. 206).

The household production of health facilitates accommodating the processes associated with health as individuals, family subsystems, family, and embedded contextual systems interact. The concept has integrating qualities for envisioning the complex factors that mediate family health, and it provides a way for various disciplines to organize thoughts about how health can be promoted.

Early childhood is a time when health habits are formed and influenced by the household. A study (Backett, 1992) was done about how children in middle-class families provided a health-promoting environment for young children and the ways they decided how health knowledge, beliefs, and behaviors should be enacted. The results suggested that members had conflict as they attempted to make sense of the social, cultural, and moral constraints of daily life. Biomedical knowledge was translated into behavior when:

- Knowledge made sense in its own right.
- Knowledge made sense in relation to daily experience.
- Knowledge had a social legitimacy in terms of cultural and moral context.

Not only are health habits largely taught and defined within the family, but decisions about when to seek health care and the types of care to seek are also part of the health construction (Denham, 1997; Thomas, 1990). Strengthening families with services, advocacy, and resources can facilitate child development and assist parents with their roles (Thomas, 1994).

The Socially Constructed Family Health Paradigm

The socially constructed family health paradigm is a lived experience that reflects beliefs, values, knowledge about health and illness, ideological views of health, and patterned behaviors. Social constructions are largely based on what has been experienced and viewed as meaningful. Those considering marriage or anticipating the birth of a child may have spent little time considering their health practices, but reasons occur at some point to compare similarities and differences. Although those with similar cultural contexts may notice fewer differences, most persons establishing a household quickly become aware of traits of the other person about which they had previously been oblivious. As individuals are united, a social construction of patterned routines is initiated that, over time, becomes the distinctive family health paradigm.

Figure 9–1 provides a way to depict the social construction of family health as a summative response to functional and contextual factors. Family members individually and collectively interpret unique life events and complex contextual variables that have the potential to affect the health and illness state of single individuals and the family as a whole. Some experiences are perceived as normative (i.e., health producing, health sustaining, health regaining), and others are seen as non-normative (i.e., health depleting, disease producing, risk increasing). Accommodations often occur incrementally as members cope with liminal events (e.g., time periods that warn of pending family developmental changes, such as pregnancy or the recommendation of hospice care for a dying family member), unpredictable life events (e.g., the birth of a disabled child, employment loss, relocation), usual developmental changes (e.g., school enrollment, adolescence, aging, death), and chronic problems (e.g., alcohol misuse, substance abuse, domestic violence, health alterations). Accommodations are often responses to threats presented by the embedded context, but they may also relate to genetics or innate characteristics of single family members or family subsystems. While the definition of family health may have many similarities to family health practices, what is said and what is practiced may differ.

Ecocultural Niche

Ecolocultural theory is intended to be valuable crossculturally and combine recent developments from several disciplines (Super & Harkness, 1980; Weisner, 1984; Whiting, 1976, 1980; Whiting & Edwards, 1988; Whiting & Whiting, 1975):

> Ecocultural theory emphasizes that a major adaptive task for each family is the construction and maintenance of a daily routine through which families organize and shape their children's activity and development. The activities of everyday routine create opportunities for development-sensitive interactions on which development partly depends. The everyday routine and the development-sensitive interaction... are shaped by the surrounding ecocultural niche (Gallimore, Weisner, Bernheimer, Guthrie, & Nihira, 1993, p. 186).

The theory gives credence to the intense meanings of family environment; assumes the family's viewpoint about goals, values, and needs; and suggests that parents' beliefs can equal or be more powerful influences than income, household size, or social supports (Bernheimer, Gallimore, & Weisner, 1990; Gallimore, Weisner, Kaufman, & Bernheimer, 1989). This theory suggests that everyday activities should be the units of analysis because they can lead to outcome assessments; are not based on single

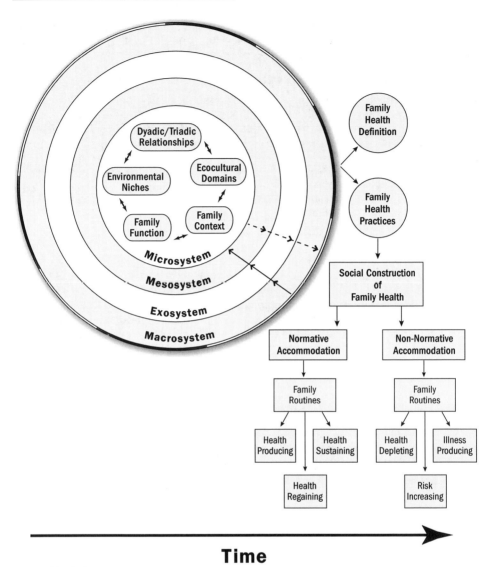

Figure 9–1 Social construction of family health definitions and practices.

individuals; are less likely to be linked *a priori* to variables such as income or social class; and are sustained across a variety of settings, times, and situations. Key theoretical points are:

- They explicitly include family-constructed meanings of circumstances and the proactive responses to those circumstances.
- The ecocultural niche is composed of the family's material conditions, values, goals, and meanings.
- Family themes and ecocultural domains provide the basis for routines.
- Daily routines or activity settings are the critical units of analysis.

■ Everyday routine is an adaptation problem common to all families.
■ Accommodation is the response process that alters daily routines.
■ Ecocultural theory is applicable to all families regardless of culture, race, ethnicity, or social strata.
■ Families should be compared based on processes of social construction of activity settings rather than family or child status alone.

These points have strong implications for family-focused care and forms of nursing practice that include household variables.

Families are not viewed as helpless victims of circumstances; rather, they regularly take individual and collective actions to modify or accommodate them. It is the premise of the Family Health Model that families strive to maintain the themes, identity, and patterns of routine that they view as meaningful. For example, a qualitative study (Kellegrew, 2000) explored the daily routines constructed by mothers in response to the emerging self-care needs of young children with disabilities. Findings indicated that the daily lives of the family members were reconstructed to accommodate the needs of the child and the mother's vision for her child's future. Values, meanings, and themes related to cultural practices for specific families are more meaningful than mere reliance on those of dominant members of a cultural group.

The *ecocultural niche* pertains to the ways families interact and organize their lives within their embedded households to address health needs. Many contextual determinants (e.g., proximity of kin, health risks imposed by the environment, stresses intrinsic to neighborhoods, employment opportunities) influence functional status and member interactions. The ecocultural niche is influenced by the unique ways that members incorporate traditions, spirituality, and symbols into everyday life. Although the niche may predominately have a hierarchical nature, it can be altered and reordered. It is the safe place or schema members use to cope with unpredictable factors and integrity integral to health. Although some may possess great latitude in choosing where to live, work, or play, others may experience constraints because of lesser education, opportunity, or marginalizing factors.

Weisner (1984) identified 12 domains (e.g., family work, public health, home safety, child-care tasks, peer groups) related to family that had some impact on child development. Families make accommodations related to careers, work schedules, jobs, and residences in order to sustain valued patterns of behavior. Members may be willing to learn new skills, participate in activities, seek assistance from those outside the family boundaries, redistribute household tasks, or attend to or neglect faith practices if the implications are strongly related to meaningful needs associated with health needs. Parents use resources and constraints to construct everyday routines that accommodate values and goals pertinent to health outcomes (Gallimore et al., 1989). Everyday routines are affected by *ecocultural factors,* positive and negative variables initiated by the context or resulting from interactions with or within the context. Ecocultural factors are themes that families use to organize daily behaviors and family health routines. For example, families often use religion or faith explanations to coordinate and arrange practices related to diet, alcohol avoidance, and activities that should be shunned. Another family theme pertains to what is esteemed as "normal" behavior. For example, some families think spanking is violent and choose to discipline by using "time-outs," taking away privileges, or "grounding." Other families may tolerate regular screaming or yelling behaviors and even hitting, shoving, and beating as "normal." Family themes may have to do with expectations about gender behaviors, acquisitions of material goods, social appearances, family togetherness, meaningful childhood, and parental behavior. Family members may not always clearly articulate their themes, but they are incorporated into the fabric of daily life and routine behaviors (Denham, 1997, 1999a, 1999b, 1999c; Gallimore et al., 1989). Those who choose to practice using the Family Health Model would consider the implications of the family's themes and routines in providing family-focused care.

Reflective Thinking

Consider your family of origin experience and think about the concept of an ecocultural niche. What are the pertinent aspects that a stranger might use to define your family's ecocultural niche? What are the family themes present in your family of origin when you were in grade school? High school? What about now? Have the themes changed over time? Are you currently establishing a family of procreation? If so, how are the themes different from those in your family of origin? Be prepared to participate in a class activity and share some of your personal experiences.

Ecocultural Domains

Based on ideas reflected in the literature (Bernheimer et al., 1990; Nihira, Weisner, & Bernheimer, 1994), 12 *ecocultural domains* have been identified as potentially influential contextual and functional categories of family life that define the themes and routines pertinent to functional roles related to health (Fig. 9–2). Resources and constraints, values and goals, and member abilities to accommodate changes impact these domains. The family-of-origin experience is often used to measure future values, roles, and practices. Some domain aspects may remain unchanged during the life course, but others are altered. Figure 9–2 presents the domains relevant to family health and the household production of health as if they were segments of an orange that appear to be unique delineations closely approximating one another. But in reality, the domains are enmeshed, integrated, and difficult to separate, making domain analysis especially difficult. However, domains provide ways to conceptualize systemic interactions among members and their contextual systems. If a biological system is envisioned, then a frame of reference for the household production of health would consider the circulatory system of health beliefs, a skeleton of health knowledge, and a musculature of health routines.

Knowledge, traditional practices, and values relevant to domains are slow to change, but accommodations are made when a reason strong enough is encountered. For example, while she was growing up, a young woman lived in a home where her parents practiced faith healing, and the daughter held fast to similar beliefs throughout her adult life. Now in her early 40s, she is faced with breast cancer. Although she always said that she would never undergo a surgical procedure, the gravity of her diagnosis, uncertainty of her prognosis, and promise of others' successes led her to choose medical pathways she never thought possible for her. Beliefs and behaviors associated with health may be resistant to change and not very pliable, but when vital family health themes are threatened and accommodations needed, openness to new information or interventions may occur. Family health themes are closely linked to rules, values, boundaries, and behaviors associated with a family's ecocultural domains.

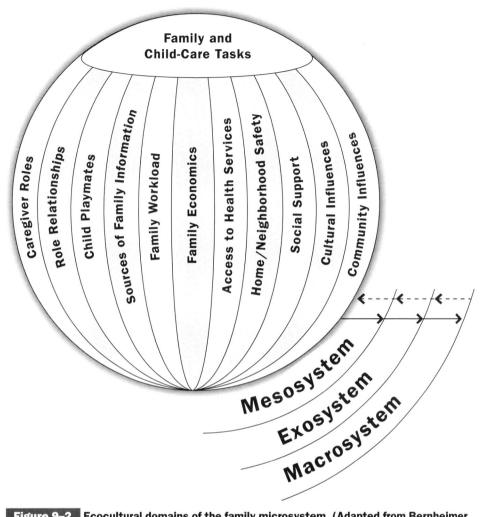

Figure 9–2 Ecocultural domains of the family microsystem. (Adapted from Bernheimer, LP, et al: Ecocultural theory as a context for the individual service plan. Journal of Early Intervention 14(3):219–233, 1990; Nihira, K, et al: Ecocultural assessment in families of children with developmental delays: Construct and concurrent validities. Am J Ment Retard 98(5):551–566, 1994.)

The Family Health Model suggests that strongly adhered to beliefs and behavioral patterns related to family themes and identity are not quickly amenable to interventions. However, when nurses collaborate with members to achieve meaningful family goals, it is much more probable that some accommodations will occur. Family-focused care implies ascertaining family needs in relation to health concerns and providing supportive assistance that enables the family members to accomplish their goals. Examples of factors that affect ecocultural domains are:

- Members' genetic predispositions
- Members' social hereditary factors

- Individual and family developmental variations
- Broad environmental conditions

These factors are antecedent to and contiguous with the ways members function, assume roles and responsibilities, interact, and organize their ideas about health practices.

👫👫👫 *Cooperative Learning*

The instructor will divide into the class into three groups. Select one of the ecocultural domains (see Fig. 9–2) and then discuss possible family themes that may affect aspects of that domain with the potential to affect functional processes, family roles, and health outcomes. What are the possible themes for a newly formed family? A family expecting its first child? A family with preschool, school-age, or adolescent children? What happens if the family seems to be trying to accomplish multiple tasks simultaneously? Your group should report your ideas to the class and be prepared to respond to questions from your classmates.

▣ Intergenerational Transmission of Family Health

Individual and family health are concerns that extend beyond a single generation. Genetically linked or inherited disorders may be of immediate concern or not realized until later in life. Options are now available for genetic testing for many single-gene disorders such as Huntington's disease, Down syndrome, and polycystic kidney disease. Genetic testing may be fraught with ethical questions and concerns about exploitation and misuse, but it also offers great possibilities for treatment and prevention of many conditions and diseases. Many unresolved questions still await answers, but the development of future medical technologies and completion of clinical trials hold great promise for the future for individuals with some intergenerational disorders.

Intergenerational Relationships

Family developmental processes, systems of knowledge, and beliefs over time have ongoing effects on knowledge, beliefs, and behaviors related to present and future health conditions. Functional processes of the individuals and family subsystems residing within the household niche are affected by concerns such as individuation, family cohesion, member resilience, and personal and family boundaries; these all affect a family's capacities and interactions with larger contextual systems. The interaction of the family membership within the household niche creates a family narrative that affects present and future generations. Members' collective memories affect functional processes that are internal and external to the household as past, present, and future events are interpreted and past recollections persuade meanings from generation to generation. The collective memory holds the potential for present and future choices. In addition, embedded contextual systems provide formal institutions (e.g., government agencies, health-care systems, religious organizations, educational settings) and informal structures (e.g., class, ethnicity, neighborhood, social networks) that influence age cohorts and generations.

Generations differ from one another, and potentials for health and risk may be related to historical periods. For example, although many parents of today's "baby boomers" were neither born nor raised during the Great Depression, their parents were and carried the memory of fears associated with the time to children born in the late 1940s and early 1950s. Many baby boomers can still recall their parents telling them to clean their plates because children in China or some other nation were starving. Many baby boomers might respond that thankfulness was not what they felt; instead, they were willing to ship those leftovers to the starving children! The earlier generation learned to "save for a rainy day" and strongly believed that if you did not work, you should not eat; maxims taught to the parents of baby boomers were, in turn, taught to their own children. However, the embedded context provided more relevant messages to the children of the 1960s and 1970s than those of their grandparents or parents as the baby boomers came of age in a time of opportunity and opulence. This generation eats at fast food restaurants and silently disposes of children's uneaten food into trash bins with nary a whisper about starving children in distant lands. A cultural context that encourages spending, materialism, and debt has convinced baby boomers that the present is important, and many have not saved for retirement. Human development occurs within a context of time, culture, and history that gives meaning to beliefs and practices. Although older generations feared infectious disease and used quarantine as a means of coping, today's families fear violence and the effects of media and social pressures on children's choices to use drugs or alcohol or to smoke. As a result of the terrorism of September 11, 2001, future fears will likely be related to other terrorist acts, distrust of diverse ethnic groups, and biological warfare. Children encounter life filtered through the experiences of prior generations and later may parent their own children in ways that respond to these earlier events.

A life course orientation emphasizes trajectories, transitions, and timing that influence not only the present generation but also connect the past with the future (Elder, 1995; Moen & Erickson, 1995). Developmental processes have been extensively studied in children, but less is known about adult developmental processes or how adults provide latent influences across generations. Although generations are greatly influenced by family-of-origin factors, they are equally affected by contextual experiences and serendipitous circumstances. The valuing of developmental processes from birth through death entails rethinking the influences and meanings on members' roles, relationships, responsibilities, and functions. Although much is known about parental influences on child development, less is known about the ways adult children continue to develop and influence the developmental processes of their peers and aging parents, how grandparents influence the development of their grandchildren, or how grandchildren affect their grandparents. As the baby boomers become the "elder boomers," much about health potentials and health constraints is yet to be learned. *Health constraints* are forces imposed by persons, structures, or systems that impede, restrict, or inhibit processes of becoming, health, and well-being that intergenerationally affect individuals and families.

Intergenerational Interactions

Social class, culture, ethnicity, family economics, and education are often cited as factors that affect individual status, but the implications are less often considered across generations. For example, in the Appalachian culture, many families have close ties to their immediate family and extended kin networks (Denham, 1997). These ties tend to be closest when members live near one another; have the lifelong opportunity for regular interactions; share similar educational backgrounds, employment status, and personal interests; and have similar value orientations. However, a person of Appalachian heritage may discover that although aspects of heritage are retained, college graduation, marriage, and employment in a high-technology position in a large city could well mean that ideas from childhood are less meaningful in new contexts. For example, a young man aspires to participate in the Olympics but finds himself far from home in a social context very different from his family of origin. He shares peer interactions that are in sharp contrast to the ones that occur with his friends at home. A young woman becomes a parent and gains new understandings about her mother and parenting activities, which creates harmony and communication in sharp contrast to what was experienced during her teenage years. Life's disruptions and changes foster new directions and opportunities that may affect intergenerational interactions, with potentials to alter health.

Earlier generations make important contributions to family health histories and the ways families define and practice health. Intergenerational relationships hold keys to genetic and health heritage; knowledge about where reservoirs of support exist; facts about stress and coping; and particulars about resilience, hardiness, and well-being. A family genogram might provide keys to complex inherited patterns intergenerationally related to member concerns and timing of events. An eco-map can provide data about family relocation, residences, social networks, employment, and other data about environment and contextual influences over the life course. A socio-map can provide facts about peer groups, supportive resources, and threats that occur over a lifetime. The Family Health Model encourages nurses to think about the usefulness of intergenerational data for understanding family health behaviors and for intervening in family health.

🏃🏃🏃🏃🏃🏃🏃 *Cooperative Learning*

Think about your family and identify three or four traits that have been passed on in the family; identify personal traits linked to parents and previous generations. One trait should be related to physical appearance, one should be related to genetics, one should be related to personality, and one should be related to a food preference. List the traits on the board by category.

When you and your classmates have listed the traits, then have a class discussion about patterns of intergenerational transmission. What happens when children are adopted and do not know anything about their parents? What about children who are conceived through artificial insemination? How do families use information related to their heritage? What information is useful for families to know? What information would be helpful for family nurses? How can nurses use information about prior generations in family-focused care?

▓ Summary

More needs to be known about the ways family function and contextual systems interact across generations to affect health processes. Greater understandings are needed about functional determinations that are influenced by the household economy (e.g., child care, child poverty, employment patterns, use of health-care services) versus those perpetrated by the household context (e.g., employment opportunities, legislative mandates, community resources). What are the key influences of family function related to health? In what ways can nurses collaborate with families to potentiate the household production of health? How do multiple generations impact and influence health processes? The Family Health Model provides nurses with ways to conceptualize practices that include household and intergenerational perspectives of families. Furthermore, the model suggests ways that these conceptualizations can become operational in clinical practice.

Test Your Knowledge

1. Describe what is meant by the *household production of health* and give an example that suggests how nurses might intervene.

2. Explain two ways that the family household can potentiate health and two ways that it might introduce negating factors.

3. Discuss how a nurse employed in home care or a community health setting might use an idea about the *household production of health* as a way to assist a patient.

4. Identify what is implied by the idea of *social construction of health*.

5. Select an ecocultural domain and compare and contrast some ways nursing practice might differ with a newly married couple, a family with two school-age children, parents sending their last child off to college, and a family facing the retirement years.

6. Parents who are concerned about risk for Down syndrome in their recently conceived child are seeking guidance about what to do. As the nurse working with them, how would you counsel them? What family interventions would you suggest?

7. How does the idea of intergenerational transmission of health factors potentially affect the household production of health?

Chapter

10

Core Processes and Family Health

CHAPTER OBJECTIVES *At the end of this chapter, the reader will be able to:*

■ Define the seven core functional processes associated with family health.

■ Describe the core functional processes and give examples about how they affect family health.

■ Identify ways the core functional processes can be used to increase the household production of family health.

You give but little when you give of your possessions. It is when you give of yourself that you truly give. For what are your possessions but things you keep and guard for fear you may need tomorrow?

—Kahlil Gibran The Prophet

This chapter provides ways of thinking about the functional aspects of family health and identifies ways to use conceptual ideas in practice. The intent is to provide nurses with some approaches for thinking about how to consider nursing practice in ways that tangibly address relationships between functional perspectives and health status. In the author's research, findings have indicated that families used seven functional processes to incorporate information, values, and beliefs into behaviors, activities, and routines relevant to family health. These concepts are described and examples are provided to identify ways they are applicable to family-focused practice.

Nurses have many ways to think about functional status from previous learning and past experiences that are applicable to family-focused practice and family health. The goal of nursing is to assist family members to optimize processes of becoming, health,

> ### Box 10–1   Assumptions about Nurses' Roles and Functional Outcomes Relevant to Health
>
> - Nurses can collaborate with families to effectively transition from social, cultural, spiritual, economic, political, or physical spaces and increase health potentials.
> - Nurses can collaborate with family members to use knowledge, space, time, and resources in ways that optimize health potentials.
> - Nurses can collaborate with families to gain access to resources needed by members that are located in the embedded contextual systems.
> - Nurses can collaborate with families to access social, cultural, spiritual, economic, and political information beneficial to health.
> - Nurses can approach families in culturally sensitive ways and assist them as they incorporate health information and skills into routines that maximize the processes of becoming, health, and well-being across the life course.

and well-being. *Optimize* implies to make as effective or functional as possible. Family-focused care targets actual problems and health potentials. *Health potentials* are inherent aptitudes within individuals, family subsystems, families, and the embedded contextual systems that increase capabilities and maximize knowledge, space, time, and resources. Health potentials are targets related to goal accomplishment, family identity and themes, and health routines. Other concepts meaningful to family outcomes (e.g., hardiness, resilience, self-efficacy, cohesion, maturation, individuation, stability, perseverance) are also pertinent to family health.

A role of nurses is to help family members interact in ways that optimize potentials, abilities, and contextual resources as they accommodate life course experiences that affect members' processes of becoming, health, or well-being. Across the life course, families use functional processes to address actual problems, minimize risks associated with health concerns, and maximize health potentials. Several assumptions have been identified that posit that nurses can collaborate with families in many ways to produce optimal health outcomes for all members (Box 10–1). The idea of *core processes* (i.e., caregiving, cathexis, celebration, change, communication, connectedness, coordination) were generated from findings in the author's family health research (Denham, 1997, 1999a, 1999b, 1999c). These core processes describe concepts that are germane to family's functional status and health that nurses can target as they collaborate with families and others to realize family health potentials. A subject from one of the family health studies (Denham, 1999b) nicely described some concerns related to functional status and family health also identified by others:

> The first thing I would think of would be an emotional state of affairs of the family. I would think of particular medical-physical problems, 'cause to me family health would be a unit of the family and how they are working with each other and how supportive they are. And that's what I'd see as a real problem in this country, because we don't have healthy families.... They don't communicate. They don't support each other. They're not a working unit. The family as an entity isn't healthy because its parts don't communicate with each other and support each other.

A family's *functional processes,* or ways members interact to potentiate, negate, threaten, mediate, and enhance individual and family health, are complicated by many factors. First, operational definitions of what family members mean by health and illness may be quite different from the ideas held by others. In fact, neither family nor professional definitions may be consistently used. Thus, needs exist to clarify what is intended, identify agreement or disagreement in interpretations, and maintain consistency in shared understandings. Second, the nature of family subsystems and interactions with embedded contextual systems makes it difficult to recognize confounding factors that complicate *helping processes*. Helping processes are the interventions used by nurses and others to provide family-focused care that assists individuals, family subsystems, and families to enhance the functional processes. Therefore, nurses and others must not limit their focus to individuals; rather, they should consider broader possibilities of causation or association. Family members vigorously interact through health routines that are modified and adjusted over time. *Health routines* are patterns of behavior, activity, or ritual relevant to health aspects that are rather consistently adhered to for extended time periods. The dynamic quality of member interactions and the potentials for constructing needed accommodations in these routines provide explicit targets for family-focused interventions.

Thirdly, member interactions involve complex networks of embedded systems beyond the immediate boundaries of the household niche. Family members may not be completely aware of their reasons for specific health routines, and they may have conflicting purposes for continuing, altering, or adhering to them. Members may differ in their valuing of processes and behaviors for attaining goals, even when the family as a whole agrees that a goal is desirable. Therefore, nurses may need to intervene in different ways with multiple family members to attain desired goals. A family-focused intervention may need to be aimed at agencies, institutions, or persons outside of the family to achieve a family goal. For example, as a result of a degenerative disease, a family member becomes blind. The family may agree that the member needs to attain the highest level of independence possible and may be willing to work with the blind member to facilitate learning skills that enhance self-efficacy. However, the family may be greatly impeded if they have no knowledge about services for blind individuals, have limited information about adaptive devices that blind people might use to accommodate losses, and lack financial resources for obtaining services or devices. Family-focused care implies assisting the family to develop routines that support goal accomplishment. Therefore, nursing interventions may include contacting services for the visually impaired to ascertain if the blind member qualifies, assist the family to identify safety risks associated with blindness, and set up a plan of care that addresses needed changes in family health routines. The plan of care would engage multiple members and probably require several interactions before goals were completely realized.

Family-focused care implies assisting families to:

1. Reduce health risks
2. Maintain optimal levels of wellness
3. Develop routines and achieve goals that enhance the processes of becoming, health, and well-being
4. Accommodate changes that maximize health potentials
5. Support family members through normative and non-normative life experiences
6. Enable family members to obtain information, resources, education, counseling, or other forms of support that enhance health routines

Although nurses might already possess some knowledge and skills related to functional status, it is posited that the core processes provide a foundation for assessing, planning, implementing, and evaluating care specifically linked to health.

Table 10–1 provides an overview of the core processes and identifies potential areas where a nurse might interact while providing family-focused care. Core processes are enmeshed, so it is often difficult to consider one process without also addressing others. Nurses who understand these processes can use them to impact family interactions, support family needs, and assist families to construct health routines that meet family goals.

Table 10–1	Functional Processes Related to Family Health	
Functional Process	**Definition of the Process**	**Potential Functional Areas of Concern**
Caregiving	Concern for family generated from close intimate relationships and member affections resulting in watchful attention, thoughtfulness, and actions linked to members' developmental, health, and illness needs	Health maintenance Disease prevention Risk reduction Health promotion Illness care Rehabilitation Acute episodic needs Chronic concerns
Cathexis	The emotional bond that develops between individuals and family as members invest emotional and psychic energy into loved ones	Attachment Commitment Affiliation Loss Grief and mourning Normative processes Complicated processes
Celebration	Tangible forms of shared meaning in which family celebrations, family traditions, and leisure are used to commemorate special times, days, and events to distinguish them from usual daily routines across the life course	Culture Family fun Traditions Rituals Religion Hobbies Shared activities
Change	A dynamic, nonlinear process that implies altering or modifying the form, direction, and outcome of the original identity by substituting alternatives	Control Meeting expressed needs Meanings of change Contextual influences Compare and contrast Similarities and differences Diversity
Communication	The primary ways parents socialize children about health beliefs, values, attitudes, and behaviors and use information, knowledge, and actions applicable to health	Language Symbolic interactions Information access Coaching Cheerleading Knowledge and skills Emotional needs Affective care Spiritual needs
Connectedness	The ways systems are linked together through family, educational, cultural, spiritual, political, social, professional, legal, economic, or commercial interests	Partnering relationships Kin networks Household labor Cooperation Member roles Family rules Boundaries Tolerance for ambiguity Marginalization
Coordination	Cooperative sharing of resources, skills, abilities, and information within the family and with the larger contextual environment to optimize individuals' health potentials, potentiate the household production of health, and achieve family goals	Family tasks Problem solving Decision making Valuing Coping Resilience Respect Reconciliation Forgiveness Cohesiveness System integrity Stress management

Caregiving

A growing body of evidence about caregiving shows that nurses and others have keen interests in relationships between caregivers and illness needs. As decreased lengths of stay continue and reimbursement systems to pay for some forms of care are increasingly limited, the need for family members to care for ill, disabled, and dying members at home will most likely escalate. The needs of those with chronic illnesses place great demands on caregivers, who are primarily mothers or other women. The terms *caregiver burden* and *caregiver strain* have been used to describe the difficulties associated with meeting long-term care needs. The terms *informal caregiver* and *formal caregiver* have been used in the literature to differentiate between professional and family caregivers (Fletcher & Winslow, 1991). If health is viewed from household perspectives, it is family members who are the care providers across the life course. For most families, it is only when the safety net of family support for caregiving fails that other systems are sought.

In the Family Health Model, *caregiving* is defined as a concern for other family members generated by close intimate relationships and member affections that result in watchful attention, thoughtfulness, and other actions aimed to support members' development, health, and illness needs. Family-focused care implies having knowledge about variations in caregiving needs and intervening in ways appropriate to meet these needs. When family health was studied (Denham, 1997, 1999a, 1999b, 1999c), caregiving was identified as a functional role with a number of associated tasks:

- Manage members' genetic and biophysical heritage.
- Support and sustain members' health.
- Avoid or reduce health risks imposed by the family context.
- Instruct and guide children toward healthy behaviors.
- Provide opportunities for family fun, relaxation, and stress reduction.
- Care for members' illness events.
- Enforce family values related to health.
- Obtain supportive resources from the embedded context.

A focus on assessment of caregiving tasks could assist nurses to plan care for the needs of multiple household members. For example, families with ill members may need a great deal of support. Over the past few decades, studies about chronic illness in children have increased our understanding of the needs related to normalizing the illness experience (Deatrick, Knafl, & Walsh, 1998), coping with critical periods of the illness (Clements, Copeland, & Loftus, 1990; Gallo & Knafl, 1998), and identifying adequate support systems (Cohen, 1997). Parents with developmentally delayed children experience a great sense of burden as they cope with children who have severe conditions or functional dependence (Mahoney, O'Sullivan, & Robinson, 1992). Evidence exists that families with the greatest needs may have the least support available to them (Greenberg, Seltzer, & Greenley, 1993; Leonard, Johnson, & Brust, 1993) and that family caregivers' support needs vary over time (Greenberg et al., 1993; Ray & Ritchie, 1993; Teisler, Killian, & Gubman, 1987; Youngblut, Brennan, & Swegart, 1994). Families with members who have extensive caregiving needs face a contextual environment with competing social demands, parental needs, and financial concerns (Turner-Henson, Holaday, & Swan, 1992).

Differences in the ways mothers and fathers of developmentally disabled children adapt have been noted. Whereas mothers' emotions seem more similar to chronic sorrow, fathers' reactions are more closely aligned with resignation (Mallow & Bechtel, 1999). The greater the dependency needs for a family member, the greater the needs for broad contextual support at certain time points during the life course (Gallo & Knafl, 1998; Hilbert et al., 2000; Walker, Hilbert, & Rinehart, 1999). Persons who provide caregiving assistance generally have some level of personal satisfaction and feelings of self-worth linked to the experience (Hilbert et al., 2000; Ray & Ritchie, 1993). Clinicians who are concerned about the burdens of caregiving on the household production of health should consider how family-focused interventions could assist members to optimize their time, energy, and resources.

Little in the literature specifically addresses the effects of long-term caregiving on parents of disabled children (Hilbert et al., 2000), and less is known about the caregiving tasks associated with well families; both areas appear meaningful for considering family-focused interventions. A surprising finding in the family health research was that families viewed as well families by health-care providers often had members with chronic illnesses or disabilities (Denham, 1997, 1999a, 1999b, 1999c). Assumptions that well families have no ill members appear to be erroneous. Increased technological capabilities, medical knowledge, and surgical skills mean that more households have members who require continual or special caregiving. Mothers usually have the primary responsibility for caregiving, but others also participate. In well families in which mothers were the caregivers of young children, mothers often described biophysical and mental health concerns (Denham, 1997, 1999a, 1999b, 1999c). The Family Health Model encourages clinicians to view caregiving as an active accommodation that family members use to assist one another with changing needs over the life course. Nurses need to carefully address caregiving tasks associated with the household production of health.

👪👪 Cooperative Learning

The instructor will divide the class into three groups. One group should focus on caregiving in well families; the second group should focus on caregiving in families with a chronically ill adult; and the third group should consider caregiving in families with a child who has a physical disability. Each group should identify someone to record key discussion points to later report to the larger group. Groups should answer the following questions:

1. What are the unique caregiving concerns?
2. What family aspects might a nurse want to assess?
3. Who might be affected by the caregiving demands?
4. How do caregivers' needs differ from those of other family members?
5. How might the nurse provide family-focused care?

After your group discusses its answers, you should report your conclusions to the class.

Cathexis

The term *cathexis* refers to the emotional bonds that develop between a person and those cared about as the developing person invests emotional and psychic energy into the loved one (Rando, 1984). This behavior has also been referred to as the development of affectional bonds or attachments that initially occurs between child and parent and later between adults that results in persons seeking to be close to a preferred individual.

This results in:

- Behaviors mediated by goal-oriented behavioral systems
- Intense emotions that affect the formation, maintenance, disruption, and renewal of attachment relationships
- Keeping persons in touch with their caregivers
- A view of caregiving as being a complementary function of attachment
- Providing a biological function related to reproduction
- Deviant behaviors when interrupted or disturbed, especially during infancy, childhood, and adolescence (Bowlby, 1980)

In the Family Health Model, cathexis refers to the warmth, love, and regard developing persons within a household experience and provide for one another. Cathexis is an essential aspect of emotional well-being. Cathexis can also refer to intellectual and affective energy invested in objects or ideas that might be actualized as healthy activities but are also risky or unhealthy. For instance, the terms *fanaticism* and *obsession* are sometimes used when persons become too attached to objects, activities, ideas, and sometimes persons. Although many have said that one cannot love too much, extremism in any form may have the potential to increase risks.

Individuals work hard throughout their lives to form attachments while the inevitability of loss looms on the horizon. As American families have had smaller numbers of children and some wait until much later in life to have their first child, parental investment in attachment processes can be profound. Today's parents often make major life investments as they bond with their children, and loss can be devastating. For example, life in a society that says problems can be solved means some would-be parents may invest great amounts of time and financial and emotional resources in attempts to artificially conceive a child. Although technology enables the process, finances may be an impediment when conception does not occur after several attempts. Although medical treatment is often effective in curing childhood cancers, the loss of a child is a great source of sorrow for many years. Grief and loss can become the unexpected or non-normative experience that results from the normative experience of attachment in families.

Decathexis is a term often used to discuss the disconnecting or disentangling needed when one is grieving the loss of a close attachment. When the decathexis results from grief associated with the death of a loved one, the concern is detaching and modifying emotional ties so that new relationships can be established (Rando, 1984). Other forms of decathexis occur when persons divorce, separate, relocate to new communities, lose a pet, accept new employment positions, see a child off to college, witness the marriage of adult children, or experience social withdrawal of close friends when serious illness occurs. Decathexis is rarely a simple process and, in cases other than death, it often means leaving the past behind and establishing new relationships. Worden (1982) discussed four tasks of mourning when death is the reason for the loss:

1. Accept the reality of the loss.
2. Experience the pain of grief.
3. Adjust to an environment in which the deceased person is missing.
4. Withdraw the emotional energy and reinvest in another relationship.

Other losses may evoke similar needs as healing occurs when the grieving person is able to think about the loss without great pain but retains a powerful, long-lasting sense of sadness.

The Family Health Model assumes that persons experience attachment and loss in many ways other than dealing with death. Family-focused care aimed at cathexis might initially identify attachments viewed as health potentials. However, because persons are severed from things they attach to over the life course, care must also target decathexis and assist families to achieve balance between the two. Tasks that might need to be addressed include:

- Acquire new roles and skills.
- Make room for a world without the person, object, or idea in it.
- Redefine one's identity so that it embraces the memories tied to the loss.
- Accept therapeutic changes in the life course.

The term *chronic sorrow* has been used to describe losses suffered by persons who are afflicted with chronic illnesses or disabilities as well as the grief experienced by their caregivers. Chronic sorrow continues in cyclical patterns of strong emotions and periods of calmer emotions with feelings of intensity that accumulate with new losses and resurge as old losses are recalled (Lindgren, 2000). The meaning of loss may differ depending on the type, age of the person experiencing the loss, and the developmental stages when the loss is experienced. As a parent of a child who developed juvenile diabetes at age 11 years, the losses felt by my daughter and myself have been different. Although she grieved losses resulting from the ways her disease management made her different from her peers and created a severe self-consciousness during puberty, my response was more associated with fears related to her brittle condition and future complications with life consequences. Now at age 34 years, she has severe neuropathy, Charcot's syndrome, hypertension, chronic renal failure, and blindness. The loss of her sight, the necessity to have dialysis three times a week, and an even more stringent need for medical management has awakened new forms of sorrow in both of us that are very different from those experienced several decades ago. However, although we both live with feelings of chronic sorrow related to her conditions, we experience it in different ways.

Using family-focused care, nurses can assess the cathexis–decathexis processes of family members to determine the relevance to health concerns. The attachment–loss experiences of family members are often deep-seated normative functions with the potential to affect members' processes of becoming and well-being. When the processes are uncomplicated, individuals and families experience normal loss responses (Bowlby, 1980; Parkes, 1972; Zissok & Lyons, 1988). Although painful and difficult, the loss experience has somewhat predictable cycles unique to individuals and families. Persons need nurturance, emotional care, and understanding from supportive others throughout the life course. If family members are unable to attach in meaningful ways or fail to provide adequate support during times of loss, it is posited that the functional capacities of the family are threatened and a need for family-focused care exists. Although family members often say that members provide their greatest support whenever loss is experienced, careful assessments may indicate that the support may be less beneficial than reported. Within households, it is likely that several members are coping with similar issues simultaneously, and the differences in their unique coping processes may be sources of misunderstandings within the household and may be areas where family counseling is needed.

Medical management or prescriptive treatments may occasionally be needed to cope with deep emotional pain, but the use of drugs should not be the primary way to respond to normative processes. When used, drugs should be short-term adjuncts to other therapeutic interventions. However, when non-normative cathexis–decathexis responses or what might be identified as inappropriate attachments or complicated grief occurs, then the family may need supportive care beyond what a generalist nurse can provide. Inappropriate attachments may occur when persons have mental illnesses, mental disabilities, or personality disorders; abuse substances such as drugs or alcohol; or participate in abuse and violence. Some incidents may be reportable to law enforcement authorities or be referred to other mental health providers, service agencies, or health-care institutions. However, nurses may still be able to provide family-focused care to some family members as they work to meet their health goals. Nurses who work with families with problems of complicated mourning must have knowledge and skills to intervene with the associated psychological, behavioral, social, and physical symptoms. Syndromes related to complicated mourning include absent, delayed, inhibited, distorted, conflicted, unanticipated, and chronic mourning. People experiencing these types of mourning often require professional help (Rando, 1993). Inadequate treatments of complicated grief can result in physical and emotional symptoms with long-term health consequences.

Reflective Thinking

Think about your life experiences. What kinds of attachments have you had in your lifetime? Who are the family members with whom you are closely bonded? What about friends? Have you had other experiences of close attachment—maybe a pet, a place, or some special object?

Have you experienced the loss of someone with whom you were closely attached? What was this loss experience like? Have you ever experienced the loss of a pet, object, or some other meaningful thing? Were your experiences the same or very different? Recall your losses; are your feelings different now from when they first occurred? Do you have any unresolved losses?

Think about your roles as a nurse. What kinds of assessment of attachment and loss have you done with patients? Can you think of times when they might have been appropriate? What therapeutic interventions might you consider related to attachment and loss that might assist families with their household productions of health?

 ## Celebration

Celebrations have existed from the earliest times and are used to observe lifecycle events, family milestones, cultural and ethnic heritage, gender differences, religious beliefs, holidays, special member events, seasonal events, and so on. In the Family Health Model, *celebrations* are defined as tangible forms of shared meaning in which family celebrations, family traditions, and family leisure commemorate special times, days, and events to distinguish them from usual daily routines across the life course. Celebrations enable intergenerational transmission of symbolic actions that signify the passing of time, provide reflective points for reminiscing about the past, enable families to share narrative histories, allow families to transfer customs and practices from one generation to another, and afford opportunities for making meaning. Celebrations embrace the past, present, and future; the tenuous and the tenacious; the contiguous and the distant; the unknown and the transcendent; and continuity and change. Celebrations capture imagination, respect history, and impress humanity with their transitory existence. Symbols are often used in conjunction with celebrations to express ideas, values, allegiances, emotions, relationships, and aspirations.

Celebrations include formal celebrations, family traditions, and family leisure and are times when family members have occasions that are different from the customary rigors of daily life. *Formal celebrations* have prescribed aspects with expectations that behaviors will be repeated and used to commemorate meaningful events tied to family identity (e.g., birthdays, anniversaries, weddings, holidays, family reunions, religious practices). Formal celebrations usually involve extended family members and close friends, are costly, and take extensive commitment and planning time. *Family traditions* are viewed as formally organized family times such as vacations, weekend getaways, camping trips, attending children's athletic events or special interest activities, and other events characteristic of a particular family. Traditional patterns may include special family entertainment, leisure, play, exercise, and recreation that provide family members opportunities for casual interaction, relaxation, laughter, fun, pleasure, and enjoyment. Traditional activities often provide memorable experiences but require planning time, organization, and money and may occur away from home. *Family leisure* is defined as informal, usually home-based, activities that have minimal costs connected to them but provide multiple members the opportunities to interact in casual, relaxed ways as they participate together. Examples of leisure activities are game playing, watching television or home videos, gardening, and cookouts.

Celebrations are unifying events for families that are important to family identity, themes, and goals that can be linked to health outcomes. The Family Health Model suggests that families need to be encouraged to participate in wellness or health promoting activities that encourage relaxed times together, foster dyadic and triadic relationships, and provide renewal experiences. Family self-care has been defined as "a specific approach to clinical practice that recognizes the uniqueness and strength of the family constellation and places primary emphasis on the family's ability to promote and protect health" (Gray & Sergi, 1989, p. 69). Therapeutic intervention aims at providing support for family members so that high levels of functioning can be attained, psychological difficulties can be prevented, and normal adjustments to health crises can be anticipated (Danielson, Hamel-Bissell, & Winstead-Fry, 1993). Family-focused care aimed at family therapeutics would include celebration, tradition, and the use of leisure time. Increased automation, mechanization, and technology have reduced labor at home and work, and the wide availability of transportation and economic resources has made leisure time a primary focus for many American families. Appropriate use of leisure time can provide common goals that are strengthening and can be measured as outcomes, but they can also be threats and divisive if they separate members for extended time periods (McGowan, Delamarter, Schroeder, & Liegler, 1989, p. 217). These authors suggest some concerns that nurses might consider in leisure care:

- Who will be involved?
- When will the activities occur?
- Where will the family go? What will they do?
- Why does the family want to participate?
- How is the family able to provide for activities?
- What costs are associated with the activities?

Families with less time and fewer resources may need more assistance in planning therapeutic family celebrations. Family-focused care encourages nurses to be creative in assisting families to use leisure as a means to potentiate health.

Celebration brings an air of expectation and the possibility of reprieve from the toils and stresses of daily life. Celebration is a time of reprieve from the usual burdens associated with life and is a chance to be rejuvenated. Celebration means that the despair sometimes experienced in the mundane and commonplace can be temporarily set aside and substituted with hopefulness. According to Miller (1986):

Hope is a state of being, characterized by an anticipation of a continued good state, an improved state or a release from a perceived entrapment. The anticipation may or may not be founded on concrete, real world evidence. Hope is an anticipation of a future that is good and is based upon: mutuality (relationships with others), a sense of personal competence, coping ability, psychological well-being, purpose, and meaning in life, as well as a sense of "the possible" (p. 52).

Miller (2000) identified three levels of hope: (1) superficial wishes; (2) hope for relationships, self-improvement, and self-accomplishments; and (3) hope for relief from suffering, personal trials, or entrapment. Family-focused care allows nurses to view these areas as important primary concerns for processes of becoming and well-being. Celebration contains the essences of optimism, expectation, and anticipation often associated with hope. Bringing the fragrance of celebration into everyday life experiences may create balms of meaning that can decrease the stress, anxiety, despair, and anguish that too often accompany the human experience.

Family-focused care may include the use of healing rituals, or self-created celebrations generated to cope with and transcend life's troubling dilemmas, debilitating conditions, and prolonged sorrows. *Healing* can be defined as "something that facilitates movement toward wholeness, suggests the impossibility of separating what is mental, from what is physical, and from issues that appear to be spiritual in nature" (Achterberg, Dossey, & Kolkmeier, 1994, p. 9). Healing rituals are forms of mind–body treatments that make one whole. A ritual is a form of empowerment that enables one to get in contact with one's being. It is a way to integrate the mind, body, and soul and transform usual events into sacred moments (Biziou, 1999). Families can create ritual behaviors that are meaningful ways to connect to others, find emotional healing, enhance creativity, usher in new life stages, and acknowledge daily routines (Biziou). Rituals include specific formulas for action, encourage positive family interactions, evoke a sense of transcendence, and empower one to care for oneself and others. Families of origin that do not include the use of rituals or minimize the values of celebration may fail to inspire their descendants with ideals about creation and continuance. Those who have minimized the use of celebrations throughout their life course may require assistance in creating meaningful rituals (Imber-Black & Roberts, 1992). The Family Health Model recognizes that celebration is an area that is not often emphasized by nurses but is one that could be used in family-focused care to enhance family functioning and promote health promotion and disease prevention.

 Critical Thinking Activity

Some say that divorce is one of the most difficult experiences in life. Take some time to think about how you might assist a family in creating a divorce ritual that is meaningful and one that will help the healing process. What would the ritual include? What would occur? When would it happen? Who should be there to participate? What things are needed to create the ritual? Is it something that is done once or something that needs to be repeated?

After you have constructed your healing ritual, share it with others. Perhaps the class could work together and write a paper or prepare a resource that others might use related to healing rituals.

How do you personally feel about this experience? Do you think divorced families might benefit from healing routines? Describe how you might use the idea of healing rituals in family-focused care.

Table 10–2	Change Process Techniques Pertinent to Family Health	
Process	**Goals**	**Techniques***
Consciousness raising	Increasing information about oneself and problem	Observations, confrontations, interpretations, bibliotherapy
Social liberation	Increasing social alternatives for behaviors that are not problematic	Advocating for rights of repressed, empowering, policy interventions
Emotional arousal	Experiencing and expressing feelings about one's problems and solutions	Psychodrama, grieving losses, roleplaying
Self-re-evaluation	Assessing feelings and thoughts about oneself with respect to a problem	Value clarification, imagery, corrective emotional experience
Commitment	Choosing and committing to acts or belief in the ability to change	Decision-making therapy, New Year's resolutions, logotherapy
Environment control	Avoiding stimuli that elicit problem behaviors	Environmental restructuring (e.g., removing alcohol or fattening foods), avoiding high-risk cues
Reward	Rewarding oneself or being rewarded by others for making changes	Contingency contracts, overt and covert reinforcement
Helping Relationships	Enlisting the help of someone who cares	Therapeutic alliance, social support, self-help groups

Source: Prochaska, JO, Norcross, JC, and Diclemente, C: Changing for Good. Avon Books, New York, 1994, with permission.
*These are primarily professional techniques used by psychotherapists.

Change

Change is an individual, family, and societal phenomenon that occurs on a moment-to-moment basis and over extended periods. It happens spontaneously in a moment and takes a lifetime to occur. Change is desired and dreaded, enduring and temporary, and predictable and unpredictable. Change begets change. Change can create personal awareness and feelings of complete oblivion. Change occurs on its own and is provoked by others. *Change* is defined as a dynamic nonlinear process that implies altering or modifying the form, direction, and outcome of the original identity by substituting alternatives. Within a family, one member can change or be affected by changes with only small impact on the family as a whole, but some changes that affect individual members intensely also affect the entire household.

Change is most productive when it is aligned with individual and family goals. According to Prochaska, Norcross, and Diclemente (1994):

> Change has remained enigmatic, and none of the several hundred different therapies can effectively explain just how it occurs. Furthermore, no therapy is any more successful than the change strategies that determined, persistent, and hardworking individuals develop for themselves (p. 21).

These authors have identified the nine processes of change as consciousness raising, social liberation, emotional arousal, self-re-evaluation, commitment, countering, environmental control, rewards, and helping relationships. Table 10–2 provides a brief comparison of the nine processes, goals, and techniques that are relevant to change. Change processes are places in which family-focused care can target goals and control change to meet expressed needs. Successful change creates feelings of control, power, hope, and greater success (Ryan, 2000).

Watzlawick, Weakland, and Fisch (1974) described first-order changes as those that affect one or several parts of the family system, with the whole remaining unaffected. They described second-order changes as those that affect the entire system. A disconnect among member perceptions about family changes is not unusual because individuals perceive things differently. Change must be considered in relationship to prior changes,

changes presently occurring, or changes desired in the future. For example, after years of studying change processes in smokers, Prochaska et al. (1994) found that people who were successful in changing their smoking behaviors used diverse processes at different times and chose change techniques that depended on the situation's demands. These researchers identified six predictable and well-defined stages of change: precontemplation, contemplation, preparation, action, maintenance, and termination.

Family-focused care begins with an assessment of the stage of the change process for individuals and families. Although stages are progressive, this does not mean that persons cannot fall back into an earlier stage, and progression through one stage does not necessarily lead to the next.

Although some persons are highly motivated toward creating positive change, many require assistance to initiate or maintain change. Techniques such as consciousness raising, reframing, goal setting, thought stopping, relaxation, and stress management can assist in making changes. Wright and Leahey (2000) suggest these ideas about change:

- Change is dependent on the perception of the problem.
- Change responds to interpersonal, intrapersonal, and contextual influences.
- Change is dependent on contextual restraints and resources.
- Change is dependent on co-evolving treatment goals.
- Change is not the result of understanding or knowledge.
- Change is not a process that occurs equally in all family members.
- Change is a major reason for family nursing to occur.
- Change is a covariant process based on the family's readiness and the nurse's abilities.
- Change is influenced by variables beyond the control of either the family or the nurse.

The Family Health Model implies that nurses can target change processes as a functional family aspect to accommodate alterations related to meeting health goals.

Communication

Communication modes differ widely from family to family, but all of them use various forms to transfer information within the household and between the household and embedded contextual systems. Communication is the way emotions are expressed and ideas, knowledge, skills, and concerns related to health are transmitted. In the Family Health Model, *communication* is defined as the primary way parents socialize children about health beliefs, values, attitudes, and behaviors and convey information, knowledge, and actions applicable to health; verbal and nonverbal forms of communication are equally meaningful. Communication is the nucleus of interactions that affects member relationships, roles, and responsibilities beyond the parenting years and across the life course. Families that use terms such as "we" and "us" rather than "I" may be viewed as healthier families, but all families have some communication needs associated with family health.

Mothers with young children often described teaching their children health-related behaviors and suggest that various family and contextual forms of communication are used as reinforcement (Denham, 1997). For example, one mother said she taught her preschool children about good nutrition by having them with her in the kitchen when she was cooking and showing them what would be healthy snacks. She described how close friends and extended family members reinforced her ideas. A grandmother caring for her young children said she had a place in the refrigerator and in a cabinet where healthy snacks were kept. She described how she thought children's visits to their mother's home threatened her teachings about personal hygiene because their mothers failed to provide clear instructions and they often returned to the grandparents' home unkempt. The mothers described in this paragraph each used a variety of communication techniques to accomplish health goals related to nutrition.

Communication is more than language acquisition, but it is tied to linguistic aspects that are acquired in the early months of life. At age 10 months, infants in a low-functioning group could understand 10 words but say none of them, but those in a high-functioning group could understand 150 words and say 10 words (Fenson, Dale, Reznick, Bates, Thal, & Pethick, 1994). At age 16 months, whereas lower-functioning toddlers understood about 90 words and said about 10 words, a high-functioning group understood about 350 words and spoke about 180 words. However, early patterns may not tell the whole story of language acquisition and may not always indicate future learning because children tend to be individualistic in language development and do not necessarily parallel the group (Bates, Dale, & Thal, 1995; Bates, Marchman, Thal, Fenson, Dale, Eznick, Reilly, & Hartung, 1994). Some children tend to be slow and steady as they develop language, but others experience bursts of expressiveness. A longitudinal study (White, 1993) found that infants who scored higher in intelligence and had more social skills had parents who directed more language toward them. Although parents influence early language acquisition, children's exposure to increasing numbers of persons and the larger society also influences their language development as they mature.

Gender differences in forms of articulation, verbal interchange, and social interactions have been noted. However, differences in the ways boys and girls interact may be more similar to ends of a continuum rather than discrete dualism. Girls choose play that involves talking and sitting together, but boys roughhouse, threaten, and clobber one another (Tannen, 1998). Two recent books about the emotional lives of boys suggest that the family, institutions, and society place distressing expectations on boys to act macho, confident, and tough while ignoring an emotional abyss that is often disabling (Kindlon & Thompson, 1999; Pollack, 1998). Although girls seem to be gaining voices as society empowers them, some boys may be emotionally crippled by gender expectations about ways to communicate feelings and express ideas. Pollack states, "We want our boys to be sensitive New Age guys and still be cool dudes" (p. xxv). What are the relationships between communication and health? How does society influence communication patterns? What are the appropriate targets, goals, and interventions that need to be included in family-focused care to address processes of becoming, health, and well-being? The Family Health Model suggests that communication is an important functional aspect corresponding to health processes. Family-focused care requires that nurses be highly skilled in areas of communication to address individual, family, and group health needs.

👫👫👫 Cooperative Learning

Get a partner and take turns sharing with one another about an experience in your family when you thought that you were misunderstood. It might be something recent or something that happened a long time ago. How did you feel when it happened? What did you do? How do you feel about it now? What might you have done differently?

Have a class discussion about family communication and identify some areas where nurses might intervene. In what areas could nurses assess needs, plan intervention, and evaluate outcomes? How does family communication influence health processes?

Connectedness

Affiliations, associations, bonds, friendships, acquaintances, and relationships are all concepts relevant to connectedness. The ways individuals coexist with peers, colleagues, neighbors, agencies, institutions, and helping others affect many life aspects, including health. In the Family Health Model, *connectedness* is defined as the ways individuals are committed and linked to family, educational, cultural, spiritual, political, social, professional, legal, economic, and commercial interests. Roles and responsibilities are often outward expressions of personal commitments, but they also provide tangible ways for nurses to discuss expectations about family relationships. Connectedness has to do with household boundaries and their modulation in response to needs for resources and supports over time and the division of labor related to family needs, and it may indicate the degree of tolerance for ambiguity. Wright and Leahey (2000) suggest that careful observation of the connections within and between systems is an important role of nurses.

In the family health research completed by this author, partner relationships and kin networks were the primary indicators of the household production of health. Family connectedness implied ways members accepted tasks related to household needs and were open or closed to supports outside the household. Families that agreed to hospice services were open to ideas and services from a variety of multidisciplinary care providers and incorporated the skills and knowledge derived into family routines (Denham, 1999b). Families with young children seemed willing to accept assistance from various providers referred to them by those who provided prenatal and well-child care (Denham, 1997, 1999a, 1999c). For example, a mother said:

> My mother-in-law helps too! If she knows that we are trying to potty train or she knows it is time to start, she'll go ahead and start without me. Like I wasn't really thinking about my daughter being old enough at the time for her to begin wiping her own self, but my mother-in-law decided that she could do that ... and so she began! She was doing it downstairs and I said, "That's fine, we'll do it upstairs too." We work together!

In Appalachian families, it is common to find kin networks in which members have daily or regular interaction. In this Appalachian family, grandparents and a great-grandmother lived downstairs, and the adult family with three youngsters lived upstairs. Information about who comprises the family network should be a concern for nurses who are interested in providing family-focused care.

Friendship circles that evolve through peers, colleagues, alliances, clubs, gangs, or other social networks are influential. The ways members connect with others inside and outside the family have the potential to affect processes of becoming, health, and well-being. Friendships affect actions, knowledge, experiences, perceptions, behaviors, and emotions. Friendships can occur because of shared interests, or they can expose people to new areas of awareness. Friendships that are health enriching or devastating may be time and content dependent. For example, a father in the family health studies (Denham, 1997) thought that it was acceptable for his preschool-age son to play with toy guns because that had been his own experience during his childhood; however, the boy's mother believed that playing with guns was not in her son's best interest. The boy's father described connections to persuade the mother it was a harmless activity:

> I think she is going to give in now because I think it is about time for him to do that. All of his other friends are playing with guns ... cowboys and Indians ... and things such as that. I think she will relinquish here shortly!

Connections also have implications for the ways families are influenced and incorporate information into the household production of health. In the first family health study (Denham, 1997), a local public health initiative had focused on lead screening. Parents in five of the eight families had been informed about lead risks, had taken their children to the health department for well-child care, and had had their children tested. The influence of the media, school systems, the public health agency, and others in the community created increased awareness about lead in these families living in older homes. One mother said:

> There is one area that kind of scares me. There is a space underneath the house, they call it grandma's basement. There is a dirt floor in one area underneath an old porch, but it has been filled in some ... but it then goes down into a very small basement area. Now that dirt area, the children like to play in it and I got rather concerned about lead poisoning and stuff. They were tested for lead at the health department. I don't know, probably a year and a half ago and they said that their lead levels were a little high.

Although a year had passed, this mother recalled what she had previously learned and continued to vigilantly monitor her children's play. Connections pertain to family rules about boundaries. The Family Health Model suggests that nurses who provide family-focused care consider connections related to health as functional processes for assessment, intervention, and evaluation.

Coordination

Coordination occurs when individuals cooperate rather than compete to accomplish goals and when family members have a sense of sharing in rewards or punishments. In the Family Health Model, *coordination* implies cooperative sharing of resources, skills, abilities, and information within the family and larger contextual systems to optimize health potentials, maximize the household production of health, and achieve family goals. Coordination requires acceptance of diversity, presence and support during critical times of family need, and interaction with social entities outside the family's boundaries. Coordination promotes shared learning but varies as members negotiate tasks, juggle time commitments, and differentiate between their willingness and abilities to contribute. Coordination concerns members' loyalties to family ideals and rules and occurs when members unite to accomplish tasks.

Coordination needs may vary, depending on things such as unique contextual circumstances, prior member and family experiences, and consensus about family goals. A perplexing dilemma in working with families is the difficulties some members might have in naming family goals or identifying important family themes because these may be rather abstract notions embedded in behaviors. Another quandary is that subsystem interactions are often silently orchestrated, and there may be unconscious behaviors that members have difficulty discussing. Another concern related to coordination has to do with innate member traits that affect the ways time is used and activities are valued.

In the family health research, Appalachian families often worked together to accomplish health goals. Coordination was implied by who had which tasks and abilities to work together. Goals were accomplished when members shared beliefs and had strong filial attachments. For example, a teenage daughter had lived in her mother's home since her parents divorced, but some problems with her mother's boyfriend meant that she decided to move to her father's household, a blended family. The stepmother said, "Her lifestyle and our lifestyle are so different from where she was raised. That was hard for her to adjust to! There are rules here."

Coordination of daily tasks to meet health needs may take a great deal of family cooperation to achieve common goals. Some family members discussed their inability to cooperate. For example, a mother in another family said:

> I have a sister, and my husband says she tries to run my life. I think she does have a role on some of my decisions. She is supportive when it comes to the kids and stuff . . . to health and things like that. She is always there for us, but a lot of other things she kind of sticks her nose in!

In a later interview, this same mother said this about her extended family:

> You know, we live so close and they would be so controlling . . . I think we have a big stress factor there. They try to run our lives, especially when it comes to the kids. I'll tell the kids "no" and she'll . . . She's got one of these swimming pools . . . And I'll tell them they can't get in it. She'll allow them to get in it! They'll get in trouble 'cause I told them no or she'll give them junk food after I told them no.

In this case, family coordination was inextricably linked to stressors internal and external to the home, and this family was challenged by the problem solving needed to maximize the household production of health. The family had limited economic resources and counted on extended family members for transportation, child care, and emotional support. Coordinating activities, retaining extended family members' supportive relationships, and limiting stress were major concerns for the family.

Coordination often plays out in decision making about daily activities. How do families decide what gets done and when? Who is responsible for doing what? What gets done today and what gets left uncompleted or postponed? Families may be continuously shuffling among choices and possibilities related to conflicts between individual needs and the needs of others. Families may lack experience, skills, knowledge, or the resources necessary for coordinating household activities. For example, if a working mother has limited time but her family thinks that it is important for school-age children to be actively engaged in social activities, then how do the parents maintain good nutrition for multiple members on the days when everyone seems to be going in different directions? Mothers may also be conflicted when coordinating demands that mean choosing between caring for themselves and caring for others. When family members are caregivers for chronically ill or dying members, they may have to do their usual tasks plus assume additional responsibilities. Coordination of multiple roles adds stress, tests coping skills, and can threaten health. The Family Health Model implies that family-focused care aimed at families' functional processes to coordinate demands relevant to daily living can threaten or potentiate processes of becoming, health, and well-being.

Summary

The core processes have to do with the functional capacities of multiple member households and are intricately related to health. Family-focused care presents nurses with challenges as they strive to work with complex families to achieve goals relevant to members' well-being. Although basic nursing education equips nurses with knowledge and fundamental skills relevant to family functional status, expert family nurses require additional experiences, knowledge, and skills for working with the complex interactions of families and their embedded contextual systems. Although nurses may focus on family's core functional processes, goals of care are aimed at outcomes related to family health. The Family Health Model encourages nursing care that targets interactional processes to accomplish family goals. Box 10–2 provides some propositions related to family's functional status and health that can be tested through practice and investigated through research.

Box 10–2 **Propositions about Relationships between Functional Processes and Family Health**

- Children who learn health values and behaviors in early life continue many of these patterns over the life course.
- Families with dyads and triads that share health beliefs, attitudes, and behaviors provide greater support for individuals' health-care needs than families that lack this congruence.
- Health interventions targeted at family dyads and triads result in more optimal health outcomes than interventions aimed only at individuals.
- Interventions that target core family processes, family goals, and contextual systems result in more optimal health outcomes than interventions aimed at solitary individuals.
- Families with intact core functional processes describe more optimized processes of becoming and well-being.
- Families with well-functioning dyads and triads have higher levels of well-being for individual members and greater health for the family as a whole.
- Health of individuals and families is increased when congruency exists between member abilities, family health goals, and supportive contextual systems.

Test Your Knowledge

1. Define and give an example of the core process of caregiving.
2. Define and give an example of the core process of cathexis.
3. Define and give an example of the core process of celebration.
4. Define and give an example of the core process of change.
5. Define and give an example of the core process of communication.
6. Define and give an example of the core process of connectedness.
7. Define and give an example of the core process of coordination.
8. Describe how core processes might be used to address family needs when a member smokes and risks related to second-hand smoke are a concern for a premature infant.
9. Explain how core processes might be used to address family concerns about risks associated with genetic inheritance of Huntington's disease.

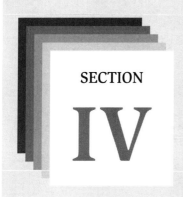

SECTION

IV

Structural Aspects of Family Health

Chapter

11

Family Health Routines: The Social Construction of Family Health

CHAPTER OBJECTIVES *At the end of this chapter, the reader will be able to:*

■ Explain ways rituals enhance family life.
■ Define what is meant by the concept of family health routines.
■ Discuss family health routines as the structural aspect of the household production of health.
■ Describe relationships between contextual and functional factors and family health routines.

> *The function of ritual is to give form to human life, not in the way of mere surface arrangement, but in depth.*
> —Joseph Campbell, Myths to Live By

This chapter provides a comprehensive view of family routines as a structure used by family members within the household niche to discuss knowledge, resources, and behaviors that address health needs. The Family Health Model posits that all families have ritual-like practices relevant to health that members can recall and describe regardless of the family configuration, member traits, or cultural context. Steinglass, Bennett, Wolin, and Reiss (1987) studied alcoholic families and found that routines and rituals were excellent clinician research tools because (1) daily routines can be observed and specific behaviors recorded and (2) family members could verbally reconstruct family rituals. Family-focused practice implies that family routines should be a central focus for practitioners who are targeting family health. Routines provide insight into the actual behaviors pertinent to health and are amenable to the field of nursing's scope of practice and nursing actions.

Ritual as a Foundation for Family Health

Rituals

Rituals are often considered from anthropological and sociological perspectives, but less attention has been given to potential biological, health, or nursing perspectives. Rituals or routines are widely discussed in some literature but have been largely ignored by nurse clinicians, educators, and many researchers (Denham, 1995). *Ritual* has been defined as "an act or actions intentionally conducted by a group of people employing one or more symbols in a repetitive, formal, precise, highly stylized fashion" (Myeroff, 1977, p. 199). Rituals are "conventional acts of display through which one or more participants transmit information concerning their physiological, psychological, or sociological states either to themselves or to one or more participants" (Rappaport, 1971, p. 63). Ritual is a social performance (Goffman, 1959); a systematic occurrence with characteristics of prescription, rigidity, and rightness (Bossard & Boll, 1950); and a stabilizing force for past patterns and "responses to changes in the present and anticipation of the future" (Cheal, 1988, p. 642). Rituals link private and public meanings and create opportunities to express acceptance or demonstrate rejection of social standards (Roberts, 1988). Whereas *secular rituals* tend to include the relationships between individual behaviors and collective ceremony without offering specific explanations, *religious rituals* provide a canon of principles to explain behaviors (Moore & Myeroff, 1977).

Ritual has a form of sanctity in human communication and is a process described as having three key properties: transformation, communication, and stabilization (Wolin & Bennett, 1984). *Transformation* is the time that precedes the actual ritual (e.g., shopping for Thanksgiving dinner, planning a vacation) and has been described as *liminality,* a time during which the fullness of what is to happen as a result of the ritual has not been completely realized (Turner, 1977). *Communication* is the dynamic interactive stage of the ritual during which participants actively engage in the experience and invite emotional involvement and interactions in ways that differ from nonritualized events. *Stabilization* has to do with the continuance or predictability of the event and provides a means for linking the past, present, and future.

Family Rituals

In a study of family rituals from 1856 to 1949, Bossard and Boll (1950) defined a *family ritual* as "a pattern of prescribed formal behavior pertaining to some specific event, occasion, or situation, which tends to be repeated over and over again" (p. 9). Family ritual is "a symbolic form of communication that, owing to the satisfaction that family members experience through its repetition, is acted out in a systemic fashion over time" (Wolin & Bennett, 1984, p. 401). Family rituals are formal repetitive patterns that enhance a family's self-image and express it to members and nonmembers (Reiss, 1981). Weisner (1984) suggested that daily routines are central to a family's drive to construct and sustain a pattern of care, supervision, and stimulation for children that fits with family goals and meanings. The household niche provides opportunities to model and reinforce family values. Family rituals sometimes include a sense of social consciousness in which family members demonstrate their family pride (e.g., entertaining guests, attending church together). "Family rituals may be perceived as being a fairly reliable index of family collaboration, accommodation, and synergy" (Denham, 1995, p. 17). Family rituals provide information about members' relationships, changes occurring within the family, the ways crises and information affect needs, things members value and believe, and ways families celebrate and live their daily lives (Imber-Black & Roberts, 1992).

Imber-Black and Roberts (1992) identified four types of family rituals. The first type is day-to-day essentials (e.g., eating, sleeping, hello's, goodbyes), meaningful actions that provide set patterns in the course of the day that provide expression of family identity and member connections. A second type of ritual is traditional times, during which usual patterns are altered to celebrate special events (e.g., anniversaries, birthdays, reunions, vacations) accompanied by memorable customs with unique family adaptations. A third type of family routine is holiday celebrations (e.g., Christmas, Kwanzaa, Passover, Halloween) or events that link a family to the outside community and culture. The fourth type of routine was noted as lifecycle rituals (e.g., baby showers, confirmations, bar and bat mitzvahs, graduation, weddings, retirements) or events that mark life course journeys and only happen once. Table 11–1 provides an overview of some other ways that family rituals have been interpreted in the literature.

Table 11–1	**Ritual Types and Dimensions**
Reference	**Ritual Types and Dimensions**
Bossard and Boll (1950)	Described 20 ritual events included in family life
Reiss (1981)	Hypothesized that links exist between family rituals and the ways families solve problems; identified four types of families: 1. Environment-sensitive or "normal" families 2. Achievement-sensitive or competitive families 3. Consensus-sensitive or rigid families 4. Distance-sensitive or families with delinquent members
Wolin and Bennett (1984)	Family celebrations Family traditions Patterned routines
Roberts (1988)	Six types of family rituals: 1. Under-ritualized families 2. Rigidly ritualized families 3. Skewed rituals 4. Hollow rituals 5. Interrupted routines 6. Flexible routines
Fiese (1992); Fiese & Kline (1993)	Eight dimensions of family rituals: 1. Frequency of occurrence of the activity pattern 2. Expectations about mandatory participation 3. Emotional investment 4. Meanings of symbolic significance 5. Demand to intergenerationally continue the activity 6. Deliberateness or advanced preparation in activity planning 7. Assigned roles and duties associated with the ritual 8. Degrees of the activity's rigidity or flexibility
Schuck & Bucy (1997)	Four dimensions of family rituals: 1. Structure 2. Meaning 3. Persistence 4. Adaptability

Family Routines

The terms *ritual* and *routine* are sometimes used interchangeably when discussed in terms of celebrations and traditions, but far fewer references are identified about relationships with health promotion, health maintenance, disease prevention, illness care, health recovery, or end-of-life care. Routines have been described as "repetitive behaviors that may or may not have symbolic significance to the family and often lack historical embeddedness" (Denham, 1995, p. 15). Family routines are behavior patterns related to events, occasions, or situations that are repeated with regularity and consistency (Bossard & Boll, 1950; Fiese, 1993; Imber-Black & Roberts, 1992; Reiss, 1981; Steinglass et al., 1987). Patterned behaviors are characterized by exactness or precisioned occurrence, a degree of rigidity in performance, and a sense of correctness in their existence (Bossard & Boll). Family routines appear to have a strong intergenerational component and are ways families teach members valued behaviors (Denham, 1997, 1999b; Fiese, 1992, 1995; Niska, Snyder, & Lia-Hoagberg, 1998; Wolin, Bennett, Noonan, & Teitelbaum, 1980) and may be a way to dialogue about family care when talking with individual patients (Rogers & Holloway, 1991). Family meals are an example of routines that reflect the ways members share their lives and their family themes (DeVault, 1991).

Family routines have been identified as key structural aspects of family health that can be assessed by nurses, provide a focus for family interventions, and have potential for measuring health outcomes (Denham, 1999a, 1999b, 1999c). Routines provide a means for family members to conceptualize and discuss the household production of family health (Denham, 1997). Family routines have "universal attributes of family life, varying only in content and frequency from family to family" (Sprunger, Boyce, & Gaines, 1985, p. 565) and provide information about predictable family behaviors (Keltner, Keltner, & Farran, 1990). Routines supply information about behaviors and their predictability, member interactions, family identity, and specific ways families use values. Patterned routines help members define their roles and organize their daily lives, but participants seldom consciously plan them (Bennett, Wolin, & McAvity, 1988). Routines are recognized with great consistency by multiple members and can be recalled, discussed, and taught (Denham, 1997; Fiese, 1995). Although routines are dynamic and evolving, after patterns are established, members usually strive to retain the patterns. Routines appear to be resilient and unique to family households, but the potential to modify them still exists.

👫👫👫👫 *Cooperative Learning*

Find a partner and brainstorm together about family routines each one can recall from your childhood. These routines may or may not have to do with health concerns. After you have created a list, prioritize the three most important routines in your family-of-origin experiences. Then share with the class how your family routines have changed over time. Discuss whether these routines are still continued within their families of origin and ways they have been altered over time. If some students are now part of another family, then discuss ways routines are different. Discuss new routines class members may have intentionally tried to initiate in their families.

Therapeutic Rituals

Although nurses have not usually considered the use of ritual as a therapeutic intervention, the concept has been used widely in family therapy. In 1977, Palazzoli, Boscolo, Cecchin, and Prata first described the use of prescribing family rituals in family therapy as a valuable intervention. Since then, many authors (Bennett, Wolin & McAvity, 1988; Cheal, 1988; Rogers & Holloway, 1991; Starr, 1989; Whiteside, 1989) have referred to the therapeutic merit of rituals. Doherty (1997) described the "intentional family" as one that deliberately creates meaningful actions associated with repeated behaviors. Therapeutic rituals can be used to assist families to resolve conflicts and resentments, negotiate roles and boundaries, develop shared meanings, and mobilize resources for healing and growth (Bright, 1990). The successful use by other disciplines of ritual as a therapeutic modality with families appears to provide support for considering the use of rituals in nursing practice and family-focused care.

■ The Concept of Structure

In the Family Health Model, the term *structure* is used to describe the ways family members use beliefs, values, attitudes, information, knowledge, resources, and prior experiences to structure behaviors that impact health. It is posited that family routines provide a structure for understanding the complex interactional patterns that affect the household production of health and give insight into family lifestyles, member behaviors, and actual practices. "Family routines provide a predictable environment and predictable timing for interaction among family members" (Keltner, 1992, p. 129). Box 11–1 provides a list of assumptions derived from the family health research and the author's knowledge and experiences about relationships between families, health routines, and family health.

The Family Health Model suggests that health routines are important ways to measure interactions among embedded contextual systems, family functional status, and member

---

Box 11–1 **Assumptions about Family Health Routines and Family Health**

- All families have systemic behavioral patterns related to family health.
- Individuals, family subsystems, and families vary in the ways they participate in family health routines.
- Members participate in individual, subsystem, and family health routines that are characterized by patterned behaviors that can be described by household members.
- Family health routines are impacted by the household's embedded contextual systems and the functional interactions of the household members.
- Beliefs, values, traditions, culture, personal experiences, information exposure, resources, and encounters with health-care professionals influence the unique social constructions of family health routines.
- Children's socialization about health processes is largely imposed by the family's social construction of health routines.
- Family households are the primary places where children learn about health, develop health attitudes, and establish health behaviors.
- Family themes and goals provide undergirding for the ways family health routines are socially constructed.
- Families use accommodation processes to create, deconstruct, and reconstruct family health routines.
- In most cultures and families, mothers are often the initiators and keepers of family health routines.
- After family health routines are initiated, members adjust the character of the patterns over time so that they retain consistency with their family health paradigm.
- Family health routines that lose their meaningfulness are dissolved.
- Families create, deconstruct, and reconstruct new health routines or alter familiar ones to accommodate normative and non-normative life experiences over the life course.

health variables within the household. The use of routines provides a way for nurses, family members, and others to discuss members' health practices, behaviors, and knowledge; identify family goals; and create plans for optimizing processes of becoming, health, and well-being. Routines also provide ways to strategize about care needs related to illness, episodic or acute conditions, health promotion and protection, and health-seeking actions. According to Jensen, James, Boyce, & Hartnett (1983), "Family routines may be viewed as behavioral units of family life which provide order and structural integrity to the course of daily events" (p. 201). Steinglass et al. (1987), researchers who have studied alcoholic families, have described routines as "background behaviors that provide structure and form to daily life" (p. 63). Daily routines reflect a family's temperament, and "the way these routines are structured is more directly determined by such properties as the family's characteristic energy level, preferred interactional distance, and behavior range" (Steinglass et al., p. 64).

Differing Perspectives about Structure

Structure has been widely discussed in the literature for decades. Structural perspectives are used to observe, measure, and illuminate processes and procedures of small groups (Cattell, 1953); provide information about family relatedness and interactions (Straus, 1964); and suggest ways to view absolute, relational, comparative, and contextual properties of complex organizations (Lazarsfeld & Menzel, 1969). Eshelman (1974) discussed structure based on power (e.g., matriarchal versus patriarchal), family form (e.g., nuclear family versus single parent family), and marital patterns (e.g., marriage within a racial group versus biracial marriage). Family lifestyle has been viewed as structural patterns of family organization (i.e., value system, communication networks, role systems, power structure) that are important when a family faces stress (Parad & Caplan, 1965). Structure has been described in terms of being closed (i.e., stability through tradition), open (i.e., adaptation through consensus), and random (i.e., exploration through intuition) (Kantor & Lehr, 1975). Family types were considered in relation to access distance regulation (i.e., space, time, energy) and target distance regulation (i.e., joining–separating, freedom–restriction, sharing–not sharing).

According to Minuchin (1974), structure refers to the ways a family is organized, the subsystems it contains, and the rules relevant to family interactional patterns. The family therapy model views family as an open sociocultural system faced with internal and external demands and change. Families are composed of subsystems with differentiated boundaries that provide indicators of family function (e.g., disengaged family versus enmeshed family), and the goal of therapy within this framework is to assist the family to restructure themselves in a more functional way (Minuchin & Fishman, 1981). The structural-functional perspective implies that members' abilities to cope with demands and change are influenced by their interactions, responses to change and demands, and family organization.

Pratt (1976) viewed family health as a result of a family energized and structured so that developing members could fully develop their unique potentials to support interdependent actions that contribute to health. A sociological perspective described family health as the "general level of health in a family so inextricably intertwined with the patterns of family relations that health itself becomes a vital aspect of the fabric of family life" (Pratt, p. 139). Pratt's energized family structure includes:

- Family responsiveness to individuals' autonomous needs and interests
- Abilities to actively cope with life's stresses and necessities
- Flexibility in task accomplishment
- An egalitarian power distribution

■ Regular and diverse forms of member interaction with the family and others
■ Positive personal and composite health practices

Pratt's view of family structure is connected with both context and functional status.

Nursing Perspectives of Structure

The term *structure* is repeatedly used in the nursing literature to discuss family organization and is identified as an important aspect of family health.

> We propose that the nursing perspective of family health should link family structure, function, and health variables (including both wellness and illness), incorporate the biopsychosocial and contextual system aspects of nursing, specify the paradigm view, and address the levels of family interaction with the nurse. This definition suggests a paradigm shift where family health embraces more than the health of individuals as parts of a family, and recognizes the family health system as the central phenomenon of the study (Anderson & Tomlinson, 1992, p. 59).

When discussing the nature of family, Gilliss (1991b) noted "there is a lack of consensus about what should be evaluated and how selected methods might access the data that make the family unit more than the sum of its parts" (p. 198). However, much in the current literature related to family structure seems more germane to therapy and focuses on members' psychosocial interactions.

In nursing, the concept of structure has been used to describe characteristics such as member roles, family forms (e.g., nuclear, single parent, blended), family subsystems, power structures (e.g., matriarchal, patriarchal), communication processes, and value systems (Friedman, 1998). Friedman uses a structural-functional approach to understand the ways families use structure and function within their systemic context to strive for equilibrium. Rather than taking a systemic view of stability obtained through feedback loops and circular causation, the structural-functional perspective "tends to resort to more 'part analysis,' linear notions of causality, and more static views of family" (Friedman, p. 165). The structural-functional approach primarily focuses on the ways family parts are arranged to form the whole and concentrates on the ways they function to meet society and subsystem needs. Friedman targets communication patterns, power structure, role structure, and family values for assessment and intervention. Structure and function are viewed as equally important content areas.

In the Calgary Family Assessment Model, family is described in relation to its internal structure, external structure, and context (Wright & Leahey, 2000). The *internal structure* consists of six subcategories: family composition, gender, sexual orientation, rank order, subsystems, and boundaries. The *external structure* is composed of the extended family members and larger systems. The *context* consists of ethnicity, race, social class, religion, and environment. These authors suggest that assessment tools such as the genogram or eco-map provide visual tools for decreasing ambiguity about the family's internal and external structure. They perceive that change is determined by the structure of the system. Structural determinism suggests that the unique status of an individual's structure determines whether interpersonal, intrapersonal, and environmental influences are interpreted as agitating or bothersome (Maturana & Varela, 1992). This implies that distinct structural aspects affect the ways change occurs across the life course.

In the Framework of Systemic Organization, Friedemann (1995) refers to family structure as persons in the household, other family members, children, significant persons of support, and persons who drain resources. The model focuses on the family's ability to maintain congruence in the midst of change. The ability to adjust to normative changes and re-establish congruence within the family as a whole, between family members, and between the family and the environment are ways to consider health in families. This systems model uses structure as a way to identify the family actors who affect and respond to health-illness needs and crises. The framework is a "structure to organize assessment data of complex situations, determine on what level to enter the system, set goals with the clients, and find ways to pursue them" (Friedemann, p. 348).

 ### Critical Thinking Activity

Think about the concept of structure and consider the ways you structure your daily life. List all of your routines that are related to health. How often do you participate in these routines? Do other members participate in these routines? Is your life highly structured, with many routines, or is it mostly unstructured, with few routines?

Choose one routine area that you would like to change. Have you unsuccessfully tried to make changes in the past? If you failed, why do you think this happened? Do others in your family think you need to alter this routine? Do other members in your family influence your routine? In what ways are you influenced? Are there things within the family context that influence your routine? What are those things?

Think about nursing practice. If you met a person with concerns similar to your own, then what kinds of interventions might you provide? What kinds of support might a family nurse provide to assist families in making changes in routines? What would the nurse need to know in order to help families in meaningful ways? How much support would families need? How long would they need it?

If you had to write a nursing care plan for yourself, what would it look like?

Structural Perspectives and Family Health

Use of Structural Perspectives in Research

Two concerns exist related to the use of structure to understand family health. The first concern is based on the fact that an extensive body of research has used a structural perspective for decades to investigate topics such as psychological processes, health and illness concerns, parenting effectiveness, substance abuse, risk behaviors, and treatment outcomes. Although findings in many of these studies may have some relevance to nursing practice, the applicability is not always clear. For example, Silver, Stein, and Dadds (1996) studied psychological adjustment and illness severity in children with chronic illness by dividing them into four different family structures (i.e., two biological parents, mother plus another adult relative, mother plus unrelated spouse or partner, mother alone). Findings indicated that greater relationships existed between children's health and adjustment when children lived with their mother and unrelated partner or their mother alone than when they lived with their mother and with either their biological father or another adult relative. Children in the mother plus unrelated partner group tended to have poorer overall adjustment than children in the other three groups. Although these findings have relevance to understanding the impact of family structure on children's health, a nurse may be able to do little about altering the partnering relationship status. Nurses may be troubled when trying to meaningfully apply this knowledge to interventions relevant to health outcomes.

Another study (Vaden-Kiernan, Ialongo, & Kellam, 1995) found that boys in both mother–father and mother–male partner families were significantly less likely than boys in mother-alone families to be rated as aggressive by teachers. Family structure gives little information about other family processes that may also be predictors of aggression, and it does not assist in choosing preventive actions. Nurses interested in impacting the health of families may not identify as useful the findings from many structural studies about families.

Although studies often provide attention-grabbing findings related to family structure and functional outcomes, the results are not extremely helpful to nurses interested in health-care perspectives. For example, a longitudinal study (Baer, 1999) of three ethnic groups identified increased family conflict over 3 years for all groups, but significant differences were found between nuclear and single-parent families. Another study (McFarlane, Bellissimo, & Norman, 1995) about family functioning and adolescent well-being compared parenting styles and family configuration and found that parenting (rather than family configuration) was the main determinant of both family functioning and well-being of adolescents.

Jenkins and Zunguze (1998) compared drug use in adolescents in grades 8, 10, and 12 who lived in single-parent (both mother- and father-headed), stepparent, and two-parent families from northeastern Ohio. Findings indicated the largest significant group differences were between single-parent, father-headed, and two-parent groups, with adolescents from father-headed families showing more frequent beer and liquor consumption at the 10th grade level.

Another study (Farrell & White, 1998) compared adolescent drug use and parent–adolescent distress in a sample of African-American 10th graders found no significant differences in the ways either gender or family structure moderated the relationship; however, peer influence and drug use increased with the level of mother–adolescent distress. Decision making of Australian adolescents from one- and two-parent families was compared, and findings indicated that those with one parent participated in a greater number of family decisions (Brown & Mann, 1990). A study (Spruijt & Goede, 1997) of families from the Netherlands examined the effects of transitions in family structure (i.e., stable intact families, conflict intact families, single-parent families, stepfamilies) on physical health, suicidal ideation, mental health, relational well-being, and employment and found that young people from single-parent families had the lowest scores. Although nurses are seldom prepared to address needs related to many aspects of family structure, they are able to assist and support family members in processes of becoming, health, and well-being.

Other examples from the family research literature also suggest that minimal application to nursing practice is derived from some structural perspectives. For example, structural analysis has been used to study families, households, and care of frail older women. Findings have indicated significant differences between arrangements between childless and other older women and less striking—but consistent—differences depending on the number and gender of living children (Soldo, Wolf, & Agree, 1990). Family structure and changes in living arrangements were compared in elderly unmarried parents, and findings indicated that those with more children are more likely to change from living alone to living with a child (Spitze, Logan, & Robinson, 1992). Although the number of children does not affect the odds of moving from living with a child to other arrangements nor does the child's gender affect the tendencies to begin co-residence, a slight increase in the movement out of co-residence was noted in families with sons. Results of studies such as these are interesting, but how do they apply to nursing's scope of practice?

How can a nurse use knowledge about family structure? Assisting families to stay intact is certainly of concern to nurses. But when the structure has already fractured before the encounter between the nurse and the family, then what interventions can the family nurse use to address the areas of practice with which nurses have the greatest concern? It seems that nurses need more tangible ways of focusing on the structural issues pertinent to nursing practice and family's health-illness needs. Merely knowing about family structure as it is usually understood does little to inform nurses about how to optimize the structure and suggests little about how to intervene in health concerns. Knowing that families with children and those that are childless may have different needs certainly is useful information, but how can nurses use this information to address family health needs?

> Family scientists and family physicians tend to use inconsistent definitions of family health and to approach the concept primarily from a psychosocial functioning perspective without integrating specific health variables of significance to nursing. In part this is a consequence of compartmentalized knowledge and methods designed to study intra- and inter-individual interactions, not systemic and ecosystem interactions (Anderson & Tomlinson, 1992, p. 60).

Perhaps it is time for nurses to investigate some alternative ways to consider structure that might be more amenable to nursing practice and aimed at health concerns.

Structural-Functional Perspectives and Family Health

A concern about the use of structural-functional perspectives to guide nurses' thinking about family health has to do with conceptual confusion in the model itself. The range of concepts included in a structural-functional perspective certainly have relationships to family health. However, historically the model has not clearly focused nurses' thinking about family-focused practice in ways that target family health concerns. The model seems to focus on analysis and linear causality of family interactions that are not always pertinent to nursing or family health.

Nursing has long used theories developed by disciplines external to nursing, as long as the application of the theory seemed appropriate and meaningful. A problem has been that the interpretation of appropriateness and value has mostly been an individual act without real consensus from the discipline. The consequence of private interpretations' being the rule rather than the exception results from a lack of empirical evidence in many practice areas. Nurses are often more willing to be followers than leaders, trusting the traditions of practice without critically thinking or judiciously weighing the quality and effectiveness of outcomes. For example, in family nursing, many available standardized measures have been based on theoretical frameworks derived from family therapy. Although the validity and reliability for family instruments have been well established, less attention has focused on critically evaluating the merit of these instruments for family-focused practice. Whall (1995) stated:

> Because each discipline has its own societal mandate and perspective, theories external to nursing were not adequate to the task unless they were reformulated. Moreover, I believed then, as I do now, that nursing could and should not just reform existing theory external to nursing but should also develop its own family theory (p. vii).

According to Friedemann (1995), the theoretical formulations presently available to nurses are still not "specific enough to serve as practice guidelines and models for family research and the formulation of hypotheses" (p. ix).

Fawcett and Whall (1991) said that the frameworks needed for family nursing practice must be distinguished from those used by other disciplines and should incorporate nursing knowledge, nursing actions, and family and member goals. Feetham (1991) indicated that "a clear and explicit conceptual or theoretical framework derived from existing family perspectives" is needed to provide a "complete and logical linkage of the framework to the empirical aspects" (p. 58) of family practice and research. As nursing increasingly focuses on outcomes, evidence-based care, and measurable interventions, attention to the ways frameworks from other disciplines are used to answer nursing questions or direct practice becomes increasingly important. Answering questions with current interpretations of structural dimensions may continue to produce knowledge that is less applicable to family-focused practice.

Friedemann (1995) has suggested several problems that are inherent in the use of linear approaches derived from structural-functional models:

- Linear models defy systemic principles and offer no provisions for exploring continuously evolving processes.
- Linear models that claim to lead to objective truth are challenged when individual views of family and health are subjective.
- Linear models lack solutions to the units of analysis for family problems.
- The focus of linear models tends toward central tendencies but neglects issues of diversity.
- Linear models fail to consider change over time (pp. 182–184).

Substantive programs of research relevant to family health are needed to extend the body of knowledge relevant to nursing. Models that include member roles, family processes, and health indicators using systematic and contextual perspectives are needed to guide family-focused practice. Nurses need to explore the continuums, dichotomies, and holistic perspectives pertinent to family behaviors and embedded household niches.

In Friedman's (1998) Family Assessment Model, the health-care function includes the following assessment areas:

- Family's health beliefs, values, and behaviors
- Family's definition of health
- Family's perceived health status and illness susceptibility
- Family's dietary practices
- Sleep and rest habits
- Physical activity and recreation
- Family drug habits
- Family's role in self-care practices
- Medically based preventive measures
- Dental health practices
- Family health history
- Health-care services received
- Feelings and perceptions regarding health-care services
- Emergency health services
- Source of payment
- Logistics of receiving care

Although relationships do exist between these criteria and family health, the generality of the topics does little to inform nurses about relationships and gives little guidance for how to use assessment data for planning interventions. Although the structural-functional model serves nursing practice well in some areas, the schema lacks the specificity needed to direct family-focused practice.

Use of structural-functional models has mostly targeted individuals with families viewed as the context of care rather than the unit or target of care. Nurses who are less prepared to address family concerns may not be able to use individual assessment data in ways that result in valued family interventions. Hoffman and Lippitt (1960) identified 11 approaches to family life and child development that may be pertinent to family health:

1. Parental background
2. Current setting
3. Family composition
4. Relationships between parents
5. Characters of the individuals who parent
6. Child-oriented parental attitudes
7. Overt parental behaviors
8. Child orientation toward parents and siblings
9. Overt child behaviors toward other family members
10. Personal character of the child
11. Behavior of the child when he or she is away from the parents

Although these assessment areas target structural-functional relationships and consider some contextual aspects, an emphasis on biophysical or specific health areas is lacking. Vagueness about structural-functional perspectives may not provide nurses with the necessary directions for attending to the breadth, depth, and scope of family health.

Structural models mainly focus on internal nature and less effectively consider powerful contextual factors that are potentiators of family health. The Family Health Model suggests that nurses consider structure as ways families receive, store, process, and respond to health information, as well as the knowledge and experiences germane to socially constructed patterned behaviors. The model implies that family routines provide structural perspectives that capture health beliefs, values, traditions, experiences, knowledge, skills, and behaviors of multiple members residing in a household niche. As structure, family routines provide ways to assess, intervene, measure, and evaluate factors related to the contextualized family's usual functional interactions that are germane to health.

Family Routines as a Social Construction

Introduction to Social Constructionism

Family health routines are basic structures of family life that can be operationalized according to cultural rules related to health and illness situations. The use of health routines is also a powerful language that gives insights into the societal notions, policy, and politics about health and illness. A social constructionist view allows for *cultural pluralism,* an understanding that truth and knowledge are culturally specific and embedded in the behaviors and routines of family life. Kuhn (1970) said science does not proceed by a slow growth of facts but instead by revolutionary shifts in which one accepted paradigm replaces another. The idea of modernism refers back to the end of the 17th century, a time often referred to as the Enlightenment period, when reason, rationality, and science—rather than religion or myth—began to be used to explain the world. For example, in earlier times, people thought that the Earth was the center of the universe and the sun moved around it. It was not until the time of Galileo (1564–1642) that this absolute truth was brought into question and the Earth was discovered to be part of the larger universe. Fact became fiction when new truth was uncovered and revolutionized thinking. Perhaps it is time to revolutionize some thinking about the nursing field's scope and methods of practice.

Arnold Toynbee first coined the term *postmodernism* in 1939, when he proposed the idea that the modern era ended somewhere between 1850 and 1875. Although the idea of postmodernism is a concept that appears in a variety of disciplines, the term is difficult to define. *Modernism* often refers to an objectivity that was once provided by an omnipotent narrator with a clear-cut moral position undergirded by faith in humankind's advancement through technology and rational planning. *Postmodernism* is an academic term used to refer to times or things that are dynamic, evolving, and changing. Postmodernism favors parody and irony and focuses on reflexivity, fragmentation, discontinuity, ambiguity, and simultaneity. It is often associated with terms such as *structuralism, deconstruction, reconstruction,* and *social construction* to describe a world that is rich with diversity; pluralism; and evolving science, information, and technologies. *Relativism,* often associated with ideas of postmodernism, argues that there is no such thing as absolute or objective truth and that reality has no meaning apart from what is viewed as real.

Deconstruction implies the need to look at systems or structures rather than at individual concrete practices because structures have points of origin, or things that created the system in the first place. Thus, one might argue that the family is the center of the household production of health and the embedded cultural context is a significant point of origin for family structures or routines that are relative to family health. The embedded context and functional processes provide the impetus for the ways ideas and behaviors related to health are formed. Routine structures or patterned behaviors are family members' social constructions through which the household production of health can be observed, measured, and evaluated and provide an entry for intervention over the life course of the family.

Health routines are complex systems, structures characterized by binary pairs or the opposition of terms placed in some sort of relation to one another (e.g., health and illness, life and death, fit and feeble, strong and weak, potentiating and negating, support and isolation). Jacques Derrida (1976), a leading figure in the thinking about deconstruction, argues that in Western culture, all binary pairs value the first term over the second (e.g., light and dark, masculine and feminine, right and left). According to Derrida, deconstruction has to do with overthrowing and displacing the hierarchy. Newly created families often need to disassemble accepted or valued practices from the family of origins as they create different systems of meaning. Claude Levi-Strauss, a French anthropologist, is known for his development of structural anthropology. In his book *The Elementary Structures of Kinship,* he argues that kinship relationships represent a specific kind of structure. Additionally, in his book *The Raw and the Cooked,* he explains how myths are structures that provide understandings about cultural relationships. He discusses binary pairs (or opposites) as the basic structures for all cultural ideas and explains that different cultural myths have some similarity because they are based on structural sameness. One might say that family routines are the structure or embodiment of a family's myths about health. Routines provide imperatives to consider health from cultural and population perspectives influenced by embedded contexts. Levi-Strauss argued that myths consist of units put together according to rules that use binary pairs or opposites to form associations and provide structure. In the Family Health Model, it is posited that binary pairs (e.g., well or sick, health or disease, pain-free or pain, dependent or independent) are culturally defined within families. Family values and themes result and inform members about ways to socially structure their lives and incorporate health routines.

If gender is viewed as a system of cultural signs, then the meanings that constitute gender have direct effects on how individual lives are lived, social institutions operate, and health is understood and practiced. Gender is an area with which we continue to have discourse. If we look at the binary opposition (i.e., masculine and feminine), masculine is almost always privileged, and privilege has the direct effect of enabling men to occupy positions of social power more often than women. *Bricolage* is the use of terms without acknowledging the whole system of thought that produced the terms and ideas. An example of bricolage is our common use of Freudian terms such as *penis envy* and *Oedipus complex* without fully understanding the whole system of thought that leads to the meaning. Judith Butler (1999), a feminist, discusses Freud's forms of psychoanalysis as a meaningful way to think about gender in a postmodern form. She questions the idea that a person is male or female, masculine or feminine, and tries to demonstrate that gender is a social construction and a performance in which persons use signs, symbols, and costumes or disguises. Butler's discourse frames questions from perspectives that are different from Freud's and suggests that many possibilities of gender arise from family narratives. She concludes that gender is neither a primary category governed by single identification with one gender nor a set of properties governed by the physiological processes. Instead, she says, gender is a set of internalized signs imposed on the mind and body.

How do cultural contexts shape everyday lives? Deconstruction is a way to show the multiple layers of meaning at work in any interactive process. Michel Foucault (1926–1984) studied history from a position of discourse and attempted to show that the ways people think about truths, human nature, and society change over time. He used *discourse,* a formal and orderly way to think and write that has no fixed rules about how language is used. Discourse is culturally determined and possesses the power to engage, but under certain conditions, some discourses are preferable. For example, Foucault suggested that the idea of madness described persons in an earlier historical time as being possessed by demons or being village idiots, but such individuals are now considered mentally ill. When society embraces a common body of thought, it is then interpreted by behaviors, actions, symbols, and ideas in a universal way. Therefore, the present discourse about health is different from that of a century ago and even several decades ago. The historical period provides a language for the discourse about health and illness, and family routines emerge that respond to the current discourse. A discourse about health might argue that the imposed context presently based on payment for medical care largely determined by insurance companies, employers' willingness to pay, reimbursement systems, managed care organizations, and policy has little to do with societal needs pertaining to health. The foci of the present discourse are illness orientations, medical management of disease, and profit; a different discourse might talk more about well-being, self-management, and population needs.

One could discuss binary understandings and the discourses as part of social constructions made by distinct cultural groups. A structuralist model argues:

- Language produces reality.
- Perceptions of reality are framed by the structure of language.
- Meaning is understood through language.
- Identity is intrinsically linked to the linguistic system.

The Family Health Model suggests that the following premises guide the family's social construction of the household production of health:

- Meaning is understood through differences.
- Opposites structure meaning.
- One knows the whole by its parts.
- Signs and symbols have attributed meanings.
- Health is constructed through the signs and symbols of the culture.
- Health becomes part of collective family experience as signs and symbols are interpreted based on cultural directives.
- Cultural signs and symbols identify ways to construct family health routines.
- Family relationships govern participation and forms of family health routines.

- Family health routines become more meaningful as they are shared.
- Meaningful family health routines are the structural language of family health.

A postmodern view suggests that society is not based on absolute truth; instead, ideas of relativity offer many explanations from a variety of perspectives. A postmodern view allows for the possibility that each question has an infinite number of answers, all equally valid, with no single paradigm providing an absolute answer. Postmodernism tolerates fragmentation of ideas, possibilities, progressive arguments, pluralism, discontinuity, and contextual indetermination. The Family Health Model suggests that:

1. Family health routines are a social construction for considering health from a structural perspective.
2. Family health is closely linked to the family household, member routines, and embedded context.
3. Family routines are socially constructed within household niches in response to embedded contextual systems.
4. Family members use functional processes to create, deconstruct, and reconstruct family health routines.
5. Social constructions of family health differ when embedded contextual systems differ.
6. Routines structure and order members' lives and serve to organize health in the household niche.

 Critical Thinking Activity

Suppose you were working with a first-time mother seeking prenatal care. Think about the things important for giving the newborn baby a healthy start. Make a list of things that the mother should know and do that will potentiate the newborn's health during the first year of life. Consider the possible variations in culture and think about what differences might imply about mother's knowledge, experience, and concerns related to parenting. Think about how those things might be incorporated into family routines.

Identify three family routines that could give the newborn a healthier start and would be health promoting for future development. For each routine, identify specific outcomes in terms of both the mother and the newborn that nursing can achieve in each routine area. Then list specific nursing interventions appropriate for routines that could be addressed during the prenatal period. When will the intervention occur? Will it need to be reinforced? If so, how often and by whom? What resources or supports will the mother need? Who else in the family might need to be involved in the intervention?

Next list assessment areas to be completed before the baby's birth. What things will need to be assessed after the birth? How and when will outcomes be evaluated? How would interventions related to routines be addressed after the birth of the child? Do you think nurses can be effective in assisting new families in forming health routines? What impediments might you foresee? How would practice need to be adjusted to include family health routines?

Routines in Early Childhood

Early childhood is a time when health information is absorbed and health practices are formed. This period of life is when family health routines with lifelong implications are socially constructed. It seems that better interventions for assisting families create meaningful health routines that incorporate empirical evidence about health practices into everyday life are needed. For a long time, it has been thought that young children do best when they have consistent care provided with regularity and in predictable ways (Bailey & Wolery, 1984; Crittendon, 1989). Although nurses need to assess the care parents provide, families also need assistance in designing routines that address nutrition, health, safety, and interactions (Lubeck & Chandler, 1990). Families with young children need to be taught about environmental, developmental, and behavioral issues, or the ecobehavioral daily caretaking tasks related to health, nutrition, and safety (Lubeck & Chandler, 1990). It has been identified that whereas families with infants were more likely to describe meaningful rituals associated with being a couple, families with preschool children described meaningful rituals centered on their children (Fiese, 1993a). Families in the early stages of parenthood with preschool children reported practicing a greater number of meaningful rituals than did families with infant children, and those with more rituals had greater marital satisfaction than those with fewer routines (Fiese, Hooker, Kotary, & Schwagler, 1993). Meaningful family rituals appear to be associated with greater marital satisfaction in mothers than fathers. Mothers use routines to facilitate children's development and sense of self (Giddens, 1991; Ludwig, 1998).

Assessment of family household, parental traits, member interactions, and related contextual systems are areas with implications for family routines. It has been identified that parents who consistently retain daily routines for child-care tasks may be better prepared to implement interventions for improving children's health, participate in family-focused interventions, and address practices that create health risks (Chandler, Fowler, & Lubock, 1986). A study about preschool children found that those with predictable home routines (e.g., meals, bedtime rituals) were more likely to be cooperative and have interest in participating in a Head Start program than children who adhered to fewer routines (Keltner, 1990). A later study by Keltner (1992) found that families with more structured home environments and family routines positively affected child health status in ways that extended beyond genetic traits or basic caregiving considerations. An interesting contrast can be made between what has been found about children and Ludwig's (1998) findings about older women. She expected to find that older women increased their routines in older age to accommodate age-related changes. Instead, she discovered that older women had fewer routines than in earlier life periods. More needs to be known about the effects of family routines across the life course.

In the author's research about family health, parents recalled some health beliefs and practices learned in early childhood and could compare some things about their family-of-origin experiences with the ways they were parenting their own children. In the family health research (Denham, 1997, 1999a), parents could describe whether their current behaviors were consistent with their childhood routines or if they had been modified over time or rejected because of childhood experiences. Health beliefs and routine practices were modified as developing persons engaged in peer and social relationships and established procreating or partnering alliances. Parents did not easily recall discussions about health practices before marriage or partnerships, but they did describe negotiations that occurred later related to prioritizing needs. Other important findings about routines were:

- The birth or presence of children meant that family routines were developed.
- Differences in intergenerational values meant some parents had conflict when new routines were different from those of their families of origin.
- Teaching and learning about health were recounted as casual, mostly unplanned, and largely aligned with parental priorities.

👫👫👫👫 *Cooperative Learning*

Spend some time discussing as a class what the term *household production of health* implies. First identify what health products a nurse might assist a family household to produce. Then identify areas a nurse might need to assess related to the household production of health. Next name some barriers (e.g., contextual, functional, structural perspectives) a nurse might encounter in trying to assist a family. Finally, decide what kinds of nursing interventions might be done to enhance the household production of health.

Discuss ways nurses might include family themes and goals into individual patient or client encounters. How could nurses use the idea of household production of health as they work with community health or take part in a health fair? Describe the knowledge and skills family nurses would need to focus on the household production of health.

Routines and Chronic Illness

As life increases in length, the potential for chronic illnesses also increases. Present and future concerns related to chronic illness have to do with the ways families are affected as they care for their members. Asthma and upper respiratory infections (URIs) are examples of conditions in which acute exacerbations mean emergency visits, hospitalization, and other forms of high-cost medical care. Family-focused care that includes interventions aimed at the family routines pertinent to the chronic condition could reduce the exacerbations and better control the chronic condition. For example, a study (Boyce et al., 1977; Hart, Bax, & Jenkins, 1984) about childhood URIs found that levels of family routines and family organization affected health status. In poor black preschool children, episodes of URIs were shorter when families had more patterned routines. When Markson and Fiese (2000) compared families that had children with asthma with families with healthier children, a lower level of anxiety was noted in the families that reported more meaningful routines. The researchers concluded that rituals could be protective for children with asthma when parents experience heightened stress. Although routines of families that had children with asthma were not significantly different from those that did not have an asthmatic child, it may be possible that routines are protective factors related to anxiety (Markson, 1998; Markson & Fiese, 2000). Chronic conditions such as asthma and URIs are of major concern and may be conditions that could respond to interventions that target family routines.

Diabetes is another example of a chronic condition with increasing numbers of affected individuals. The condition is greatly influenced by adherence to a medical regimen, an activity program, and a dietary plan. The trajectory of the disease is affected by household practices as members reinforce behaviors that can increase control and reduce complications. A qualitative study (O'Connor, Crabtree, & Yanoshik, 1997) about the attitudes and views of diabetic patients and their responses to diabetes interventions found that responders differed in the ways diabetes care was incorporated into daily routines. Not only the diabetic individual, but also the family, could benefit from interventions that enable them to make changes that support care needs.

An interesting case study (Seppanen, Kyngas, & Nikkonen, 1999) focused on parental coping and social support in two Finnish families with diabetic daughters. The study found six phases of parental coping used by the families to gain control and accommodate the changes presented by the chronic disease. Family functional status, composition of household, family resources, and the larger context all have the potential to affect the diabetic member's ability to accommodate needed changes and modify routine patterns. Variations in perceptions and the use of time may enhance interventions related to health routines. For example, a study (Boland, Grey, Mezger, & Tamborlane, 1999) about diabetic control in adolescents found that a lack of consistency in summer routines resulted in worsened metabolic control and higher Hb A_{1c} levels than when school was in session. A family may need assistance in constructing routines that enable the diabetic family member to incorporate a medical regimen into daily practices. For example, in a study (Drozda, Allen, Standiford, Turner, & McCain, 1997) about personal illness models, parents of pre-adolescents and adolescents with diabetes mellitus reported that the major problems caused by the disease were related to the increased need for structuring daily health routines. Presently, education and counsel for diabetic care involves instructing individuals about specific care practices that are needed, but assessment of customary family practices may be ignored. Family-focused care suggests that the routines of the household need to be assessed with interventions planned that assist members to deconstruct old routines that might be detrimental and construct or modify ones to incorporate behaviors that potentiate health and well-being.

Summary

The Family Health Model suggests that routines are vital parts of the lived health and illness experience and need to be included in assessments, care plans, interventions, and outcome evaluations. The social construction of family health is a maze of complex contextual, functional, and routine structures that are interactive and not easily separated. Paradoxically, the household production of health attempts to be a coordinated and systematic structure of ordinary daily events that are in continual flux as change is encountered. Considering routines as the ways members socially construct the household production of health provides a concrete way to observe, assess, and measure behaviors and implies that interventions must fit with family values, themes, and goals. Routine behaviors appear to be a logical structure for thinking about nursing practice in which family is the unit of care. Nurses can use routines to think critically about family processes and develop interventions that affect decision making and behaviors that are germane to health. More needs to be known about the merits of using routines as measures of health knowledge and behaviors. Compelling evidence is needed to ascertain the relationships between (1) family routines and member health, (2) the embedded context and health routines, and (3) family functional processes and the household production of health.

Test Your Knowledge

1. Define the term *ritual* and give three examples of rituals that might enhance health.
2. Define what is meant by the term *family health routine*.
3. Discuss what the structural-functional aspects of family care are.
4. Explain how the idea of family health routines might be considered a structural aspect of family health.

5. Discuss the concept of social construction and identify what this might mean for young parents who are considering their parenting roles while expecting their first child.

6. Choose a chronic illness that you are well informed about and describe how a nurse could use the family health routines to improve care for the individual and family.

7. Give three examples of ways a nurse might use family health routines in practice.

Factors That Affect
Family Health Routines

CHAPTER OBJECTIVES *At the end of this chapter, the reader will be able to:*

- Describe what an *ecocultural niche* is.
- Discuss factors involved in acquiring and learning health behaviors.
- Explain how health behaviors are modified.
- Identify how family themes and ecocultural domains affect family health routines.

> *The only way to keep your health is to eat what you don't want, drink what you don't like and do what you'd druther not.*
> —Mark Twain

In the family health research (Denham, 1997, 1999a, 1999b, 1999c), routines were characterized by highly ritualized individual practices and complex multiple member interactions. Some routines appeared quite resilient, but others were more irregular and were created in response to immediate needs. Some routines were highly ritualized, but others occurred less frequently and with less regularity. Routines had dynamic elements that were affected by individual characteristics, household factors, and member values. Although common patterns and themes were noted, there were also unique variations among families and among members within families. This chapter provides descriptions about potential effects on family health routines.

Key Variables Related to Family Health Routines

The family health construction is affected by several contextual and functional categories that were initially identified in the dissertation study (Denham, 1997) but have been modified as additional research was completed (Fig. 12–1). The categories are: (1) parental beliefs, values, and traditions; (2) temporal patterns; (3) the ecological context; (4) exposure to health information; (5) member interactions; and (6) accommodation of life events. Nurses and other health-care providers may influence family health routines at times, but behaviors are mainly socially constructed through member interactions within the embedded household niche across the life course. Family behaviors are directly and indirectly influenced by conflicting value systems and ideas, diverse faiths and religious perspectives, dynamic cultural traditions, advancing information technologies, and media that introduce different lifeways. Exposure to changing ideas that occur within a day of some individuals' lives exceeds what many in previous generations experienced in a lifetime. Making sense of the information and experiential input can

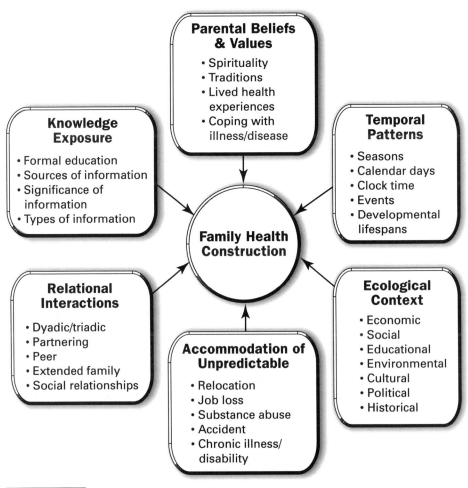

Figure 12–1 Factors Affecting the Modification of the Family Health Construction.

be a mammoth task as families try to hold fast to important values and traditions while integrating the old and new in meaningful ways.

In the family health research (Denham, 1997, 1999a, 1999b, 1999c), members' communication styles, levels of cooperation, patterns of interpersonal caregiving, and valuing affected the structure and practice of health routines. Family members differed in their:

- Levels and specificity of participation in various health behaviors
- Consistency and rigidity in following routines
- Exact content and style of routines
- Flexibility in modifying routines

Subjects said health routines were modified as:

- Members' beliefs and values changed
- Individuals' experiences differed from those of the family of origin
- Developmental changes occurred
- Alterations in the embedded context occurred
- Unpredictable life events were accommodated
- Boundaries of member interactions shifted
- New information and experiences were valued

Family members encounter a profound number of variables with the potential to enhance or threaten the health-illness experience. It is easy to focus on isolated factors and overlook the complex dynamics of interacting issues that impact family health. It is neither the contextual nor the functional processes alone but the equivocal nature of their interactions that impacts the household production of health. As family members engage within their embedded contexts, they encounter many alternatives that shape their social constructions. The quandary of complementary and contradictory messages about health and illness is continually faced. The Family Health Model suggests that looking at family routines is a viable way to assess household use of health information, member experiences, and contextual resources of unique families.

 Critical Thinking Activity

You are a family case manager assigned to a new family. The Lopez family has three children who are 6 months, 2 years, and 5 years old. This southern California family immigrated here before the birth of their first child. Although the two younger children appear to be healthy, the oldest child has had repeated bouts of asthmatic attacks over the past 6 months, with each one seeming more severe. The family has visited their family physician on several occasions and has brought the child into the emergency department a number of times during the past few months. The parents have been instructed about medications, the use of inhalers, and the possible causes of asthmatic attacks and have been advised about prevention. Mrs. Lopez usually brings the child in for care. On the present visit, she reports that her husband has recently lost his job and they are not sure how they will pay for their son's medications.

Develop a series of interview questions that you might use in a family assessment that will help you plan effective care. Mrs. Lopez speaks some English, but she looks perplexed at times when you try to explain things to her. Make a list of questions for each aspect of family health (e.g., embedded context, family functional processes, family health routines). You should have a minimum of 15 assessment questions. After you have listed your questions, provide a rationale for why each question is pertinent and explain how you might use the information in your role as case manger.

After completing the exercise as an out-of-class activity, gather in groups of three in the classroom and compare your questions in each assessment area, discuss your rationale for the questions, and compare ways to use the information. After the discussion, develop a single list of questions for each of the three dimensions, discuss the choices, and determine how a case manager could use information obtained through assessment for family-focused interventions.

Family Identity

Family identity implies "the family's subjective sense of its own continuity over time, its present situation, and its character" and refers to an "underlying cognitive structure, a set of fundamental beliefs, attitudes, and attributions the family shares about itself" (Steinglass, Bennett, Wolin, & Reiss, 1987, p. 58). Family identity is a "gestalt of qualities and attributes that make it a particular family and differentiate it from other families" (Steinglass et al., 1987, p. 58). These researchers viewed family identity as challenged throughout the life course, with one of three fates resulting:

- Continue unaltered into the next generation
- Blend with aspects of the identity of the other spouse's family of origin
- Disappear as the new family embarks on a new and novel family identity

A family can "establish a set of traditions and shared beliefs that are powerful enough to demand full adherence by all family members across multiple generations" (Steinglass et al., 1987, p. 61). Individual identity is weakened or subjugated when the family identity is of high caliber. In the study of alcoholic families (Steinglass et al., 1987), the researchers concluded that daily routines and family rituals provide ways to view the regulatory processes of family temperament and identity.

Temporal Patterns

Time factors are ongoing influences on family routines that create stress, direct choices, and influence perceptions. "Time is a major organizational principle that structures and regulates social life" (Ludwig, 1998, p. 169). Time "shapes daily schedules, commitments, and priorities; gives concrete shape to a family's collective history; lies at the core of our personal biography; and serves as the basis for anticipating the way that events will unfold in the future" (Daly, 1996). Alan Lightman (1993), in his fictional work titled *Einstein's Dream*, paints word pictures that describe multiple interpretations of time as it links the past, present, and future.

> In this world, time is like a flow of water, occasionally displaced by a bit of debris, a passing breeze. Now and then, some cosmic disturbance will cause a rivulet of time to turn away from the mainstream, to make connection backstream. When this happens, birds, soil, people caught in the branching tributary find themselves suddenly carried to the past (pp. 13–14).

Lightman later describes what he calls *mechanical time,* or time that is "rigid and metallic as a massive pendulum of iron that swings back and forth, back and forth, back and forth," and body time, or time that "squirms and wriggles like a bluefish in the bay"

(p. 23). He suggests that persons are mostly stressed when the two times meet, but they are content and at peace when they go their separate ways. He proposes that time is visible everywhere:

> Clock towers, wristwatches, church bells divide years into months, months into days, days into hours, hours into seconds, each increment of time marching after the other in perfect succession. And beyond any particular clock, a vast scaffold of time, stretching across the universe, lays down the law of time equally for all (pp. 33–34).

He concludes that time is absolute and "a world in which time is absolute is a world of consolation" (p. 37). Although the predictability of time allows us to recognize its motion, people in motion seem to be more obscure and complicated.

Time marks history that can be recalled and gives evidence that the past and future are entwined with the present. Time is a paradox rarely contemplated and mostly deciphered according to events and circumstances across the life course. Time gives order to life and organizes beginnings and endings. Lightman (1993) notes:

> Children grow rapidly, forget the centuries-long embrace from their parents, which to them lasted but seconds. Children become adults, live far from their parents, live in their own houses, learn ways of their own, suffer pain, grow old. Children curse their parents for trying to hold them forever, curse time for their own wrinkled skin and hoarse voices. These now old children also want to stop time but at another time. They want to freeze their own children at the center of time (pp. 73–74).

It is the individual and collective memory of time that provides shared meanings of history. Although some cling to the past and nostalgically view earlier times as most meaningful, some hope for a better future, and others see the present as most valuable. Humanity moves in response to time—some want to hasten it, others want to slow its hands, and some deny its existence.

Time is a visible dimension of family and family health. It is impossible to fully understand individual behaviors or family health routines without including temporal meanings. Time is linked to perceptions and energy rhythms that vary within members in single households and among families within a cultural context. Time has significance because family members perceive differences between health and illness. Daly (1994) suggests that families internalize time and schedules and are mostly taken for granted until a crisis occurs. Friedemann (1995) identified the six rhythms of time that can be described and assessed as activity and rest, sleep and wake, time orientations (past, present, future), social time and private time, structured versus unstructured time, and developmental stages. Time might be viewed as reversible or nonreversible. In other words, there are times when events are repeated and have the possibility of being altered, but there are also times when events can neither be overturned nor altered. For example, in a study by Crouter & McHale (1993), parental work patterns affected parental involvement, child monitoring, sibling caregiving, and child involvement in summer activities. The authors concluded that summer recess and the school year represent different family ecologies with vastly different social processes occurring. Use of time is culturally conditioned, influenced by subjective meanings that, in turn, are reflected in the social constructions of daily life and have economic value (Ludwig, 1998). Families that have children with special needs tend to fit family and child needs into culturally relevant contexts (Gallimore, Weisner, Kaufman, & Bernheimer, 1989; Segal & Frank, 1998).

In the family health research (Denham, 1997, 1999a, 1999b, 1999c), seasons, clock time, calendar days, traditional times, developmental stages, and significant events were all times that impacted family health patterns (Box 12–1). Time influenced the ways

---

Box 12–1 **Definitions of Clock Time**

Seasons

Periods of the year (e.g., spring, summer, fall, winter, past, present, future) clearly demarcated by the calendar. Meanings, roles, and family expectations are often associated with seasonal times.

Clock Time

Associations tied to actual measured minutes and hours (e.g., morning person or night person, activity or rest, sleep or wake). Many health routines are tightly associated with clock rhythms.

Calendar Days

Differences attributed to particular days of the week (e.g., weekends, Monday mornings, Friday afternoons, "Hump Day," social time, private time). Family members often attribute special meanings and activities to specific days, with the potential to alter routine behaviors.

Traditional Times

Days given special meaning by one or more family member (e.g., holidays, celebrations, special instances) during which interactions may include multiple members, extended family, close friends, peer groups, or others with shared values and ideals.

Developmental Stages

Specific points in time when relationships among members diverge from prior experience (e.g., marriage, childbirth, transitioning from school age to adolescent or adolescent to adulthood). Sometimes these times are clearly separated, but they are usually evolving, with more than one stage experienced simultaneously.

Significant Events

Times that are out of the ordinary (e.g., hunting season, vacations, school starting or ending) that signal exceptions to usual behaviors. These variations may be brief or prolonged over days, weeks, or months and have different boundaries and expectations from other times. Events may require active involvement of several members or a solitary member, but the consequences of the events have broad family implications.

---

routines were structured and prioritized. Subjects often described ideal routines but then explained reasons to veer away from the ideal. For example, families with preschool children often described optimal dietary routines but explained that on busy days, it was usual to alter ideal routines by eating at fast food restaurants or fixing less nutritious meals. After-school activities, work schedules, and family activities often interfered with meals and resulted in poorly planned meals with food eaten in a hurry. Subjects said activity patterns, stress levels, schedules, and family relationships were often based on seasons, with some mothers viewing summer as a healthier time, one that is less stressful, and one with more chances for casual family interaction (Denham, 1997). Clock time affected sleep and rest patterns, ways members spent time together, and stress levels. Weekends were often prized as favorite calendar days because such things as leisure, relaxation, hobbies, and spiritual ties brought the family closer together. Families with school-age children had routines based on the school calendar.

Holidays, celebrations, and traditional times were viewed as events and often meant variations from usual family patterns. Events were often tied to family identity and valued as special times the family could spend together. Some subjects said vacations were times when family members shared new experiences and found renewal (Denham, 1997). In bereaved families, the terminal phase of the loved one was an "event," a time when family members were together more than usual, recalled shared memories, and provided support for one another (Denham, 1999b). Health routines of those providing support to the terminal member were often out of control, and some family members were especially affected when the dying person's symptoms were severe and poorly controlled, when caregiving demands were prolonged or intense, immediately after the family member's death, and during bereavement.

Developmental stages also affected family routines. Family members described changes in health practices influenced by family transitions (e.g., marriage, birth, death, school attendance, adolescents). Mothers were actively engaged in health teaching of young children during the preschool years and continued to reinforce teaching and provide new information for school-age children (Denham, 1997, 1999c). However, adult children often consulted their mothers as they wrestled with decision making about nonacute health issues and family health decisions (Denham, 1999a, 1999b, 1999c). Developmental tasks or stages seem to have universal qualities as families are faced with the challenges of sequential life cycles over the life course, a process Steinglass et al. (1987) called *systemic maturation*. Regardless of culture, ethnicity, race, or family characteristics, families are confronted with rather predictable developmental tasks. Although individual developmental tasks vary according to age, properties, and experiences of family members, family developmental tasks often arise in response to individual needs. According to Steinglass et al. (1987), families have three fundamental developmental issues; it is posited that these issues can become organizing factors for family routines:

1. Define internal and external boundaries.
2. Choose a limited number of major developmental themes (e.g., use of resources, care of chronically ill members).
3. Develop a set of shared values and views about the world and identity of the family.

Assessment of routines should include these criteria.

Time has many perspectives and is a continual force impacting family life. Its emergent properties unfold in expected and unexpected sequences throughout family life. Daly (1996) suggests that time is subjective and a social construction affecting individual courses of action in an emerging present that helps define ways that past events are interpreted and made meaningful. More needs to be known about the ways that public time (e.g., school, work, social engagement) affects private time (i.e., individual, family) and ultimately impacts the household production of health. In time, members face attachment, stabilization, and loss that cause members to construct health routines in response to organizing family themes. Routines of children first become synchronized with those of the family, later with the schools where they attend, and finally with the larger society (Monk, Flaherty, Frank, Hoskinson, & Kupfer, 1990). The Family Health Model suggests that time is pertinent whenever routines are considered; it is a crucial factor too often overlooked when considering lifestyle variances.

 ### *Reflective Thinking*

Consider how time affects your personal health routines. What variations do you experience based on clock time, seasons, or calendar days? Do you view the variations as mostly positive or negative? Provide an example of a positive variation and a negative one. What about your family of origin? Can you think of variations in the ways time affects various members? Describe how the differences are positive. What are some negative variations? What things might a nurse do to assist a family to address the effects of time on health routines?

Cultural Factors

All persons and families have culture and ethnicity, even when they are not consciously aware of the impact. In the mainstream culture, it seems increasingly difficult to identify discrete familial roots. Many families are less focused on generational heritage and identify as American, with few references to ethnic tradition. Few citizens recognize that mainstream values are derived from legacies associated with early settlers that have been reshaped as history evolved. The face of the United States' people continues to be amended as persons from diverse cultural and ethnic contexts continue to immigrate to the country, settle throughout the land, become citizens, and challenge past viewpoints. For many new citizens, assimilation of mainstream values while living with the customs of their ethnic, racial, and religious heritage means that they become bicultural. Unfortunately, their biculturalism does not always serve them well, and many live as marginal societal members who are unable to satisfy the expectations of either culture.

Consciousness about needs to become culturally competent continues to increase in nurses and other health-care professionals. *Cultural competence* is defined as a set of congruent behaviors, attitudes, and policies that come together in a system or agency or among professionals and enables the system, agency, or professionals to work effectively in cross-cultural situations (Cross, Bazron, Dennis & Isaacs, 1989; Isaacs & Benjamin, 1991). Cultural competence is a process with incremental levels: cultural destructiveness, cultural incapacity, cultural blindness, cultural pre-competence, cultural competency, and cultural proficiency. Davis (1997) said cultural competence implies assimilation and transformation of knowledge about individuals and people into standards, policies, practices, and attitudes for appropriate use in sundry settings to increase quality and produce better outcomes. The National Center for Cultural Competence at Georgetown University's Center for Child Development stated:

> Despite recent progress in the overall health status of the nation, all segments of the U.S. population have not equally benefited. A long-standing and well-documented pattern of disparity continues to plague racially and ethnically diverse populations in this nation as it relates to the incidence of illness, disease and death. This pattern of disparity is evident both in health-care outcomes and utilization. While the complex array of causes for health disparity are neither well documented nor well understood, it is evident that disproportionate poverty, discrimination in the delivery of health care and the reluctance of health-care organizations to provide culturally and linguistically competent care are indeed contributing factors (Goode & Harrisone, 2000).

The ability to work within culturally diverse communities (e.g., neighborhood advocacy associations; ethnic, social, faith-based organizations; public media) and support natural helping networks is a key of cultural competence (Cross et al., 1989) Understanding the contextual experience and the events that maintain and promote health are essential ingredients for appropriately planning health services (Boyle, 1984). Alternative belief systems, intuitive health experiences, and health myths often contradict the institutionalized or formally sanctioned health-care delivery system (Thorne, 1993). Culture is at the heart of family values, themes, routines, and health.

Culture, along with spirituality and ethnicity, is one of the core requisites of rituals; core requisites along with their associated variables (i.e., behaviors, traditions, values, patterns, rituals) are the antecedents of family health routines (Denham, 1995). In many families, it may be nearly impossible to separate the enmeshed cultural, spiritual, and ethnic influences that affect patterned behaviors. These influences give rise to language and perceptual meanings that affect family identity and alter family themes. Culture is not dormant; rather, it is a continual integration of knowledge and experiences into life patterns that are transmitted intergenerationally. Health is partially a human response to cultural experience. Conflict often arises between the dominant and subordinate culture when those in the dominant culture view others as marginal, ineffective, or less valuable. Although the dominant culture assumes to take a helpful or assistive mode, it often distorts other cultures and approaches them in pejorative ways.

Casual and formal interactions of persons with different life perspectives mean that routines are continually being shaped and reinterpreted. American rituals are similar to a tapestry of changing social rules and cultural meanings that are increasingly reorganized on the basis of theatrical metaphors and anonymous elites (Deegan, 1998). When the embedded context supports ethnic and cultural patterns because they are perceived as functional and beneficial to the family, they can be retained in a rather pure state (Friedemann, 1995). However, patterns viewed as traditional and normative continue to be challenged by change. Although the cultural context might imply that certain behaviors and traditions are expected, media, societal, and developmental influences persist in altering patterns. However, even in the face of change, some cultural patterns remain resilient and enduring. The enduring qualities often instill stereotypical images in society's collective memory that remain even when behaviors are altered.

Cultural routines are associated with birth, death, religion, valued traditions, and other meaningful family behaviors and usually involve complex behaviors of multiple members. The ethnicity and religion of a family are closely aligned with actions taken in some families' daily routines. A study (Meyers, 1992) about Hmong children with developmental problems studied families' cultural beliefs because choices that families make about health and educational services are influenced by their beliefs. Weisner, Beizer, and Stolze (1991) studied the effects of religious beliefs and those who were nonreligious on the support systems used by U.S. families with children who had developmental delays. They found that religious families focused more on family for support and that nonreligious families focused more on outside resources. Religious families were more likely to see their child's problems as opportunities rather than burdens, receive more interpersonal support, and use their faith to interpret their circumstances. Family-focused care implies that assessments of the household niche; appropriate use of interpreters; and family reports about faith, values, and traditions provide information about cultural meanings of health behaviors.

👪👪👪 *Cooperative Learning*

Work in small groups to identify desirable characteristics of a culturally competent nurse. Each group should develop a list of characteristics and provide a rationale to support each of the ideas. In a class discussion, identify the top five traits needed to be a culturally competent nurse. How does being culturally competent differ from being culturally sensitive? How can a nurse's performance be evaluated to determine if he or she exhibits these qualities? How does one obtain and maintain proficiency in cultural competence? Why is cultural competence important for understanding family routines?

An Example of Cultural Experience and Health Routines

In the family health research (Denham, 1997, 1999a, 1999b, 1999c), family members and community participants were mostly identified as Appalachian. Some argument exists about how one defines an Appalachian person and whether it is truly a culture or subculture of American society. In this research, families were identified as Appalachian because they lived in Appalachia, had multiple generations of extended family located in the area, and could describe a family history of many generations tied to the region. Most highly valued their heritages and kin, were intimately connected to the community, and expressed a strong sense of place and love for their homeland. Subjects shared some similarities with others identified as Appalachian and were similar to many others in the mainstream culture, but they differed somewhat on the topic of family health.

These families focused more on present needs and had less interest in wellness or future health. Cultural influences were important in decision making about when to seek medical care. Cultural context better explained the similarities in family health definitions and practices than socioeconomic indicators explained differences. Although family health was somewhat influenced by the availability of medical services, health insurance, and health knowledge, member beliefs, values, traditions, and past experiences were more important. Some parents could recall folk practices and home remedies used by their families of origin, but few currently used any and instead described the use of mainstream medical practices similar to those of other Americans. Appalachians have been described as fatalistic or behaving as if they were powerless in some situations. These families accepted life as it was encountered but still strove to find answers and obtain help related to pressing medical concerns, especially those involving children. Appalachians are often characterized as being nonconfrontational. Although this may be true in some life areas, family members provided numerous examples about how they were, indeed, confrontational when health needs were at stake. Although many Americans tend to be future oriented, some cultural perspectives tend toward a present orientation, valuing the past and present more than the future. Appalachian families may possess some cultural uniqueness, but they have many qualities similar to others. Close social ties to extended family, a sense of pride and independence, and a reverence for faith and religious heritage were familial factors also characteristic of other cultures. Most had little interest in relocating and were strongly rooted to a familiar place where their families had lived for generations with extended kin nearby. Although the slower pace of life may be somewhat different from what occurs in more urban regions, these people still shared many similarities with others in the nation.

Culture often affects dietary patterns. In these Appalachian families, cultural heritage shaped food preferences, meal patterns, and roles associated with food preparation. For example, although men in parts of the United States enjoy cooking, a home economist in the studies said: "Men just aren't as likely to cook because food is women's work." She further explained:

> You'll occasionally run into somebody who will throw things on the grill. You may find someone who likes to cook wild game. I think food is not looked upon as much as an eating experience as it is something you need to do in order to be healthy and keep going. Although the social aspects of food are important too, when you look at home comings, you look at a lot of meetings . . . they have food attached to them, but it's not a dining experience. It's more of "breaking bread together" and "sharing what you have rather than a dining experience . . . you frequently see the covered dish."

Fathers generally viewed food preparation as woman's work, but some were willing to assist with meals when their wives worked or cooked when the wives or partners were absent. For example, a grandfather in one family frequently cooked for the family and prided himself in his gourmet preparations. Additionally, this man's adult son described his ability to make homemade noodles and times when he enjoyed cooking.

Some dietary patterns were influenced by ethnicity, a farming heritage, and times for family sharing. Most families purchased meat at the grocery store rather than raising animals, but the hunting and gathering past seemed to be a continuing influence for some Appalachian families. Even when parents held full-time employment, some families continue to farm. Many took pleasure in the family garden and enjoyed growing vegetables and fruits; sharing their crops with family, neighbors, and friends; and freezing or canning foods for later use. Several families still butchered their beef and raised chickens for eggs and meat. Some male members enjoyed hunting and fishing and obtained some meat by hunting deer, rabbit, squirrel, and wild turkey. Most families planned meals around meat and potatoes, and many enjoyed simple fare such as cornbread and beans or biscuits and gravy, much like their ancestors. A community informant described childhood practices:

> We lived on a farm, so you have big meals. The men were out working and mom was always fixing fried potatoes, we had a lot of . . . of course, the only kinda meat that I remember butchering was a hog. Now the older ones [siblings] say that there was occasionally beef, but beef couldn't be kept like pork could. You could salt it down and keep it. And so we had hogs . . . and chicken! Mom was always gett'en chickens and kill'en it and fix'en it for us . . . But the food, I guess . . . I know by today . . . would be considered not good for you, maybe. Because maybe gett'en too much fat and everything, but I don't think that any of that hurt any of us.

Cultural traditions were significant influences on family routines. However, it should also be noted that these families enjoyed fast food restaurants and eating out in ways similar to others. Although family members were not always adept at discussing their culture, individuals gave narrative descriptions about daily routines. Intracultural differences are important; stereotypical views ignore the diversity that survives within race and culture and wrongly conclude that a uniformity of beliefs, values, and practices exists. Although some aspects of the stereotypical caricature can most likely be identified, it fails to allow for the prevailing diversity. Family-focused care implies a need to carefully consider within group variations whenever family health routines are considered.

🛉🛉🛉🛉🛉🛉🛉   *Cooperative Learning*

Volunteers should share some specific differences they have personally experienced related to cultural variations. Examples can be from family-of-origin experiences; from interactions with friends, neighbors, or acquaintances from other cultures; or from patient care experiences. How might these variations be pertinent to family health? In a class discussion, identify:

1. What nurses need to know about culture and family health
2. How nurses should be prepared to provide care to persons from diverse cultures
3. Things nurses can do to increase cultural competence and avoid stereotypical assumptions

---

Family Themes, Member Interactions, and Family Health

Family members interact based on valued themes. For instance, a family that earns a modest income may be very content with their material state, but a family making a six-figure income may desire more wealth and a higher standard of living. Money may mean the ability to meet daily needs, or it may be linked to social status, personal achievement, success, or greed. Themes about money, finances, economics, and resources within families govern interactions and provide a basis for understanding some routines. When new situations occur, established family routines perceived effective at earlier times may have their utility tested and force families to adapt and create new patterned behaviors (Campbell, 1991; Thomas, 1990).

Family's ecocultural domains were discussed previously, but it is important to remember that valued themes juxtapose with domains and are enmeshed with family interactions and routine behaviors. Domains include variables imposed by contextual resources, constraints, family values, goals, and accommodations. Members often interact based on themes associated with ecocultural domains. For example, if the domain of concern is social support and the family values individuation, then they may be less likely to offer or seek support from others outside the immediate family. If a family has strong "familial values" or believes that extended family should be close and involved, then expectations about kin roles will be placed on extended family members. If a family believes that the village or the community, however it is defined, should act like a family, then they may be open to receiving support from others, expect others will help in times of need, and recognize personal responsibility to assist others in times of need. Another example related to the ecocultural domain of caregiver roles might affect themes related to ways a family with a member who has a developmental disability or a member with a chronic illness seeks help. If the family theme is strong familial values, then the family might expect kin to share in caregiving responsibilities. If the theme is individuation, then the family may be independent and refuse help from others outside the immediate family. However, a family that views themselves as part of a community might expect that others outside the family circle will assist. Family's themes guide interactions and the ways routines are socially constructed.

Different themes cause families to interact differently and develop rules and routines that support valued themes in each of the ecocultural domains. Steinglass et al. (1987) stated: "Themes are found in the family's implicit directions, its notion of 'who we are' and 'what we do about it'" (pp. 58–59). The term *family rules* is binding directives that obligate members to one another and the outside world (Ford & Herrick, 1974). A study (Kelley & Sequeira, 1997) examined the changing structure of American families and found that family rituals and togetherness was one of eight dimensions of strong families. Knowledge about valued themes provides a basis for creating and implementing interventions related to family values and goals. Routines "may be perceived as being a fairly reliable index of family collaboration, accommodation, and synergy" (Denham, 1995, p. 17). Members are usually unaware of the large number of accommodations they make regularly within the household as they simultaneously balance the limitations and resources related to the ecocultural domains, adapt to continuous unfettered demands from many unrelated sectors of the embedded context, and use members' functional processes to interact as a household unit to meet the unending needs of individual members.

Accommodation of Life Events

The accommodation process was discussed earlier, but it is important to reiterate that it is an active process that can be contrasted with the passivity found in adaptation. *Adaptation* is less intentional and is often an unconscious response to circumstances, events, or situations that disrupt, threaten, change, or alter usual household patterns. *Accommodation* is "proactive efforts of a family to adapt, exploit, counterbalance, and react to the many competing and sometimes contradictory forces in their lives" (Bernheimer, Gallimore, & Weismer, 1990, p. 223). Accommodation not only occurs as a response to distress or problems but also happens when members are motivated to achieve particular goals or attain something that is highly prized. Family accommodation is a response to "serious concerns and mundane problems in daily life" (Gallimore et al., 1993, p. 188). Family-focused practice aims at accommodation processes and targets them as potentially enabling actions to increase coping, modify behaviors, and plan changes.

An assessment of family interactions and core functional processes reflects past accommodations and adaptations presently incorporated into daily life. The Family Health Model posits that patterned behaviors generally continue as long as they are perceived as meaningful or satisfactory ways to address needs and goals. Family problems occur when adaptations or accommodations inadequately deal with concerns. Ineffective patterns may need to be deconstructed and new ones reconstructed to better fit changing themes, goals, dilemmas, or crises. Family-focused care provides opportunities to assist families with these social constructions that accommodate health and illness concerns. The model suggests that the availability of resources may predict whether families can make accommodations to meet goals.

Family health routines are visible patterns of behavior with which nurses and others can assist families to plan and structure meaningful actions within households to address health and illness needs. Although nurses or others may view some family routines as inadequate or impacting the family in health-negating ways, it is probable that the members view them as meaningful or adequate to accomplish goals. Most families do not intend to be deviant or dysfunctional but often choose adaptation or more passive methods to address the immediate needs rather than planning what nurses might view as more effective long-term measures. Although outsiders may not view some family adaptations as positive or optimal, it is speculated that family members have used their functional processes and resources in ways they view as appropriate. It is possible that other families embedded in similar contextual systems and faced with comparable concerns might adapt in equivalent ways. It is also conceived that families from similar cultural contexts experiencing similar dilemmas might choose actions or routines similar to others. Family-focused practitioners are challenged to think more systemically about population-based family health needs and assist families to accommodate specific health concerns or risks. As families encounter problems that require special knowledge, skills, and resources to construct health routines, nurses can assist by facilitating functional processes and working with contextual systems. Family-focused practice targets family as the unit of care and family routines, even when single individuals present the health need. Family adaptation of atypical routines or aberrant behaviors that compromise health or threaten well-being are particularly challenging for family nurses.

Parental Beliefs, Values, and Traditions

In the family health research, participants used family stories to describe health behaviors, influences from various media formats, social and health policies, and legislative influences. Compliance with immunizations, seat belt use, well-child care, and use of hospice services were examples of behaviors that were responses to contextual influences. However, knowledge alone was not a predictor that health information was incorporated into routine behaviors, the level of consistency in behaviors, or consistent adherence to behaviors. Although maternal beliefs and values mostly influenced young children's health routines, developmental processes, peer influences, and social contexts also influenced the ways routines were modified. For example, many described ways friends, the news, and extended family members influenced dietary patterns, exercise and activities, smoking behaviors, and substance abuse.

The Family Health Model suggests that parental beliefs acquired within families of origin have great stability and influence over the life course. However, patterns of behavior continue to evolve and are subtly altered by complex embedded factors that are not easily discerned. Parental influence does not occur within a vacuum but within a household niche that is regularly impacted by varied and unpredictable contextual forces. Teaching about values and ideals may be incorporated into children's beliefs and behaviors, but impact by the larger environment also plays subtle roles. Social norms, peer expectations, and media influences create synergistic effects with great potential to negate or potentiate parental influence. Although researchers have been studying the impact of parenting on youth outcomes for decades, less investigation of relationships between parenting behaviors and health outcomes has been completed.

Empirical studies (Bloom, 1981; McClanahan, 1983, 1985; White, 1982) provide evidence that family composition, marital categories, quality of family lifestyle, and daily activities affect the variances in households and family practices. The implicit assumptions that better education, higher income, or living in a two-parent family produce better developmental consequences and consequences are widely documented. However, traditional views of home environments have mainly focused on (1) the environmental process or effects of home on a learning environment, (2) the psychosocial climate of the home perceived by family members, and (3) variations between parents' child-rearing attitudes and child development (Nihira, Weisner, & Bernheimer, 1994). When families are faced with children who have developmental delays, they often reorganize their households, everyday lives, and ways to measure family dimensions differently from more traditional home measures (Nihira et al., 1994). Discussions about the ways family restraints and resources are coupled with member values, specifics about the household context, and actual member routines may provide better ways to understand and impact family health. A pressing need in preparing a professional workforce to provide family-focused care is educational preparedness that succinctly emphasizes the impact of family themes and goals, the household context, and ways unique members interact and shape the household production of health.

Using Routines as a Measure of Family Health

Accommodating Changes Across the Life Course

Individual and family development is erratic across the life course, but many might view normative times as periods when great energies are expended in activity and change followed by longer stability periods during which usual lifeways occur. Family life is dynamic, but most seek stability or homeostasis in which patterns of behavior become more ritualized and constant. The potential for constructions of new patterns of behavior occur whenever individuals encounter new information, acquire skills that challenge prior knowledge, face unpredictable life events, or when ambiguity prevails. In the family health research (Denham, 1997), six factors pertinent to modifying health routines were noted:

1. Parental beliefs and values
2. Experience beliefs and behaviors different than the family of origin
3. Family and community context
4. Ability to accommodate unpredictable life events
5. Family interaction patterns
6. Value information and experiences

Families identify individual and collective actions to respond to constraints and concerns that sustain valued routines or modify ones less desirable (Gallimore et al., 1993, p. 187). Families do not create problem-solving methods every time they confront a challenge; instead, "the family, over time, develops a characteristic style of problem-solving, a style that is distinctive enough as to be recognizable by an outside observer—a kind of family trademark" (Steinglass et al., 1987, p. 68). Three important dimensions related to family problem solving are:

1. Predictability of the family's response to destabilizing events
2. Affective expressiveness associated with problem solving
3. Degree of family cohesiveness during the problem solving

Members of parental dyads may each prefer adhering to health beliefs, values, and behaviors learned in their families of origin, but negotiation occurs in committed relationships that implies intimacy, mutuality, and continuance. According to Golan (1981), optimal transitional processes imply:

- Continued opportunities for personal development
- Role changes that minimize discord
- Reorganization of behavioral patterns learned in the family of origin
- Development of harmonious mutuality that balances stresses and strains

Family rules pertain to what family members view as acceptable, and these rules are guided by family values or themes that "provide the stability, commonality, and guidance" that members use in daily lives (Friedman, 1998b, p. 329). Family rules provide information about family function and the things valued, and they give information about how routines are maintained and changed. Accommodation is a life course process with the potential to positively shape routines in ways that maximize health outcomes. Accommodation is a place where family-focused care can be targeted.

Factors That Influence Routines

Family health routines created in accord with members' values and beliefs tend toward greater stability. Daily routines are organized so that they are "sustainable, meaningful, and congruent with individual needs of all family members" (Gallimore et al., 1993, p. 188). Steinglass et al. (1987) identified two constructs significant to family routines as systematic maturation and developmental distortion. *Systematic maturation* is the idea that all families have life cycles in which they "proceed through a developmental process that can be conveniently divided into three phases (early, middle, and late) based on the sequential emergence of a set of developmental themes" (p. xiii). For example, alcoholic families, families with a member who has a developmental delay, families with a member who is coping with diabetes, and families with a terminal member might have similar forms of developmental themes that affect routines in some similar ways. Consideration of whether a family is in an early, middle, or late stage may provide explicit information about the concreteness of family themes and the resilience of routines. Developmental distortion refers to "those changes and alterations in the customary shape of systemic maturation that are the consequences of specific unique experiences with which the family is forced to deal" (pp. xiii–xiv). In other words, a family may be similar to other families, but it also has unique characteristics derived from its membership and embedded context that significantly impact routines in different ways regardless of the phase of development. As one learns more about specific population-based needs, understandings about systemic maturation and developmental distortion on family health routines can be better understood.

Routines significant to family health may have arisen from rather passive indiscriminate actions or be characterized by planning, precision, and predictability. Behaviors are individual and mutual traits affected by the presence of others used to maintain family stability and balance growth, maturation, and change. Although families mostly strive for homeostasis, equilibrium, and balance, they are faced with how to actualize potentials, optimize possibilities, and transcend boundaries. Routines are affected by things such as member participation, tasks to be completed, motivation of members, goals to be accomplished, effectiveness of the core functional processes, and constraints or resources in the embedded context. Families use routines to regulate behaviors and care mechanisms and have these defining qualities:

- Routines are strongly related to family themes and are associated with ecological domains.
- Routines are bound by time and have beginnings and endings.
- Members recognize routines as special behaviors with associated member expectations.
- Routines have correlated symbolic aspects.
- Routines have predominance and often preempt or interrupt other activities.
- Routines are connected to family heritage and transmitted across generations.

Steinglass et al. (1987) found that family temperament and identity are regulatory structures of routine behaviors. *Temperament* is defined as "a psychological construct that refers to a set of enduring behavioral response styles and activity patterns that have their origins in an individual's early life" (p. 53). *Family temperament* is defined as "characteristic activity levels and response styles exhibited by families as they go about shaping their daily routines and solving problems," and it is also "the unique fit between individual temperaments" (p. 53). For example, nine temperamental dimensions identified in newborns are activity level, rhythmicity, approach–withdrawal behavior, adaptability, threshold of responsiveness, intensity of reactions, quality of mood, distractibility, and attention span and persistence (Thomas & Chess, 1979). Steinglass et al., when they studied alcoholic families, noted three dimensions of temperament:

1. The family's typical energy level
2. The family's preferred interactional distance
3. The family's characteristic behavioral range

"Families whose temperament allows them a greater range of behaviors, a greater tolerance for uncertainty, a greater flexibility in the patterning of behavior will probably accommodate new members in a more flexible fashion" (Steinglass et al., 1987, p. 54). In family-focused care, family's systemic maturation, developmental distortion, temperament, and the relationships with family routines all need to be understood.

 Critical Thinking Activity

Recall a clinical situation in which your patient interactions were such that you wanted to label the patient as "noncompliant." What were the qualities or circumstances that made you think the person was noncompliant? List them on the board.

In a group, examine the possible reasons that might cause the patient to behave this way. Explore examples related to the family's context, functional interactions, and family routines. Discuss the steps family nurses should take if noncompliant behavior is suspected. Examine possible nurse factors that may be relevant to identifying someone as noncompliant. How would a nurse's behaviors affect the outcome of patient compliance? What should nurses do to ensure that they limit their judgments and provide equitable care?

Summary

Family-focused care needs to incorporate family health routines as usual parts of practice, but more needs to be known about the best practices in using them to address chronic illnesses, developmental disabilities, caregiver needs, health promotion, disease prevention, and health maintenance. The timing and types of interventions must fit with family composition and context; member ages and developmental stages may represent distinct differences in needs. Using family routines provides a target for family-focused care that can direct assessment of health behaviors, assist members to identify values and set goals pertaining to health, plan interventions related to valued family themes, identify resources to support family goals, measure members' health outcomes, and evaluate family health outcomes. Although medical care is an important part of the health equation, family care seems at least equally important during transitional times (Doherty & Campbell, 1988). Unfortunately, care approaches are often shortsighted, fail to include multiple family members, and neglect ascertaining the concrete household routines pertaining to family health. The Family Health Model suggests that medical services aimed solely at single individuals diminish the likelihood that health outcomes of multiple members or the household production of health will be impacted. Incorporating routines into therapeutic family interventions could provide meaningful ways to assist families to construct behaviors that potentiate the household production of health. More needs to be known about the effects of competing family needs, resource distribution that optimizes member health, factors that affect the usefulness of resources, resources most predictive of family health outcomes, and cost-effective ways to use resources to benefit the family household.

Test Your Knowledge

1. Identify three factors that influence the ways children acquire health behaviors.

2. Discuss ways families modify health behaviors and explain how nurses can positively intervene in this process.

3. Give an example of a health behavior that might need to be modified if a person has recently been diagnosed with a chronic illness. Describe how a nurse might use information about family themes to assist the family establish routines to assist the ill member.

4. Identify three ways a family's embedded context might affect family health routines.

5. Explain how family functional processes and embedded contextual systems might affect family health routines.

6. Discuss three different ways a nurse providing family-focused care might use family health routines to promote health.

7. Identify five skills or areas of knowledge that a nurse might need to acquire in order to most effectively use family health routines as a target area for practice.

Categories of Family
Health Routines

CHAPTER OBJECTIVES *At the end of this chapter, the reader will be able to:*

- Identify attributes of the six categories of family health routines.
- Discuss ways nurses can use family health routines to meet individual health needs.
- Describe a plan of family care that includes family health routines.
- Identify family health routines as ways nurses can target family-focused care that can potentiate the household production of health.

> *Time is neutral and does not change things. With courage and initiative, leaders change things.*
> —Jesse Jackson

Although the family health studies (Denham, 1997, 1999a, 1999b, 1999c) were not explicitly about routine behaviors, family narratives obtained through the interviews and observations in family homes provided rich data about routines. Family routines were regularly practiced behaviors with varied degrees of member ritualization that were important to family identity and appeared to hold the potential for health-related outcomes (Denham, 1995). Family routines provided understandings about the ways members interpret health knowledge, beliefs, and traditions into patterned behaviors and have the potential to increase health and wellness as well as protect members against disease and illness. This chapter discusses the six categories of family health routine identified in the findings about family health (Denham, 1997, 1999a, 1999b, 1999c). The Family Health Model suggests that nurses and others interested in providing family-focused care should target the household production of health by viewing family health routines as primary objectives.

Emergent Understandings about Health Routines

The Emergent Categories of Family Health Routines

Family health studies (Denham, 1997, 1999a, 1999b, 1999c) have provided support for a care model that includes daily lives in an embedded household in which members interpret personal experiences and knowledge into health behaviors. *Health routines* are described as interactions affected by biophysical, developmental, interactional, psychosocial, spiritual, and contextual realms, with implications for the health and well-being of members and family as a whole. Family health routines are complex, evolving social constructions used by families to interpret their perceptions about health into structured behaviors. Table 13–1 compares the categories of family health routines from the three research studies. In the dissertation research (Denham, 1997), seven categories of routines were identified, five categories were noted in the study about health in hospice families, and six categories emerged from the study of economically disadvantaged families with young children. Important factors about health routines noted in the research are:

- Families varied in the types and number of patterned behaviors in their routines.
- Individuals and families did not equally value all routines.
- Individuals and families did not equally value all aspects of family routines.
- Individuals had some unique variations in the ways they practiced health routines.
- Families had different expectations about member roles and the rigidity of routines.
- Health routines were modified over time.
- Routines were sometimes enmeshed with one another.

In the dissertation study (Denham, 1997), members indicated they practiced patterned behaviors that were adhered to with great regularity (Table 13–2). Parents recalled some behaviors from families of origin and compared past and present patterns. They could describe:

- Differences in past and present health beliefs and practices
- Member health behaviors

Table 13-1   **Comparison of Health Routines in Family Health Research**

Study No.1 Health Routines	Study No.2 Health Routines	Study No.3 Health Routines
Dietary practices	Self-care routines	Dietary
Sleep and rest patterns	Member caregiving	Self-care routines
Activity	Medical consultation	Mental health
Dependent care	Habitual high-risk	Family care
Avoidance behaviors	behaviors	Preventive care
Medical consultation	Mental health behaviors	Illness care
Health recovery		

Source: Denham, SA: An ethnographic study of family health in Appalachian microsystems. Unpublished doctoral dissertation. University of Alabama at Birmingham, Birmingham, Ala., 1997; Denham, SA: The definition and practice of family health. Journal of Family Nursing, 5:133-159, 1999; Denham, SA: Family health: During and after death of a family member. Journal of Family Nursing, 5(2):160-183, 1999; Denham, SA: Family health in an economically disadvantaged population. Journal of Family Nursing, 5:184-213, 1999.

Table 13–2 **Family Health Routines in Families with Preschool Children (Study No.1)**

Family Health Routine	Aspects of the Routines	Description of the Routine	Examples of Routine Aspects
Dietary routines	Cultural variations	Factors from the cultural, ethnic, racial, and social context influencing diet choices and food preparation	Food procurement Food security Food choices Food preparation Food selection
	Nutritional consumption	Actual amount and type of food consumed by individuals	Meal patterns Snacking patterns
Sleep and rest patterns	Family rest patterns	Individuals' usual sleep and rest patterns	Individual rhythms Family rules Member age
	Temporal patterns	Patterns of sleep and rest that vary based on time and events	Work schedules School schedules Weekends
Activity patterns	Purposeful activities	Usual tasks necessary for meaningful family life and health	Specific tasks Time frames for completion Role expectations
	Functional activities	Behaviors associated with work, school, or play	Organized activities School attendance Employment
	Social activities	Interactions that occurred between individuals and others	Friendships Volunteering Community involvement
	Exercise	Intentional activities to increase individual and family wellness	Deliberate exercise Family fun
Avoidance behaviors	Health risk related	Protection from risks known to cause illness or disease	Illness and disease Smoking Alcohol use Substance abuse Social situations
	Safety related	Avoiding high-risk behaviors, persons, and situations that might cause trauma or injury	Household safety Environmental risks Physical interactions
Dependent care activities	Nurturant care	Activities that enhanced members' physical, emotional, and spiritual well-being	Anticipating needs Tolerating difference Emotional support Transition and growth Foster attachment and independence
	Assistive care	Assistance directed to meet self-care needs	Personal hygiene Toileting activities Social skills
	Resource care	Family members as resources to one another	Caregiver Teacher Counselor Coach
Medical consultation	When to consult	Determine when care should be sought	Symptoms observed Mother decides Prior experiences Member willingness Perceived risks
	Who to consult	Determine who could provide care	Availability Accessibility Reputation
	How to consult	Means used to obtain care	Health insurance Affordability Informal interactions

Table 13–2 *(Contd.)*

Family Health Routine	Aspects of the Routines	Description of the Routine	Examples of Routine Aspects
Health recovery activities	Individual responsibilities	Immediate recovery and return to usual roles as quickly as possible	Illness Injury Trauma
	Family responsibilities	Family responses to individual needs	Extended family Friendship circles Family resources Supportive others

Source: Denham, SA: An ethnographic study of family health in Appalachian microsystems. Unpublished doctoral dissertation. University of Alabama at Birmingham, Birmingham, Ala., 1997; Denham, SA: The definition and practice of family health. Journal of Family Nursing, 5:133–159, 1999.

■ Consistency in performing health behaviors
■ Health behaviors taught to children

Family's functional status affected (1) the receptivity to differences in members' health behaviors, (2) the degree of involvement in routines, and (3) flexibility in the modification of health behaviors. The second study (Denham, 1999b) identified routines of multigenerational families using hospice care after a member's death (Table 13–3).

The third study (Denham, 1999c) provided findings about family health routines in economically disadvantaged families (Table 13–4). Families used health routines to:

■ Support health processes related to child and family development
■ Avoid illness, disease, and injuries
■ Cooperate to attain, sustain, and regain health
■ Communicate with health experts
■ Obtain resources for individual health needs
■ Distribute family health resources
■ Structure the household production of health

Adults could recall some childhood health patterns and compare past and present behaviors. Individuals could describe member behaviors with great consistency. Mothers

Table 13–3 Categories of Family Health Routines (Study No.2)

Family Health Routine	Aspects of the Routine
Self-care routines	Dietary Sleep and rest Personal hygiene Exercise Safety and protective behaviors
Member caregiving	Support for members with health alterations Compliance with medical regimen
Medical consultation	Diagnosis of health disorder Interaction with health-care providers
Habitual high-risk behaviors	Smoking Substance abuse Work
Mental health behaviors	Family fun (e.g., relaxation activities, hobbies, vacations) Traditions and special events Spirituality Pets

Source: Denham, SA: Family health: During and after death of a family member. Journal of Family Nursing, 5(2):160–183, 1999.

Table 13–4	Categories of Family Health Routines (Study No.3)
Family Health Routine	**Aspects of the Routine**
Self-care routines	Personal hygiene (e.g., toileting, dental care)
	Physical activity
	Sleep–rest patterns
	Health promotion
	Sexuality
Dietary	Nutrition
	Shopping
	Preparation
	Meals
	Snacks
Mental health	Substance abuse (i.e., drugs, alcohol, smoking)
	Family stressors
	Self-esteem
	Maintenance of personal integrity
Family care	Family fun (e.g., vacations, holidays, traditions, special days)
	Humor
	Individual or group activities
	Coping with chaos
	Creating special times
Preventive care	Health protection (e.g., immunization, seat belts)
	Neighborhood risks
	Risky behaviors (e.g., alcohol, drugs, smoking)
	Abuse and violence
Illness care	Medical consultation
	Health care services
	Medical regimens

Source: Denham, SA: Family health in an economically disadvantaged population. Journal of Family Nursing, 5:184–213, 1999.

were reliable sources of information about members' health routines. When information from absent members was later checked with mothers' reports, it was consistent. Family members described exchanges with one another that were connected to member beliefs, values, and perceptions. Contextual and functional aspects of the family household influenced families' social constructions of health patterns, but the embedded context was a powerful determinant for the creation and retention of health routines. Regular interactions between individuals, family subsystems, families, and embedded contextual systems created feedback loops in which bi-directional exchanges occurred across time and space. Feedback loops provided information and experience that influenced the family's health perceptions and routines.

Cooperative Learning

Take a few minutes to think about your personal dietary routines and identify how the routine varies from day to day. Which routine aspects are consistent? What causes variances to occur? Are the variances mostly positive or negative?

Consider the dietary routines of another family member and think about how the routines are similar and different. Are they more alike or more different? What causes the differences? Do the differences imply that one member incorporates more or fewer nutritional guidelines into behaviors than the other member?

> In groups of three, discuss your findings. Are family experiences more alike or more different? Each group should then describe the major findings from their discussions to the entire class and discuss the implications of dietary routines as a way to think about family health.

Childhood Socialization about Family Health

In the family health studies, parents recalled childhood as times when some health beliefs and practices presently viewed as important or practiced were learned. Households were the places where children learned health information and were socialized about health practices. Parents' health beliefs and routines continued to evolve as they interacted with others, obtained new information, responded to specific member health needs, accessed health resources, and were influenced by other contextual factors. Parents not only taught children about health behaviors, but they also modeled behaviors that influenced future beliefs, values, and traditions. In all families, mothers assumed the primary role in establishing the patterned behaviors for children's health needs. The birth or presence of children was a strong key in the ritualizing of family health routines. Fathers and mothers described the value of life experiences as aids to health learning. Although fathers participated in family health routines, they described less consistent and active participation in directing children's behaviors.

Parents could describe whether their current behaviors were consistent with personal childhood routines, modified over time, or rejected because of childhood experiences. Teaching and learning about health were recounted as casual, mostly unplanned, and largely aligned with parental priorities. Parents could also discuss a congruency between their family-of-origin experiences and what their children were being taught. Parents did not easily recall discussions about health practices before marriage or partnerships, but they mostly described negotiations that occurred as ways to balance differing member needs. Families with close adult members, extended family members, and relatives from more than one generation described differences between what was experienced in their families of origin and what was practiced in the family of procreation. Second- and third-generation family participants said they retained some aspects of health routines learned in the family of origin, but new health patterns were constructed when primary households were established. Participants did not easily identify the effects of the embedded household or community on health routines, but family stories provided data that described media, social policy, and legal influences.

Self-Care Routines

Six categories of family health routines emerged from an analysis of the three family health research studies (i.e., self-care, safety and prevention, mental health behaviors, family care, illness care, family caregiving). Table 13–5 provides an overview of the six family health categories discussed in this chapter, defines each routine category, and explains some aspects of each routine.

All families had health routines related to diet, hygiene, sleep and rest, physical activity and exercise, gender, and sexuality; these were identified as self-care routines. Nurses are encouraged to envision practice roles and use previous learning to critically think about meaningful ways health routines might be targeted if family is viewed as the unit of care.

Self-care routines involved patterned behaviors related to usual activities of daily living experienced across the life course that were initially guided and strongly reinforced by parents. Routines differed across and often within families, depending

Table 13-5	Synthesis of Family Health Routines	
Family Health Routine	**Aspects of the Routines**	**Description of the Routines**
Self-care routines	Dietary Hygiene Sleep–rest Physical activity and exercise Gender and sexuality	These routines involve patterned behaviors related to usual activities of daily living experienced across the life course.
Safety and prevention	Health protection Disease prevention Smoking Abuse and violence Alcohol and substance abuse	These routines pertain to health protection, disease prevention, avoidance and participation in high-risk behaviors and efforts to prevent unintended injury across the life course.
Mental health behaviors	Self-esteem Personal integrity Work and play Stress levels	These routines have to do with the ways individuals and families attend to self-efficacy, cope with daily stresses, and individuate.
Family care	Family fun (e.g., relaxation activities, hobbies, vacations) Celebrations, traditions, special events Spiritual and religious practices Pets Sense of humor	These routines include daily activities, traditional behaviors, and special celebrations that give meaning to daily life and provide shared enjoyment, pleasure, and happiness for multiple members.
Illness care	Decision making related to medical consultation Use of health-care services Follow-up with prescribed medical regimens	These routines are the various ways members make decisions related to health-care needs; choose when, where, and how to seek supportive health services; and determine ways to respond to medical directives and health information.
Member caregiving	Health teaching (i.e., health, prevention, illness, disease) Member roles and responsibilities Provide illness care Supportive member actions	These routines pertain to the ways family members act as interactive caregivers across the life course as they socialize children and adolescents about a wide variety of health-related ideals, participate in specific health and illness care needs, and support members' individual routine patterns.

on members' developmental stages and other temporal factors. Health routines related to hygiene practices included such things as cleanliness, dental care, and toileting activities. Mothers with preschool children said they knew little about infant and child-care needs before pregnancy and that they either learned through trial and error or sought guidance from their mothers. Many mothers had received prenatal care through local public health programs, where they had also gained additional information and support through well-child clinics and the Women, Infant, and Child (WIC) programs.

The depth and breadth of data obtained about self-care routines were extensive, but only diet and sleep and rest will be discussed here. Dietary practices were the most complex health routines identified, and they were usually mentioned first as a key family health factor. Dietary routines were strongly rooted in family-of-origin patterns, varied greatly within and between families, and were often modified because of members' schedules and events as well as family traditions. Family members described dietary practices in terms of (1) individual and family food selection, (2) food procurement and storage, (3) types of food preparation, (4) meal consumption patterns, (5) snacking patterns, (6) member roles, and (7) resource availability. Families differed in the freedom allowed members regarding selection and consumption of foods that conflicted with the mothers' ideals. Although mothers mostly prepared meals and children in a single family were usually provided the same foods at meals, the nutritional value of foods consumed by members within the same family was different. Even when mothers were consistent in planning and preparing meals, individual eating patterns and members present for meals varied. When work or activity schedules conflicted with meals, mothers were apt to allow family members to consume less healthy or even unhealthy food items. Dietary patterns were largely influenced by (1) mothers' knowledge about nutrition, (2) personal choices and food preferences, (3) dietary beliefs and values, (4) work and school schedules, and (5) member cooperation in caring for one another's needs. Families had different dietary rules, including eating what is prepared; tasting new foods; ways food should be prepared, served, purchased, and stored; when and where foods could be eaten; and who had to have what for breakfast, lunch, and supper. Most adults said they tried to be consistent about adhering to healthy diets. Several described reasons for dietary inconsistencies tied to observations of ancestors and family friends who had lived to be 80 to 90 years of age without watching their diets, worrying about exercise, or seeking medical care.

Nutrition has been widely recognized as a key modifiable lifestyle factor with broad health implications. *Healthy People 2010* has identified being overweight and obese as a leading health indicator pertinent to broad public health issues (US Department of Health and Human Services, 2000). The intention of leading health indicators is to increase understandings about health promotion and disease prevention and encourage wide participation in health improvement in the next decade. Nurses have some education about nutrition and understand dietary relationship to diseases and illness, but they most often educate and counsel people about nutrition while placing little emphasis on the lived household experience or routines. Diet histories are often used to assess nutritional intake, but family patterns that influence diet are less likely to be considered. Family-focused care implies a holistic response to nutritional needs that includes things such as member values, family meal patterns, cultural and ethnic influences, personal preferences, family rules about diet, finances, knowledge about nutrition, and special dietary needs. In order to assist families to construct routines they will value and ones beneficial to health needs, families need knowledge and skills to alter behaviors and maintain changes over the life course.

Sleep and rest patterns were affected by time, role demands, work schedules, seasons, and special events, but they were affected less often than dietary routines. Preparation for sleep often occurred in close proximity to other routines such as dietary practices and hygiene care. Although snacks and baths were often closely aligned with sleep, routines, the activities were actually parts of other health routines. Unique variations in sleep and rest patterns were related to (1) bedtime and awake time, (2) sleep or rest time requirements, (3) sleep locations and persons slept with, and (4) strings of sleep-related behaviors. Sleep and rest patterns were influenced by (1) biological rhythms, (2) personal time demands, (3) family patterns, (4) developmental stages, and (5) seasons. Families living with unpredictable life events (e.g., children with special health-care needs or developmental delays, terminal illness) most often expressed concerns related to interrupted sleep routines. Mothers were the most likely to experience sleep deprivation when members were ill or unpredictable life events occurred. Inordinate stress levels with potential "pile-up" effects seemed to place these mothers at risk for depression, lowered self-esteem, and other health risks. Several mothers reported stress symptoms caused by sleep deprivation. In fact, several parents indicated that when routines were out of sync, personal stress and family discord occurred.

Safety and Precaution

Safety and prevention routines were primarily concerned with (1) health protection; (2) disease prevention; (3) avoidance and participation in high-risk behaviors such as smoking, abuse and violence, alcohol and misuse of other substances; and (4) efforts to prevent unintended injury across the life course. All families practiced some routine behaviors associated with safety and precautions, but families had different concerns and practices. These families were intergenerationally linked to kin and were well advised about familial risks for genetic disorders and diseases linked to heredity. Some described concerns about genetic predisposition to disorders for themselves or others, but they also told stories that described inconsistencies between their beliefs, knowledge, and actual behaviors. For example, one mother said multiple extended family members had problems with diabetes and voiced concerns about her own risk. Although she said that her diet needed to be controlled and exercise was needed regularly, her overweight condition and descriptions of inactivity indicated that knowledge does not ensure behavioral changes in the household experience.

Personal health values and beliefs indicated that the ability to perform usual life roles and actively participate in daily life had strong themes related to safety and child protection. Mothers were vigilant in teaching preschool children about keeping safe inside and outside the household, avoiding illnesses and diseases, and evading situations that might result in injuries. Mothers' knowledge about children's developmental stages was associated with safety concerns, both inside and outside of the house. For example, nurses in the health department had been doing active community teaching about the risks associated with lead poisoning; children in several families had been tested for lead poisoning and were found to have marginal risk levels (Denham, 1997, 1999a). A state law regarding child car seats and seat belts and an aggressive law enforcement agency ensured that these mothers buckled preschool children into car seats and seat belts, but the same law seemed far less effective in ensuring that teens and fathers also complied. Mothers with preschool children were all conscious about safety needs and cautioned children about risks, guided play activities, and warned about neighborhood concerns.

Many family members discussed routines related to actual or potential health risks such as smoking, alcohol or drug use, and non-adherence to medical routines. Some members said that they desired members to alter their high-risk behaviors and described levels of participation in risky activities as ongoing concerns. In the hospice study (Denham, 1999b), community informants and family members described how they or others neglected their health when caring for a dying member. One mother said that she had neglected to take her medications when her husband was sick. Others reported stress, weight loss, poor eating habits, physical exhaustion, and mental anguish as they assumed caregiving roles. Kin households were affected by the death of a family member.

Smoking is a habit generally viewed as deleterious to health. Participants discussed risks and negative attributes associated with smoking and drinking alcohol. One mother said, "Neither of us smoke and I don't want my kids to do it. We don't drink. I don't want to introduce my kids into that kind of life." Two mothers who smoked described long histories and pack-a-day habits but were not concerned about health risks. Several parents who were raised in households where their own parents had smoked were well informed about smoking risks and actively taught their children avoidance at early ages. In several families in which one parent smoked and the other did not, young children were often given mixed messages about the benefits and hazards of smoking. Some parents who smoked described times when they had tried to quit; one mother said: "The times I've tried to stop, I didn't like myself. I'd be real hateful! I didn't want to be around nobody. I just kind of like went into a little depression." Having knowledge about health risks related to smoking behavior was not enough to deter some individuals from smoking.

Mental Health Behaviors

Mental health behaviors were family routines that dealt with self-esteem, personal integrity, work and play, and controlling stress. Routines in this category are related to the ways individuals and families attend to self-efficacy and cope with stress. These routines are important for both individuation and family identity. Parents carefully nurtured their children, attempted to use available resources for a broad spectrum of family needs, and appeared concerned for meeting a variety of well-being needs for individuals and the family as a whole.

Family concerns often included extended family members in these Appalachian families, and many regularly provided support to kin. In some families, active participation and care for extended family members was viewed as a sign of care and viewed as beneficial, but some members said expectations created additional stress. Mental health care often meant anticipating needs; providing emotional support; redefining unique boundaries; balancing patterns of attachment and independence; and determining boundary affiliations with extended family, close friends, neighbors, and outsiders.

Mothers usually assumed the greatest responsibility for the emotional care of family members, but fathers also played roles. These families were not likely to seek professional assistance for emotional needs because doing so was often viewed negatively within the larger community. Several members of families using hospice care discussed the emotional pressures of caregiving but viewed these activities as needful. Other families described frustrations when some members did not meet their expectations in fulfilling caregiving responsibilities. Mental health routines, such as shared humor and family fun activities, individual relaxation techniques, stress management styles, participation in family celebrations, pet interactions, and religious practices, were described by members as ways to contribute to health.

Family Care

Family care routines were described as a variety of daily activities, traditional behaviors, and special celebrations that provided shared enjoyment, pleasure, and meaning to family life. These routines included things such as family fun (e.g., relaxation activities, hobbies, vacations); celebrations, traditions, and special events; spiritual and religious practices; pets; and having a sense of humor. Mothers often played key roles in decision making and problem solving related to the use of family assets and resources (e.g., time, money, insurance, knowledge, others), but other family members also participated when it came to family care.

Family cooperation was viewed as an important tactic in supporting individual members' mental health needs and spiritual well-being. Many of these parents viewed church-related activities as principal social activities, but mothers usually had the prime responsibility to oversee adherence to religious practices and church attendance. In the studies, many families were regular churchgoers, but more were not. Parents who did not attend church still encouraged their children to participate in some church activities. Faith, prayer, and belief in God were important to these families even when they did not attend church regularly, and everyday conversation was often sparked with ideas related to spiritual or religious beliefs. In some families, faith was an organizing theme for family routines. Participants often said that good communication, family and friends, and a household where members shared laughter and tears contributed to family health. Most close friendships in these Appalachian families were with persons they had known for many years, close relationships with kin or extended family, friendships with parishioners at their church, and close connections with neighbors. Although outsiders were treated warmly, they were seldom quickly welcomed into lifetime networks of close friendships.

An important aspect of family care routines was associated with creating meaningful rituals that provided opportunities to establish their separateness and yet identify with the family. Culture, religion, ethnicity, and ancestral traditions played important roles in constructing these routines. Unlike many family routines that included regular repetitive actions, family care routines were more intentional and often included decision making, a period of planning, and emotionally charged symbolic member interactions. Family care routines included special times when members spent time together engaged in behaviors that were mutually valued. Although these times may have been elaborate celebrations, families also organized their usual activities into family events. For example, one family had several evenings a week when the whole family worked together in the garden. As the crops were ready, they shared in the cooking, canning, and sharing with family and friends. Although some traditions and celebrations involved gift giving, signaled a transitional life period, or involved ancestral heritage, other family care routines related to family solidarity and indicated the value of member attachments.

👫👫👫👫 *Cooperative Learning*

Form discussion groups of three members. Choose three family routine categories and assign a category to each group. Each group should discuss the aspects that they view as important characteristics. Group members should share examples from their own families that fall in this category.

Consider how each of the category of routines can be used for health promotion, disease prevention, and medical management of a condition such as chronic obstructive pulmonary disease. Create a list of assessment questions for each area (i.e., health promotion, disease prevention, medical management). What needs to be known about individual behaviors, and what information is needed to understand family routines? Answer the questions who, what, where, when, and how related to routine category.

Each group should then report to the class the key areas they would choose to assess. Discuss the implications of assessment data on planning interventions and evaluating outcomes. How might you use family health routines in your present clinical practice?

▪ Illness Care

The routines in the illness care category relate to ways members make decisions related to health-care needs; choose when, where, and how to seek supportive health services; determine ways to respond to medical directives and health information; and actively provide for individual care needs. These routines are related to acute and chronic illness needs, diseases, rehabilitation, and trauma incidents. Key routine aspects are associated with decision making about who to consult for medical care, how members use health-care services, and ways prescribed medical regimens are followed.

In the family health research, families had routines that were sometimes described as obligatory member roles and responsibilities; kinship rules for care of ill members; and expected patterns for compliance with professional care, self-directed care, or family prescribed care regimens. Families had routines related to decisions about which incidents required expert care, if incidents required immediate medical responses, whether symptoms should be observed before action was taken, how long was acceptable to wait before taking action, whether illness trajectories would resolve themselves, and how an emergency response should be handled. Mothers mostly decided who to consult for medical care, but others, including extended family members, often gave input into the final decisions. Member valuing, the availability of resources, support, the type of health concern, and perceived benefits often influenced the use of health information. Knowledge alone did not predict that health information about illnesses or diseases would be incorporated into family health routines. Conflicting media reports about health issues and care regimens sometimes troubled parents, even when the information was not related to specific family issues. Uncertainty about the trustworthiness of media reports seemed to weaken a family's confidence about the reliability of health information.

In the Appalachian families, illness seemed to carry an underlying message to members that being ill had an associated responsibility for the ill person to get well as quickly as possible. Healthy members understood that they had roles to play in health recovery by assisting ill members to overcome health alterations and regain usual functional abilities. Ideally, individuals were expected to recover without passing the illness to others. Parents often suggested to sick children that they needed to get well so that they could go play. Family members worked cooperatively to assume caregiving responsibilities that ensured use of family resources to attend to members' prescribed illness care needs. Although other members were permitted sick days, mothers were more likely to perform usual roles even when they were ill and often reported tending to some family tasks even on days when they experienced sickness. Although some Appalachians may still use folk medicine or home remedies, the study families knew little about such treatments. However, they were inclined to self-prescribe, use over-the-counter medications, and share prescriptions left over from other family members who had suffered similar illness experiences.

In the hospice study (Denham, 1999b), many family members described having concerns about physical symptoms of the ill member for a long while before actually contacting medical experts. Sometimes symptoms became quite severe before medical care was sought. One mother whose husband had died said that she had regularly urged him to see a physician for rectal bleeding for several years before he went for care. By the time of diagnosis, the disease was far progressed. In another family, a mother ignored symptoms that included vaginal bleeding even though her husband and children encouraged her to see a physician. By the time she sought medical care, the disease was too advanced for effective intervention. Even when seriously ill members had health information and understood the associated risks, many still delayed seeking medical care. For example, a grieving wife with knowledge about the importance of following her medical regimen for diabetes repeatedly referred to her obese condition, diabetes, and severe arthritis, but she did not seem to believe that non-adherence to her medical regimen was deleterious. She did not seem to connect the fact that her routine of poor nutrition, inactivity, and laxness in taking prescribed medications was harmful to her health.

Families in which a member had a chronic illness or a developmental delay had more rigid forms of family routines than those coping with acute conditions. In the family health research, it was surprising to identify that in supposedly well families that so many had members with chronic conditions requiring prescribed medications and illness care regimens. Persons with chronic conditions such as diabetes or hypertension and even children with developmental delays often viewed themselves and were viewed by others as healthy. The family routines appeared to support individual needs based on the severity of their functionality and the unpredictability of the condition. The more able adults were to participate in usual activities, the less likely others appeared concerned about adherence to a medical regimen. However, some families were especially concerned with children's symptoms and were attentive to medical needs. Families with members who had chronic conditions often talked about "healthy" versus "less healthy" days. It was during acute episodic conditions that other family members viewed members as ill. In disadvantaged families, many had one or more members with conditions that required medical or professional care. However, these families had fewer resources and seemed to report greater difficulties following prescribed regimens than other families (Denham, 1999c).

Member Caregiving

Family caregiving required a great amount of energy and effort, whether the needs were for normative conditions or unpredictable situations. These routines pertained to the ways members interacted as mutual caregivers across the life course. Parents socialized children and adolescents about a wide variety of health-related care modalities that included participating in health and illness care needs and supporting others when they had needs. Aspects of family life pertinent to family caregiving included things such as health teaching, member roles and responsibilities, balancing the use of family resources, and providing support for illness care. Caregiving seemed to assume different characteristics when the family encountered normative conditions versus what might be considered unexpected or unpredicted life events. Members were likely to define parameters of care and assume caregiving roles associated with systemic maturation in ways similar to their families of origin. However, when family caregiving demanded more than what was usually expected, then it seemed that families deconstructed old routines and reconstructed new ones.

Mothers with preschool children played more active roles in child caregiving and were more involved in caring for life aspects with health potential than fathers. Mothers had many sources of information that supported child needs, but mothers were often unprepared to assume the complex responsibilities related to the household production of health. Family caregiving also included member actions needed to assist others comply with medical regimens; these routines included obligatory roles, responsibilities, and sometimes kinship rules. Members described greater stress burden when caring for individuals with chronic or terminal conditions and for members with disabilities. Some family members noted that family misunderstandings sometimes occurred related to the provision of physical or medically prescribed needs that resulted in less adherence to the prescribed regimen. For example, one family had a toddler who had experienced seizure activity. Her father wanted to withhold her medicine because he did not think she really needed it and wanted to avoid the lethargy he had observed in two other children. The girl's mother thought that the medication was necessary. The result was frequent heated family discussions about whether to use the medicine, increased internal tension within the family, and missed doses. Families with chronically ill or disabled members often discussed member conflict and household stress as members vacillated between being supportive and indifferent and when family routines had to be restructured to adhere to prescribed regimens. For example, when caregiving involved a dying member, many caregivers reported interrupted sleep, dietary changes, weight loss, and personal stress that occurred simultaneously with multiple family members. Responsibilities that extended for prolonged time periods sometimes meant that adult children had roles and expectations to meet in the family of origin while they retained those in their primary households. Many spouses discussed variations in personal health routines and extreme

---

Box 13–1 **Propositions about Family Health Routines and Family Health**

- Families that tend toward moderation in family health routines are healthier than families who are highly ritualized and those that lack rituals.
- Families with clearer ideas about their goals are more likely to effectively accommodate health needs through their family routines than families who are less certain about their goals.
- Families and individuals are more likely to effectively accommodate changes related to health concerns when family routines are supported over time by embedded contextual systems than families who are not supported.
- Family routines that support individual health-care needs are more likely to achieve positive care outcomes in the individual with the health concern than families that do not have routines that support the needs of family members with health concerns.
- Children who are taught health routines in the home and are supported by the embedded context are more likely to practice healthy behaviors over the life course than children who are taught health routines in the home but are not supported by the embedded context.

---

stress during the time of the member's illness and dying that continued into the bereavement period. Caregiving routines are an area where most families seemed to need the kinds of support and interventions that might be delivered through family-focused care.

Future Research

Using family's narrative dialogues is a potentially useful method for ascertaining health beliefs and family practices, but the technique is costly in time and effort and requires highly skilled practitioners. However, additional research focused on family health routines could more clearly identify routine categories, dimensions that characterize them, and interventions most predictive of potentiating the household production of health. The development of psychometrically sound instruments normed on various family groups would be useful for assessment, intervention, and evaluation of outcomes. Future research and practice should:

1. Identify within and between family variations in the ways routines are created, deconstructed, reconstructed, and maintained.
2. Determine patterns of intergenerational transmission of routines related to enduring concerns and chronic illnesses.
3. Clarify pertinent routine aspects related to health promotion, disease prevention, injury and risk reduction, health maintenance, and health recovery.
4. Identify interventions for unique health behaviors applicable to health and illness needs.
5. Compare and contrast routine dose rigidity, pattern regularity, and member participatory factors with desired outcomes.

Box 13–1 provides some propositions that might be considered in practice and investigated through research. Cultural variations within groups and family populations may assist measurement of within-group similarities and differences. Finally, greater attention needs to be focused on relationships between community context and family health routines.

Summary

This chapter provides an overview of the six categories of family health routines (i.e., self-care routines, safety and precaution, mental health behaviors, family care, illness care, family caregiving). Examples from the family health research (Denham 1997, 1999a, 1999b, 1999c) supply instructive illustrations about some family themes that nurses might identify in each category. Routines afford the family nurse with opportunities to identify individual and family behaviors pertaining to health outcomes and present areas of family life that may be responsive to nursing interventions. Although the notion of family health routines has not yet become a target for action by most clinicians, it is an area ripe for future practice and research.

Test Your Knowledge

1. Select one of the family health routine categories and describe how a family nurse might use it in the assessment process to do health promotion with a family.

2. A nurse is interacting with a family that has a toddler with a developmental delay. Identify two categories of family routines that might be related to care needs. Describe why the routines might be important and provide three specific examples of how you might use them in planning and providing care.

3. Choose a category of family health routines pertinent in your personal family life and discuss how a nurse working with your family as the unit of care might target the routines.

4. Explain ways that you might assess family care routines and intervene more effectively in your present practice roles.

5. List four things that you would need to change in your personal practice in order to incorporate family routines as a way to think about family health care.

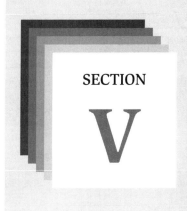

SECTION

V

Family-Focused Practice

Chapter

14

Family Theories

CHAPTER OBJECTIVES *At the end of this chapter, the reader will be able to:*

- Describe the values and contributions of various family theories to nursing.
- Identify ways nursing theories are applicable to family-focused care.
- Use a family systems perspective to understand family relationships.
- Identify ways lifecycle frameworks and other family theories are used to understand family relationships.
- Compare and contrast the Family Health Model with other family theories.

*Start by doing what's necessary, then do what's possible, and
suddenly you are doing the impossible.*
—St. Francis of Assisi

Over several decades, an expanding body of literature has grown to provide
many perspectives about family. This chapter describes an ecological
model to conceptualize a life course perspective of family health with
contextual, functional, and structural dimensions. Nurses who aim to view
family as the unit of care and practice as family-focused need some
understandings about family theory. This chapter presents an overview of
esteemed theoretical views by scholars from a variety of disciplines who have
provided perspectives relevant to nursing practice and research for many decades.
Although many nurse theorists have not emphasized the importance of family in
their theoretical frameworks, many are still applicable.

Development of Family Theory

It is vital that family theories relevant to nursing practice and research are uniquely
related to a knowledge base that is distinctively nursing (Donaldson & Crowley, 1978).
Many family frameworks used by nurses are not nursing models, but nurses have effectively used them. Gale and Vetere (1987) identified several criteria related to family
theory development that suggest a basis for considering how family theories should
look. They have suggested:

- Family theory should be clearly stated and identify relationships of key variables.
- Variables likely to influence family behaviors or events should be clearly
  specified and explained.
- Theories should identify family needs viewed as central features and describe
  ways to make them accessible and available for self-report.
- Family conflict issues should be identified by the source, type, and means for
  resolution.
- Family roles and functions should be described in terms of emotional impact,
  decision making, socialization, and other salient factors.
- Various member perspectives should be recognized.
- Systematic exploration of members' explicit and implicit values and beliefs
  should be tied to belief structures of extrafamilial structures and institutions.
- Families should be viewed over time from various perspectives that differentiate
  between predictable changes and stressors that impact developmental periods.
- Repetitive family behaviors should be made explicit.
- Family taxonomy should differentiate between acts and actions.
- Family interactions should be described in terms of individual, dyadic, family,
  and larger group interactions.
- The family taxonomy devised should describe various family atmospheres and
  lifestyles and classify family behaviors, family events, and interactional
  sequences.

If these criteria are used to measure the adequacy of family theory, then those cri-
tiquing the proposed Family Health Model will likely find gaps and areas that still need
to be more fully fleshed out. However, the Family Health Model is not intended to
be a comprehensive theory of family but instead a framework to steer family-focused
practice.

Family Theories

According to Gilliss (1991a), theories used to attend to health and illness in family nursing are largely borrowed from other disciplines, with the term *individual* often replaced with *family*, but the complex family unit and scope of nursing practice are often not addressed. A *theory* is a set of propositions about defined and related constructs that describe the relationships among the variables in order to systematically describe the phenomena of interest (Kerlinger, 1986). Theory involves concepts closely tied to individuals, groups, situations, or events and tries to explain relationships between them (Fawcett, 1993). When ideas are less concrete, the ways phenomena are viewed and organized is sometimes referred to as a *conceptual model*. Conceptual models have some of the same components as theories, but they are more loosely constructed and generally lack the propositions that identify the existence of relationships between concepts. For several decades, nurses have attempted to identify the knowledge that underpins family nursing and provides a foundation for practice. What theories do nurses use with families? How much of the knowledge taught in family nursing courses is derived from nursing research, and how much is based on borrowed theories? What about family health—do theories to guide practice exist? Which frameworks and theories provide the underpinnings needed to enable nurses to provide family-focused care? Many questions still need to be answered.

Usefulness of Theories

Presently, family theories provide only weak explanations for behaviors and often lack needed empirical findings to demonstrate how variables should be measured and evaluated. Some authors (Cheal, 1991; Coontz, 1992, 1997; Silva & Smart, 1999) suggest that evidence challenges strongly held ideas about the ways families are viewed. Theories must be formal, systematic, and operate at several different levels to be useful in understanding the complex range of behaviors and environmental relationships that affect families and family health. The usefulness of theory is based on its ability to explain a wide range of relationships and an ability to generalize them. In order for theory to be sensitive to today's families, it must consider the inequalities found in their embedded contexts—things such as "oppression, racism, sexism, heterosexism, classism, ageism, ethnocentrism, and nationalism" (Allen, Fine, & Demo, 2000, p. 2). A family theory meaningful for educators, practitioners, and researchers must:

- Describe and explain family structure, dynamics, process, and change.
- Describe invariant interpersonal structures and emotional dynamics within the family and the transmission of distress to individuals.
- Account for the family as the interface between the individual and culture.
- Describe the processes of individuation and differentiation of the family members.
- Predict health and pathology within the family.
- Prescribe therapeutic strategies for dealing with family dysfunction.
- Account for the seemingly antithetical functions of stability and change, particularly when viewed within the family's developmental cycle (Vetere, 1987, p. 27).

In order for a theory to be useful in guiding family research, Vetere (1987) suggested these questions to consider:

- Does the theory integrate and explain the available research data and generate a common research language?
- Does the theory operationally define purposive behavior and the dynamics of change?

■ Does the theory specify the conditions under which the elements will be observed and determine how novel observations are collected in order to increase the understanding about the underlying principles?

■ Does the theory provide common units of measurement that allow cross comparisons of research at different systems levels? (p. 21).

Theoretical frameworks organize thinking and give form to our understandings, but they are based on different points of view. Mistaken assumptions about conceptual constructions can result in practice that is ineffective in addressing family health concerns or results in using inappropriate or poorly chosen interventions. It is unlikely that a single theory can fully describe family or capture all of the variables relevant to family health. Some may assume that an eclectic theoretical viewpoint is needed to comprehend the many perspectives, worldviews, and paradigms of the world's families. Although competing points of view might offer opportunities to explore diversity, it is possible that openness to too many points of view can result in a schizophrenic perspective that is unable to guide practice or explain conflicting phenomena.

Theory is needed that enables practitioners to consider confounding variables pertinent to family health and ask questions that are aligned with the field of nursing's scope of practice. For example, how does being old, black, and having a physical disability differ from being young; white, Hispanic, or Asian; and having a physical disability? What member variables are affected by the embedded context? In what ways do interventions need to be altered to meet the needs of diverse family groups? How can practitioners best use family routines to optimize the household production of health for diverse family groups? What happens over time? At what points do theoretical frameworks assist ideas about practice to attain more optimal health outcomes?

♦♦♦♦♦♦♦ *Cooperative Learning*

Mark each corner of the room with one of four points of view (it may be helpful to make signs to place in each of the corners):

1. Models and theory have little meaning and little use.
2. Models and theory are important as part of education but have little value in family nursing practice.
3. Models and theories are important in education and family nursing practice, but I personally have little idea how to use them.
4. Models and theory are important in practice and research, and I want to learn how to make them practical in my own practice.

Choose the corner that best represents how you feel right now and go to that part of the room. When the groups have assembled, each group should choose a recorder. Have the recorder make two lists—one that reflects how the group members feel and one that reflects the potential effects their feelings might have on nursing practice.

After that is complete, you should choose the position that least reflects your feelings or beliefs at the present time and move to that corner. Choose a recorder for each group and again create two lists—one that reflects how the group members feel and one that reflects the potential effects their feelings might have on nursing practice.

Each group should present their findings and discuss the similarities and differences in group responses and implications for family nursing practice.

▓ Usefulness of Nursing Theories in Family Care

Fawcett (2000) has identified nursing's conceptual models as Johnson's Behavioral System Model, King's General System Framework, Levine's Conservation Model, Neuman's Systems Model, Orem's Self-Care Framework, Roger's Science of Unitary Human Beings, and Roy's Adaptation Model. Many nurse theorists responsible for the development of these conceptual models have updated their original ideas and more carefully addressed family and related phenomena. Educators, practitioners, and researchers have used these theories to better understand family perspectives. Some nursing models are discussed here.

Martha A. Rogers' Science of Unitary Human Beings (1970) focuses on beliefs about persons, energy fields, causality, patterns, homeodynamics (i.e., resonancy, helicy, integrality), well-being, and nursing. Rogers views nursing's role as promoting human betterment through focusing on the irreducible human being and environment as energy fields. When discussing energy fields, Rogers (1992) said that they "constitute the fundamental unit of both the living and non-living" (p. 30). Winstead-Fry (2000) has noted that several of Rogers' ideas are quite consistent with the questions family scientists have been asking about the predictability of patterns in healthy families, questions of normalcy, and concerns about family interventions and outcomes. She concluded that Rogers' perspectives are helpful in viewing chaos, change, disorder, communication, sense of rhythm, energy, and unpredictable patterns of families.

> Rogers would be quite comfortable with an unconventional or unpredictable definition of normal. She did use the word harmony to suggest health at one point. If one needs a definition of normal, it would be probabilistic harmony between members of the family and between the family and its environment, manifested by patterns of behavior that is rhythmic but not repetitive (Winstead-Fry, p. 278).

Rogers' ideas agree with those of many family scientists in the view that causality is not linear. Research is seldom able to account for more than 50 percent of the variance in a research study, and Rogers' theory seems a helpful way to grasp the idea that "human behavior contains probabilistic and unpredictable, non-repeating elements that linear models cannot grasp" (Winstead-Fry, p. 279). It appears that much of what has been suggested in Rogers' theory is consistent with current thinking about families and is compatible with the Family Health Model being proposed.

Dorothea E. Orem's (1971) self-care framework focuses on individual needs and deficits, abilities to meet personal self-care needs and those of dependent others, and nurses' intentional actions to assist. Orem's model has been widely used by nurses in practice, education, and research. From Orem's perspective, self-care is learned within the family, family is the origin of self-perceptions, and members interdependently function to assist one another to meet their needs. Orem (1995) stated:

> The good of order is dynamic, leading individuals to consider how their own actions are conditioned by existent arrangements, including patterns of relationships, and how their own actions to fulfill desires conditions the fulfillment of desires of other. The good of order is viewed as an aspect of human intersubjectivity (p. 166).

Orem identifies that a first step in provision of nursing care is problem identification, and a key part of this identification focuses on individuals' self-care deficits. Next, the nurse finds ways to assist in meeting stated goals that are often caused by a lack of resources or a change in roles. Finally, the nurse assists the individual and supportive family members to overcome or compensate for deficits and limitations and provides abilities that can assist the patient to overcome environmental restrictions and effectively use assets and agencies. Orem's framework encourages views of persons as biological and physiological beings with psychological responses. Orem's perspectives certainly have implications for family care and provide ways to conceptualize individual member and family needs and consider environmental interactions.

Sister Calistra Roy's (1980) nursing model emphasizes the human adaptive system and the environment. Individuals and families are continually interacting with various forms of stimuli and using a variety of behaviors to cope. The nurse's goal in using this model is to assess behavior and factors that influence adaptation and use of the four adaptive modes (i.e., regulator coping subsystem, cognator coping subsystem, stabilizer subsystem control process, innovator subsystem control process) as ways to contribute to health, quality of life, and dying with dignity. The nurse not only enhances adaptive abilities but also aims to integrate environmental interactions by enhancing conscious awareness and choice (Roy & Andrews, 1999). Nursing intervention is a key aspect of this model, and this often occurs as the nurse assists the individual or the family increases, decreases, removes, or alters environmental stimuli.

Roy has expanded her theory of adaptation over the years to include what she calls veritivity and encourages the use of the model with groups of persons in relation to one another (Hanna & Roy, 2001). *Veritivity* pertains to purposefulness of human existence, unity of purpose for humankind, activity and creativity for the common good, and meaning of life (Roy & Andrews, 1999). Roy's model has been widely used in research with families and within clinical family practices (Hanna & Roy, 2001).

Rosemarie Rizzo Parse's Theory of Human Becoming has been referred to as *grand nursing theory* (Fawcett, 2000). Parse (1997b), in discussing the purpose of her theory, stated that it was to be a "journey in the art of sciencing, a process of coming to know the world of human experience" (p. 32). Among the key terms used in Parse's theory are *human becoming, meaning, rhythmicity, transcendence, cocreating, imaging, valuing,* and *languaging.* Nursing's role is to be present with people while they cocreate quality of life based on the family's unique perspective. Parse (1981) defined family as "the others with whom one is closely connected" (p. 81). According to Cody (2000), Parse's view of family "is unbounded by structural, functional, or systematic assumptions" (p. 281), and she does not propose a particular dynamic of family health. Instead, Parse views the process as cocreated as the family process is lived. Fundamental beliefs of this theory are:

1. The human and environment are mutually and simultaneously interrelating as a unity.
2. The human-universe-health process is more than and different from its parts.
3. Health is a continuously changing process (Parse, 1987).

Parse's focus is a perspective of quality of life from the point of view of those living the life.

> The nurse does not know what kind of family life would be comfortable or rewarding for the persons involved, but is there with persons of the family as they focus on the meaning of the family life situation, dwell with the ebb and flow of the family relationships, and reach beyond the now (Cody, 2000, p. 283).

It seems that family-focused care is congruent with Parse's ideas.

According to Fawcett (2000), Watson's Theory of Human Caring (1985, 1988) is a middle-range theory. Watson (1997) originally wrote her ideas about nursing as a response to her beliefs that a clearer distinction was needed between the practice of nursing and the ideas entrenched in medicine's paradigm of diagnosis, treatment, disease, and pathology rather than caring and health. Key terms in the theory include *carative factors, caring moment, transpersonal caring relationship,* and *caring consciousness.* The theory emphasizes that humans are not objects, but instead possess a spiritual dimension uniquely linked to the self, others, nature, and the larger universe. This humanistic theory, suggesting that caring is the essence, or "core," of nursing, is contrasted with the "trim" of nursing, "the practice setting, the procedures, the functional tasks, the specialized clinical focus of disease, technology, and techniques surrounding the diverse orientations and preoccupations of nursing" (Watson, 1997, p. 50). The theory has broad implications for interactions between nurses and families.

Current development of nursing theory offers a variety of perspectives from which to conceptualize nursing science. Although the focus of many theories has been on individual care rather than family or community care, many are now considering applications to family and community health. Nursing has taken some major steps forward in conceptualizing practice in terms of families, but the majority of nurses continue to consider practice from an individual perspective. Family nurse clinicians, practitioners, and family nurse scientists prepared to address complex family health needs will be increasingly in demand.

👥👥👥👥 *Cooperative Learning*

The class should make a list of nursing theories from which the students can choose and then divide into groups of three or four students. Each group should select one of the theories. Groups will each prepare a presentation on the theory and focus on these points:

1. Identify how family is defined in the theory.
2. Describe important concepts of the theory relevant to family-focused care.
3. Discuss the points of the assigned theory pertinent to family as the unit of care.
4. Identify how the theory has been used in education, practice, and research in regard to families.
5. Suggest ways this theory needs to evolve or be tested to further its usefulness for family-focused practice and research.

Systems Theories

General Systems Theory

Systems theory gives a view of the whole that functions through interdependence of its multiple parts, a logical perspective for understanding family interactions. von Bertalanffy (1956) is usually credited with the origins of General Systems Theory. A *system* is often defined as "a set of objects together with the relationships between the objects and their attributes. The objects are the component parts of the system, the attributes are the properties of the objects and the relationships tie the system together" (Hall & Fagen, 1956, p. 18). Systems theory describes the whole by classifying the ways its parts are organized, interrelated, and defined. General Systems Theory supplies a way to describe the solar, economic, environmental, and molecular system, as well as the human or family as systems with interdependent parts.

Discussions about systems theory are often abstract and do not include clear descriptions of the concepts or fully explain the complexity of interrelated systems. Systems thinking implores considering hierarchical order and increasing complexity, so the biological system may be viewed related to its systems, organs, tissue, cells, and genetics. In families, hierarchy might deem an individual as a separate entity, an individual as part of a family, and family as part of a community. In General Systems Theory, open systems allow for the flow of information, energy, and material goods into the system as either an exchange or feedback system between the system and the environment. General Systems Theory implies that an environment exists and that it affects and is affected by feedback systems.

General Systems Theory includes thinking about open and closed systems. Whereas an open system has greater exchange of information, energy, and material between it and its environment, a closed system is more isolated and has fewer exchanges. Terms often associated with general systems theory include *negentropy, entropy, steady state, equifinality,* and *equilibrium. Equilibrium*, or *homeostasis*, is the system state usually targeted and is influenced by the openness or closedness of the system. For example, whereas an open system can be more greatly influenced by present events and independent of past conditions, a closed system is more likely to have tighter links between the initial conditions and the final state. Although open systems can be influenced by cause-and-effect relationships, the degree and direction of these relationships is complex and not easily predicted. Hanna and Roy (2001) stated: "The most useful aspect of systems theory is that it is a process-oriented theory that fosters growth, development, maturation, and the achievement of integrity and transformation of the human person whether that person is an individual or a group of related persons" (p. 11). Ideas grounded in systems thinking have greatly influenced many nursing and family theories.

Family Systems Theory

The theory of family systems emphasizes the whole of family but focuses on member relationships and interactions and the functional status of the system to address needs, goals, and sustain its members. Family systems theory has evolved over the past few decades out of sociology, psychology, and family sciences. Although sociologists were initially concerned with describing what they discovered from structural, functional, or developmental perspectives, the ideas have now melded, and family systems theory has become a more general approach. A key feature of the family systems approach, especially when it is used in family therapy, is that of a unitary conceptualization of family, a whole that is different from the sum of its parts (Whall, 1991).

Reuben Hill (1949), a sociologist, described a family as a group of interrelated persons forming a living system and changing over time as they acted; reacted; and met the challenges of separation, loss, and reunion that resulted from wartime challenges. This early research identified a family stress experience of adjustment that often resulted in a decrease in family functioning, disorganization, and crisis. Hill (1965) later developed the ABCX model of family stress and noted that the key factors were the stressor, definition or interpretation of the stressful event, and effectiveness of resources that determined whether life circumstances were viewed as crises. McCubbin and Patterson (1983) later expanded Hill's model with the Double ABCX Model to address coping aspects as predictors in the postcrisis period. McCubbin and McCubbin (1991, 1993), building on these former models, suggested what is called the Resiliency Model of Family Stress, Adjustment, and Adaptation. This model is built on several assumptions about families (McCubbin & McCubbin, 1991):

- Families face hardships and change as natural predictable aspects of family life.
- Families develop strengths and capacities to foster member and family growth and development.

- Families develop unique strengths and capacities to cope with unexpected and normative stressors and foster adaptation after crisis or change.
- Families benefit from and contribute to networks of community relationships and resources.

Hanson and Kaakinen (2001) suggest that the "resiliency model provides a way for nurses to facilitate family adjustment and adaptation by looking at family strengths and capacities for responding to stress" (p. 54).

The resiliency model identifies the ways family systems use balance and harmony to meet demands and protection factors that affect family adjustment, although vulnerability and resiliency factors are viewed in relation to family adaptation. Family stress is certainly a concern that is central to most families and is important when working with coping, change, and crisis. Some family stress models emphasize the importance of interaction of the community in facilitating high-level family health and the importance of members' abilities to reformulate the embedded social context (McCubbin & McCubbin, 1993). Systems models often address the larger systems, but the predominate focus is often more on the internal nature of the family.

The Framework of Systemic Organization

A gap between grand theories and practice models has resulted in the development of several nursing models aimed at family systems. The Framework of Systemic Organization originated at Wayne State University and suggests a way to understand the nature of families and their members, as well as functional processes within the family's environment (Friedemann, 1989a). This framework expands the nursing metaparadigm to include family and family health concepts and is a conceptual approach for working with individuals, families, and social systems such as organizations and communities (Friedemann, 1995). This theory differentiates nursing's focus on family from that of other disciplines by:

1. Considering environmental influences on family health and nursing outcomes related to actions taken on the family's behalf
2. Emphasizing a comprehensive and holistic perspective of health that includes biopsychosocial factors
3. Focusing on well-being rather than pathology (Friedemann, 1989b)

Families are viewed as open systems that strive for congruence and balance with the potential for health as energy flows between them and other systems with which they interact. Family is defined as an interpersonal system that individual members view as family and includes the functional relationships between single individuals and others who are emotionally connected to individuals. The Framework of Systemic Organization describes family health as a dynamic process in which family members respond to various systemic changes and continually seek to reestablish congruence between the family system and the environment in the areas of stability, growth, control, and spirituality (Friedemann, 1995). Strengths of this theory are the well-defined concepts related to family health, a focus on health rather than illness, and the inclusion of functional and environmental factors germane to nursing practice.

The Intersystem Model

The Intersystem Model was developed at Azusa Pacific University and is based on the evolution of thinking over several decades about systems (Artinian & Conger, 1997). This model is a way of conceptualizing interactional processes whether the client is an individual, family, institution, or community. *Persons* are viewed as the recipients of care and may be biological subsystems, psychosocial subsystems, or an aggregate (e.g., an individual who is part of several family related subsystems). "For example, we could examine the relationship of a family to a health care provider and how both the family and that provider relate to other health agencies in the community" (Artinian, 1997a, p. 7). The environment is addressed from both developmental and situational points of view. Health and disease are seen as a continuum. The model strongly leans on Antonovsky's (1987) thinking that suggests a person's sense of coherence affects his or her ability to cope and manage stress. The goal of nursing in this model is to "assist the person to increase in the situational sense of coherence when confronted with stressors that cannot be managed independently" (Artinian, 1997a, p. 9). The situational sense of coherence "describes the response that occurs in the period of time in which a client is attempting to deal with a serious life event" and measures potentials for understanding a situation and ability to organize resources (Artinian, 1997b, p. 23). In this model, family is defined as "a system of interacting persons who live together over time developing patterns of kinship and who hold specific role relationships to each other, characterized by commitment and attachment, and who have economic, emotional, and physical obligations to each other" (McGowan & Artinian, p. 130). Family subsystems are viewed as biological, psychosocial, and spiritual. The strength of this model appears to be its positive orientation toward health and resiliency and the opportunity to conceptualize the needs and motivations of autonomous subsystems that interact. This model enables the nurse to envision the family as a system interacting with its many contextual systems.

Calgary Family Assessment Model

The Calgary Family Assessment Model (CFAM), initially introduced in 1984 by Janice Wright and Maureen Leahey, was revised in 1994 with an added intervention model, and was again revised and amplified in 2000. This model provides undergraduate, graduate, and practicing nurses with guidelines for assessment and intervention to address the family as client. This framework emphasizes structural, developmental, and functional aspects of nursing care and is based on a theoretical foundation that includes systems, cybernetics, communication, and change theory "embedded within larger worldviews of postmodernism, feminism, and biology of cognition" (Wright & Leahey, 2000, p. 16). Concepts similar to other systems models are incorporated into the model, and the family is perceived as individual systems embedded in a larger suprasystem. The strength of the model is its unique way of integrating widely understood theories into a practical guide that nurses can use in clinical practice for family assessment and intervention.

Family Systems Theory and the Family Health Model

The strength of General Systems Theory is in the ease of understanding its interacting systems. The latitude and scope of the theory are far-reaching and meaningful. However, the breadth and freedom of systems thinking is accompanied by the risks of trivializing and failing to make distinctive links related to interactions and feedback systems. The strengths of the model are often turned into weaknesses when generalizations are vague, unable to be quantified, infinite in possibilities, and difficult to measure. Although systems thinking allows one to view the whole as well as the parts, it is difficult to hold both in mind concurrently and weigh the endless possibilities of independent, intradependent, and interdependent actions. Concentrating too much on the whole can result in overlooking the implications of the parts, although attention to the parts risks the possibility of overlooking the effects of the whole. Although some of these concerns are also true with the Family Health Model, the family model includes things such as time, sequence of events, historical and collective experiences, family behaviors, social circumstances, perceived meanings, and other specifics relative to health. The use of environment in systems theory is often loosely interpreted and lacks clear delineations.

The Family Health Model suggests that precise identification of factors related to the embedded contextual systems is essential to fully comprehend family health. Unless entities are made explicit, it is difficult to clearly ascertain intentions when things are sometimes viewed as systems and other times viewed as environment.

A problem with systems thinking is the assumption that variables viewed independently from the whole remain the same as when they are part of the whole and that there are clear-cut rules that govern the way parts are assembled (Vetere, 1987). Even if the parts can be viewed and understood singularly, questions remain about the ability to use reductionist methods to explain the complexity of the whole. If the whole is more than the sum of the parts, then how does one explain or fully understand the complexity of the whole without fully understanding the complexity of the multiple interrelated parts? If humans and families have behavioral systems, then is it truly possible to understand the complexity of these systems without also considering the effects freedom of choice has on entities themselves and the outcomes that result from the choices? It seems that a situational or ecological analysis is needed to fully understand the relationships and variables associated with the environmental systems and that general systems laws may be ineffective. For example, although individual or human and family systems have freedom of choice, the choices are limited by perceptions about availability and environmental factors that may be predisposing factors for individuals or family. Although freedom of choice might be viewed as a system attribute, varied situations suggest that the possibilities of choices and potential outcomes are predicated on contextual factors. Systems thinking might overlook unique values and attributed meanings related to subtle innate influences embedded in feedback systems and contextual systems. For example, a family may have well-educated members who have financial capacities that exceed the ability to provide for their usual needs. However, if the family lives in a geographically isolated region where medical specialists are unavailable, then they may never gain access to some existent medical options that are not locally available. If medical professionals do not share information about other options or fail to refer to other providers and the family system has limited information about other choices, then the perception might be that the family is doing everything possible when other knowledge or options could result in different choices. When family members are unaware of limitations, then members and even practitioners may be unaware of the restricted choices. Furthermore, systems theories often ignore the impact of changes over time even when they may seem to be accounted for in referring to feedback systems.

The main flaws in systems theory are inadequate methods of analysis, lack of synthesis of systems, and inadequate formulation of rules for applying system principles (Vetere, 1987). Vetere identified several problems in using systems theory as the way to understand families:

- Individuals are more than physical objects and possess nonphysical attributes (e.g., self-reflection) that also modulate behaviors singly and with others.
- Families are living systems with modulating boundaries that result in changing memberships, family roles, and relationships.
- Levels of family change based on feedback loops are often anecdotal and fail to consider the variety of complex alternatives possible (e.g., a family may respond to output related to child disobedience but may be immobilized if faced with substance abuse).
- Clear conceptual and operational definitions are often lacking, with loose definitions leading to empty conclusions (e.g., concluding that biological and social organizations are similar in some ways fails to encompass the many parameters of family behaviors).

■ Empirical research only provides weak links between abstract systems concepts and the reality of family interactions.

Although systems theories contribute much to understanding about the ways systems interact, they have some shortcomings when the issue of concern is family health because they lack focus on health parameters, variables, and dimensions. Although family health can be included in a systems analysis, the balance of functional and contextual variables relevant to family health and the household production of health are less easily conceptualized.

Structural and Developmental Theory

A large amount of overlap of ideas occurs when theoretical perspectives are examined and the interactions resulting from decades of thinking in single disciplines influence other disciplines as well. Minuchin (1974) is often credited with the foundational thinking that has lead to structural-functional models. He based his structural ideas about families on his clinical work with families in distress and developed a framework consistent with systems theory. His theory is an open systems approach to the family as a unit rather than the sum of individuals. Optimal family functioning occurs when the family has the ability to flexibly adapt and restructure itself as new demands are encountered. This theory has several principal features:

■ Family is a system with transactional patterns.
■ Family system functions are affected by their subsystems.
■ Family subsystems are composed of individuals, either temporarily or permanently.
■ Family members can be part of one or more systems and have different roles in each one.
■ Subsystems are hierarchically organized, with power structures within and between them.
■ Stress in one part of the system affects other parts of the system.
■ Families are characterized by qualities of cohesiveness and adaptability.
■ Changes in family structure relate to changes in individual behaviors.
■ Individuals are influenced by and influence constantly reoccurring interactions.
■ Individuals reflect the system of which they are a part.

Minuchin suggests that the whole family must be approached and that understanding must include ideas of evolving and unpredictable patterns as change occurs in response to internal and external forces. From his viewpoint, change is more probabilistic and less a cause-and-effect process because growth and change are experienced simultaneously. The theory has been widely used in family therapy with larger family systems to achieve individual changes.

In structural theory, the spouse system is generally antecedent to the development of other subsystems and includes decision making, gender roles, power, economics, and affectional relationships. The hierarchy of the spouse system is expressed with parents having power over children. The family nurtures and socializes members and is the seat of transactional interactions that influence the growth and development of individuals and the family as a whole. Subsystems include the parental subsystem, the parent–child subsystem, and the sibling subsystem. These categories are not mutually exclusive, and some functional overlap exists among the subsystems. Minuchin (1974) uses terms such as *boundaries, adaptation, stress, equilibrium, enmeshed, disengagement, alignment,* and *underorganization* to describe member interactions.

Minuchin described systems' boundaries necessary to maintain functional roles in terms of their clarity, rigidity, and diffusion and by subsystem rules intended to protect integrity and limit interference. Clear boundaries are explicit statements and understandings about what is and is not permissible; rigid boundaries are firm, less flexible, and immutable; and diffuse boundaries are variable, inconstant, and changeable. Minuchin also emphasized ideas about family cohesion, degrees of enmeshment, and levels of disengagement.

The Circumplex Model used to describe marital and family systems has evolved from Minuchin's concepts (Olson, Sprenkle, & Russell, 1979). This model uses the two central dimensions of cohesion and adaptability, but Olson (1986) later suggested that communication is a facilitative factor for the central dimensions. The model identifies a total of 16 marital and family systems. Key constructs of the Circumplex Model are:

- The dimensions of cohesion, adaptability, and communication
- A taxonomy of family types (balanced, midrange, extreme)
- Aspects of family adjustment (stressors, family coping, family resources)

The Circumplex Model focuses on normal patterns of family interactions and emphasizes family strengths rather than weaknesses (Olson et al., 1983). *Cohesion* refers to boundaries, space, bonding, decision making, and interests and is defined as "the emotional bonding members have with one another and the degree of individual autonomy a person experiences in the family system" (Olson et al., 1979, p. 5). *Adaptability* refers to power structure, role relationship, and relationship rules. *Communication* is a facilitating dimension and includes both positive (e.g., reflective listening, empathy) and negative (e.g., criticism, double messages) dimensions. Developmental stages viewed in family are courting couples, couples with children, childbearing families with preschool children, families with school-age children, families with adolescents at home, launching families, empty nest families, and retirement families (Olson et al., 1983).

According to this model, families can be disengaged, separated, connected, or enmeshed. *Enmeshment* has to do with the degree of intensity in system relationships and a closeness among members that tend to discourage individuation, autonomy, and difference. In contrast, disengaged families live together within a context but have divisive communication and tend to have more independent members who view themselves as more detached from the family. Based on this model, adaptable families that use communication to alter roles and relationships when change is needed are more likely to be viewed as flexible and willing to negotiate changes, and they usually cooperate more effectively in problem-solving tasks.

Marilyn Friedman (1998a) stressed that many theories applied to family are what she calls *structural-functional theories*. This perspective "is comprehensive and recognizes the important interaction between the family and its internal and particularly its external environment" (p. 99). The structural-functional approach views families as open social systems and a subsystem of society. Relationships between the family and its social systems are understood as family organization and ability to function. Friedman sees the usefulness in a structural-functional framework as its ability to assess family life holistically, in parts, and interactionally from a systems perspective. She has used structural-functional theory as the organizing framework for her family nursing text, one widely used in many nursing education programs. Friedman emphasizes four structural dimensions in her assessment model: role structure, value system, communication processes, and power structure. She defines function as "outcomes or consequences of the family structure" or "what the family does" (p. 102) and identifies five important functional areas: affective functions, socialization and social placement functions, reproductive functions, economic functions, and health-care functions.

Comparing Structural Theory with the Family Health Model

In some ways, structural theory has limitations as a useful way to conceptualize family health. Diminished abilities to separate the roles and functions of one subsystem from another make it troublesome to draw conclusions about attribution of subsystems to the whole. Although independent measurement of family's specific subsystem attributes can be helpful in some cases, it can also become an obstacle when trying to understand the whole. For example, individuals learn relational behaviors that may be characteristic of the ways they act in the presence of others, but these behaviors may not manifest themselves if some members of the subsystem are not present. If an individual is not engaging in the activities relevant to a specific subsystem and is isolated from the family context, the characteristics observed or reported may not include the full repertoire of behaviors available within the whole of family relationships.

Today's allowance for negotiated roles within families means that fewer distinctions exist, making it increasingly difficult to generalize which family roles are actually optimal. More and more women are employed outside the home, with most only taking time off for pregnancy and then returning to work. At one time, American men were viewed as the primary economic providers for the family. Even though men's salaries still exceed women's, traditional families are increasingly dependent on dual incomes and would experience great disparities in comfort without earnings from both wage earners. When families depend on the woman's income, the sharing and distribution of household tasks may look different from those of families in the past.

Structural theory has less focus on normal family processes and seems to have some limitations regarding what explains functional behavior in families. Minuchin (1974) developed his theory out of his work with problem families, so many of his ideas seem aligned to reinstating the hierarchy of family subsystems, member roles, and power in the parental role. The theory mostly describes the present state of family and is less able to foster understandings about causative or underlying processes and seems to have limited scope for predicting future states. The theory has limited scope for predicting future states. This theoretical perspective might mean approaching the family as an observer or participant observer, but it mainly focuses on internal processes while overlooking the effects of the embedded context. For example, the theory seems to possess somewhat limited ability for envisioning family care related to prevention or health promotion.

Friedman's (1998a) structural-functional assessment provides a wealth of information about a variety of family needs. The integration of developmental, general systems, and structural-functional theory to see family from many perspectives is the strength of the model. However, when family health is the concern, the model is less clear about which assessments should be made, and it might encourage nurses to collect assessment data that may not be pertinent to the health concern. In some ways, assessment using this model is a bit like fishing in strange waters, never knowing for sure what might bite on the hook and uncertain about what might be dredged out of the waters. Although expert family nurses may use this model to assess and analyze data applicable to health concerns, novice nurses may collect a great deal of data that prove useless or poorly connected to the problem. This model has only a piece that directly addresses the health-care function. Although other aspects of the framework might be useful for counseling and education, the model fails to provide nurses with clear directions regarding the scope of practice and the health-related interventions. The model fails to clearly link the family to its embedded context and does not suggest how the dynamics of time affect the development of multiple interacting members or how complex variables affect the household production of health. The model's emphasis on traditional families or nuclear forms may be restrictive when considering ways to use the framework to address the world's many family types and needs throughout the life course related to processes of becoming, health, and well-being. Societal changes that have prolonged longevity imply that nurses need models that assist them to better conceptualize childless years, how parenting relationships are transformed to new forms of caring relationships over the entire life course, caregiving and coping with chronicity, and health promotion that spans all of the individual and family developmental stages of the life course.

♚♚♚♚♚♚♚ *Cooperative Learning*

List the family theories on the board. Form groups of three or four students. Each group should select a theory and collectively prepare a class presentation that focuses on these points:

1. Discuss the theoretical perspective and the fit with family.
2. Explain how theory differentiates individuals from the family.
3. Describe the important concepts of the theory and their pertinence to family health.
4. Identify how this theory has been used in education, practice, and research in regard to families.
5. Suggest ways this theory needs to evolve or be tested to identify its usefulness for family-focused nursing practice and research.

■ Developmental and Lifecycle Theories

Lifecycle Theories

A number of theories relevant to family include perspectives that might be viewed as lifecycle approaches. Examples of individuals who have provided lifecycle perspectives widely included in practice, research, and education are Erikson's (1959, 1965) developmental theory, Piaget's (1971) social learning theory, Freud's personality theory, and Kohlberg's (1981) stage theory of moral adjustment. Theorists describe lifecycles in terms of critical developmental phases thought to contain important elements that increase the understanding of individuals.

- Individual development means passing through stages during which sensitivity to particular types of stimulation and experience occur.
- Individuals are open to certain experiences for specifiable time periods.
- Individuals who have interacted with others in appropriately stimulating ways acquire specific skills that enable them to move to the next stage.
- Inappropriate stimulation leads to maladaptive behaviors or developmental stunting (Gale & Vetere, 1987).

A common idea in lifecycle theories is that a sort of checkoff list exists that enables one to identify stages of developmental progress at specific time points in months and years of life. For example, Erikson (1965) identified eight stages of development for understanding challenges, risks, and achievements. Although these life-cycle theories are valuable to the life of the family, clear linkages with family health are often lacking and most models fail to fully develop perspectives that plainly address older adults, generativity, and late life viewpoints.

Comparing Lifecycle Theories with the Family Health Framework

Present concerns with diversity, culture, and global communities mean that the value of norms based on life stage thinking may be less meaningful as variations in family health are considered from racial, ethnic, religious, or regional perspectives. Lifecycle theories are often bound to norms viewed from a Western perspective and are less helpful for envisioning development in "untraditional" families. Lifecycle models seem less helpful for life perspectives beyond childbearing and parenting and fail to consider the entire life course. Gale and Vetere (1987) recommended that models:

- Include clear definitions.
- Show the ways key concepts are related.
- Provide a formal way to operationalize the model's key constructs.
- Answer questions about whether a model's measurement tools allow for a formal analysis of the model's key constructs.

Although lifecycle models aid thinking about family processes, these models often focus on distinct areas of individual or family life but do not necessarily encourage comprehension of the whole as much as parts of the whole. Models sometimes seem to approach the family as a homogenous group, fail to account for member differences, and ignore conflicting member needs. Lifecycle theories are helpful for assessing stages and development, but they do not account for the impact of interpersonal relationships, interactions between persons and environments, the vast number of alternative contextual influences, and the effects of time. It seems that neither individuals nor families are passive actors but are better viewed as transitional participants oscillating within contexts for periods of time.

Aggregation of family data to understand lifecycles has often been related to single dimensions (e.g., moral choices, language, physical growth). Attempts to be scientific have resulted in studies that have looked at isolated variables while ignoring effects of the whole. For instance, it is difficult to consider family strengths or coping in terms of static characteristics because these variables are only pertinent when interactions and contexts are considered. Lifecycle theories can mistakenly give the impression that it is possible to move smoothly from one stage to another or that one stage is completed before another commences. Life seldom offers such efficient transitions! Although developmental cycles are important for understanding member interactions, the context and interactions of biophysical or health factors relevant to multiple member households across developmental period must not be ignored. Although family health can be understood at single time points, it also needs to be considered over the life course. Longitudinal designs rather than cross-sectional analyses are needed to capture the multiple influences and transitions that occur at different time points of the family life course.

Other Theories Used with Family Nursing

Symbolic Interactionism

The basic tenet of *symbolic interactionism* is that the world is both physical and symbolic and individuals interact within the larger society based on meanings attributed to symbols. Individuals learn these meanings based on the values a specific culture affirms and then socially construct their reality. Credit for this model is given to George Herbert Mead (1934). The model suggests that individuals begin to know who they are and how they fit in the world based on their interactions with others. An infant is born without any attachment to symbols, but birth implies an immediately active and ongoing interaction with surrounding symbols. Interaction with symbols and others enable the developing child to acquire personal identity, differentiate from others, and ascribe meaning to the world. Characteristics of symbolic interactionism are:

- The importance of symbols and their meanings
- The notion of the public and personal self
- Concepts of role, role enactment, role transition, and role strain
- Human beings as actors as well as reactors (Gale & Vetere, 1987, p. 47)

Symbolic interaction theories imply that change occurs as persons are exposed to symbols, but that they also change the meanings of the symbols. Hence, when operational definitions differ based on persons and situations, methodological difficulties are created. Accounting for the validity of observation and the interpretation of the transaction is based on perceptions and constructions. Although this theory is useful to family nurses because of the focus on "internal processes of social interaction within families, rather than on the outcomes of these interactions," the theory is problematic in that "the family is seen as existing in a vacuum, with no consideration of the environment or the family's history, culture, or socioeconomic status" (Hanson & Kaakinen, 2001, p. 44). However, the theory has utility for understanding communication processes within family units and affirming the possibilities of family meanings' being socially constructed into family routines and patterned behaviors.

Gedaly-Duff and Heims (1996) introduced the family interaction model derived from symbolic interaction and developmental theory. This model focuses on a variety of concepts related to family such as career, aging, marriage, middle age, launching, and school age. However, individual development is also viewed in relation to patterns of health, disease, and illness. Family career includes family tasks and parenting of children but also embraces ideas about the diverse life that occurs across the life course. These authors considered eight stages of family development (Duvall & Miller, 1985b) as ways that nurses can plan with families related to reorganization needs at various family life stages to accomplish family life tasks related to food and shelter, develop emotionally healthy members, meet members' socialization needs, contribute to the next generation, and promote member health and care during illness. Transitions are viewed as predictable changes congruent with movement through the family lifecycles, but families are unique and may not follow anticipated trajectories.

Social Exchange Theory

Exchange theory is a rational theory based on costs and rewards (Thibaut & Kelley, 1959). The general premise behind exchange theory is that persons and families are attracted to pleasurable experiences and agreeable roles and seek to avoid distasteful experiences and loathsome roles. In relationships, individuals aim to maximize their resources and benefits and to minimize the possibilities of losses. Perceptions about costs and rewards of experiences and roles drive the choices made and the satisfaction derived. Key features of the theory are:

- The concept of rational choice
- A set of rewards that family members seek
- The costs of efforts members seek to avoid
- The means individuals use to derive the type and kind of reward believed to be deserved
- The notion of reciprocity in interpersonal relationships (Gale & Vetere, 1987)

A key idea in this theory is that persons generally continue engaging in a given experience, remain in a relationship, or maintain a particular behavior as long as it is not viewed as too costly. Costs and benefits of relationships are dynamic and continually re-evaluated in light of change and conflict. Research about economic changes that affect families is embedded in a social exchange framework in which "couples in intimate relationships organize themselves to adapt to their social and economic surroundings" (Teachman, 2000, p. 34). Rewards may come in many forms, including affection, social support, status, power, security, money, and satisfaction. Costs include things such as financial concerns and debts, undesirable personal attributes, social skills, discomfort related to lack of material goods, and poor health conditions. The worth and supportiveness of the relationship is continuously weighed against the costs associated with continuing the relationship. The theory recognizes variations among the ways individuals and groups value rewards and costs.

Distance Regulation Theory

The Distance Regulation Theory is a systems theory through which family can be viewed as complex, open, adaptive, and continuously processing new information (Kantor & Lehr, 1975). This model uses distance in both literal and metaphorical ways to describe ways information is processed. Components of this model include (1) family subsystems, (2) target family goals, (3) dimensions for achieving goals, (4) mechanisms for implementing the target and access dimensions, (5) a taxonomy of family types, and (5) roles family members may play.

Family behavior takes place within a social space through target dimensions (i.e., affect, power, meaning) and access dimensions (e.g., space, time, energy). Although for any given interaction, one of these dimensions may be predominate, all six dimensions interface when members interact. *Affect* has to do with individual needs for nurturance and positive support. *Power* is related to members' expressions of rights, status, responsibility, dominance, and submission. *Meaning* has to do with valuing, sense of purpose, and personal identity. *Space* is the boundaries and distances between individuals and groupings. *Time* identifies individual and family views about the importance of the past, present, and future. *Energy* is viewed as the overall intensity of the family experience in terms of uptake, storage, and discharge and provides a dynamic mechanism to understand biobehavioral processes, activities, and change.

Families can be viewed as open, closed, or random in style. Four family roles are mover, follower, opposer, and bystander. Movers propose actions, followers use the actions of others to support personal needs, and opposers may propose action or resist change. Both movers and opposers require the support of followers. Bystanders reflect on the actions of movers and opposers but remain independent and free to express beliefs or act without aligning themselves with either movers or opposers. As events change, individuals may change roles. The theory has many strengths, but in gaining access to the observation of usual life experiences of families, the discomfort some feel about personal disclosures and the subconscious, undisclosed, and private worlds of family life might limit the use of this theory in understanding family health.

Reflective Thinking

Reflect about the ideas of feminism and list reasons why you mostly agree or disagree with this point of view.

View several feminist sites on the Internet such as:

The National Organization for Women (NOW): *http://www.now.org/*

Feminist Women's Health Center: *http://www.fwhc.org/*

Feminist Majority Foundation Online: *http://www.feminist.org/*
Women in American History: *http://women.eb.com/*
Military Women Veterans: *http://userpages.aug.com/captbarb/*
Aviva: Women's World Wide Web: *http://www.aviva.org/*
Women's International Center: *http://www.wic.org/*

After reviewing the Web sites, identify your arguments for or against a feminist point of view. Write two or three paragraphs about what you learned from reviewing the feminist sites and describe the implications for family nursing.

Feminist Theories

Feminist theories assume that privilege and power are inequitably distributed based on gender, race, and class. A discussion about feminism begins with sexism, a picture of social reality in which male perspectives have ruled in shaping the social, political, economic, and intellectual environments (Eichler, 1988). According to Ackelsberg and Diamond (1987), feminism aims to transform our ways of knowing so that male and female qualities, reason and emotion, thought and experience, and individuality and connectedness are integrated into the life experience of men and women. Core assumptions about age, class, race, ethnicity, the presence of disability, and sexual orientation underlie feminist perspectives. Responses to the multiple realities viewed through a feminist lens are often met with political or social action aimed at prompting change and justice.

Beginning in the 1960s and 1970s, the feminist movement primarily focused on the consciousness raising of younger women, but it ignored some important issues related to mothers' caregiving roles across the life course and how aging, gender, race, and social class affected caregiving roles. A feminist perspective assumes that gender, vocation, race, and class should have equitable distributions of power and benefits. As awareness of women's caregiving responsibilities began to shift because of the issues of caring for those with disabilities, chronic health problems, and the oldest-old, feminism has taken on some different perspectives (Hooyman & Gonyea, 1995). Although family care as a women's issue was an important step in raising the awareness of policymakers, researchers, and service providers, early discussions emphasized the stress and burden associated with tasks and ignored women as a group. A feminist perspective that clearly articulates the needs for basic structural changes in the ways society is organized is necessary in order to achieve gender justice (Hooyman & Gonyea, 1995). "Family diversity must include individuals' subjective perceptions about oppression and privilege, such as their right to define and describe their own experiences in the world" (Allen et al., 2000, p. 6). Feminist theory assists in reframing the current structure of the world and family life in order to scrutinize it from more impartial and less biased points of view. When family-focused care and family health are the concerns, it appears appropriate to include feminist theory to increase understandings about the effects of social imperatives on the family life course and gender.

Summary

Theories that are germane to family and family health continue to be developed and evolve. Many theories presented in earlier times have served nursing well as the discipline has described its scope of practice. When care was mainly centered in the relationship between patients and nurses, many lifecycle theories were especially pertinent. As holistic views of patient–environment became greater concerns, systems thinking was an asset for conceptualizing practice. Today a new wave of thought has to do with embedded systems and ecological contexts. Theories used in the past continue to have meaning, but nurses also need models that reflect the discipline's ethos and provide a framework to consider the vocation and goals of nursing. Although singular perspectives and causal effects still predominate much thinking, needs exist to include potentially powerful dynamic interactions, alternative hypotheses, and unpredictable phenomena related to family health. The proposed Family Health Model uses a nursing perspective to reflect on family as the unit of care, conceptualize the impact of dynamic embedded contextual interactions on families and their members, consider the complex factors that shape social constructions of family health, and reflect on the implications of the household production of health across the life course.

A paradigm shift to family-focused care does not entail disregard for theoretical ideas that have previously served the discipline well. However, it does imply that frameworks used to address family health consider the impact of complex embedded interactions over time, value multiple viewpoints, encourage reflection about paradoxical under-standings, and not only exhibit tolerance for diversity but also respond to it in morally just ways. Family nursing needs models that incorporate the complex relationships among health, families, nursing, and the environment.

Test Your Knowledge

1. Identify a nurse theorist and describe how that theory is applicable to family-focused care.
2. Define *family* from structural and functional perspectives.
3. Describe what a *family systems perspective* means.
4. Explain the ways a family systems perspective might assist a nurse to provide family-focused care.
5. Discuss the different ways a nurse might approach family care using a family system theory versus a lifecycle model.
6. Discuss the benefits and risks of using non-nursing theories in family health care.

Chapter 15

Mothers as Family Health Leaders

CHAPTER OBJECTIVES *At the end of this chapter, the reader will be able to:*

- Identify gender-specific roles that affect mothers' health.
- Describe mothers' health roles from contextual, functional, and structural perspectives.
- Explain mothers' roles as the orchestrators of family health.
- Differentiate among mothers as gatekeepers, sentinels, stewards, and caretenders.
- Discuss the implications of mothers' roles on family-focused practice.

> *You will not grow if you sit in a beautiful flower garden,*
> *But you will grow if you are sick,*
> *If you are in pain, if you experience losses,*
> *And if you do not put your head in the sand,*
> *But take the pain as a gift to you with a very, very specific purpose.*
>
> —Elisabeth Kübler-Ross

This chapter provides a comprehensive view of family routines as a structure used by family members within the household niche to discuss knowledge, resources, and behaviors that address health needs. The Family Health Model posits that all families have ritual-like practices relevant to health that members can recall and describe regardless of the family configuration, member traits, or cultural context. Steinglass, Bennett, Wolin, and Reiss (1987) studied alcoholic families and found that routines and rituals were excellent clinician research tools because (1) daily routines can be observed and specific behaviors recorded and (2) family members could verbally reconstruct family rituals. Family-focused practice implies that family routines should be a central focus for practitioners who are targeting family health. Routines provide insights into the actual behaviors that are pertinent to health and are amenable to the field of nursing's scope of practice and nursing actions.

The literature reflects that mothers play key roles in influencing health for family members. Although nurses and others are clearly aware of the important roles mothers play in family health roles, the issue is not often addressed when interventions are planned or implemented. The family health research completed by the author (Denham, 1997, 1999a, 1999b, 1999c) identified that mothers often assumed major responsibilities for family health; played key roles in decision making about health concerns; taught, directed, and oversaw health behaviors; coordinated and supervised activities associated with health needs; and provided most caregiving tasks. Mothers are often the primary health-care providers, medical consultants, and gatekeepers for health-care services, as well as being most accountable for socialization needs related to health practices. It is posited that mothers' health roles have implications for nurses working in family-focused practice.

Gender and Family Health

Mothers were present for and participated in all family interviews when the family health studies were conducted (Denham, 1997, 1999a, 1999b, 1999c). In all 24 families, mothers played prominent roles related to health protection, promotion, and maintenance; illness care; and resource use. Mothers were primary care resources, health teachers, and decision makers. Roles that emerged from the findings of the research were gatekeeper, steward, sentinel, and caretender. Mothers orchestrate the family's health routines, determine how some resources are used for health needs, and provide the major portion of caregiving when family members are ill. Mothers' family health roles also include:

- Protecting against illness and disease
- Teaching health promoting behaviors
- Instructing risk reduction and safety promoting behaviors
- Modeling health-related behaviors

Mothers with preschool children were likely to have primary care roles for children and the household, hold jobs outside the home or be busily engaged in family work, and be actively involved with family health tasks (Denham, 1997, 1999a). The second family health study (Denham, 1999b) included families that had used hospice care when their loved one was dying; findings about members from various familial generations supported previous conclusions about mothers' roles and afforded insight about times of transition and loss. When a family member was dying, mothers and other female family members assumed primary caregiving roles, directed family care activities that often included extended family and friends, and were generally unwilling to leave the terminal member's bedside for even short periods. If the dying person was the mother, then the father was strongly supported by the children and close family members, but it was often the daughters or female relatives who assumed leadership in managing the household to care for the ill member and ensure that other family needs were met.

In the final study (Denham, 1999c), the subjects were lower-income families with less organized lifestyles, but mothers still described family health roles similar to others.

However, these mothers were more bent on merely getting through each day, described fewer safety nets or support networks, had fewer resources (i.e., kinds and amounts), were less apt to discuss goals for which action plans had been created, had more casual interactions with neighbors, and seemed generally less hopeful about the future than other mothers. Although most families in all three studies were present oriented, mothers in the more disadvantaged families had fewer goals and mostly focused on present needs. They often described health as an ideal and frequently expressed despair when they perceived stressors and environmental threats outside their control. Although all mothers described some personal stress associated with their roles and responsibilities, low-income mothers reported more stress and illness and seemed to have more complex family health needs.

Gender and Family Health Roles

Until the past few decades, gender was not often associated with health-care needs. In recent years, however, knowledge and understandings about differences between the health-care needs of men and women have increased. Deepened awareness about gender orientations has also informed us about the variations in cultural expectations about gender and roles. Women in American society are largely responsible for meeting health needs in families. Although a rapidly growing body of literature reflects extensive study of maternal roles in children's health and illness needs, fewer studies have examined roles with spouses, domestic partners, adult children, extended family members, dying members, and older members with chronic illnesses or disabilities. Although much is known about mothers' parenting roles, less is known about mothers' health roles related to well families, health promotion, prevention, well-being, and the household production of family health.

In the three family health studies, whereas mothers were primarily responsible for roles related to the household and children, fathers or male partners were more responsible for outside tasks. Whereas mothers' household roles were complex activities that started when they awakened and lasted until bedtime, fathers' tasks were more often occasional events. Men who were employed considered their work their primary roles, and most participated in few household chores and minimal child care. Men were likely to be responsible for yard work, automobile maintenance, household repairs when they were skilled, and taking out the trash. One father said:

> Yeah, I generally take care of the car and do the maintenance on it. Growing up on a farm you learn to work with your hands and think things through as far as fixing something... and that's what I've been trying to do all of my life.

Women employed outside the home still had the primary responsibilities for children and the household. Fathers who were home while mothers worked or when they were briefly away from the home did assume responsibility for child care and assisted with some selective household tasks. However, when mothers returned, the responsibilities reverted back to them. One mother described her husband:

> His job is to come in and sit down and crash. We don't argue about that too much! If I ask him to... like I'm in a hurry or something, he will take the trash out on Wednesday morning, but only if it is necessary. Otherwise it is up to me!

Another mother explained the activities of her live-in domestic partner:

> Yes he does have a few jobs. He knows there is certain things he has to do. We don't drink the water around here. So, he goes down to his parent's house, we have plastic

jugs that he takes and makes sure that we keep...have a water supply. If I get groceries, he helps me carry them in and he will take out the garbage. I still can't get him to pick his dirty clothes up off the floor. He tries to clean. His clean and my clean are two different things.

Another mother explained that her husband strongly believed that women should care for the house and do the cooking, but he consistently fixed breakfast for the grand-children and was willing to vacuum. Another husband was willing do some child-care tasks if necessary and fix lunch, but he refused to prepare breakfast. It is interesting that many of these mothers were teaching their sons as well as their daughters to participate in some household chores such as sweeping, dusting, washing dishes, and food prepa-ration activities. Fathers often saw themselves as "pitching in" when women needed assistance; mothers usually saw themselves as doing "everything."

Parents recalled that in their families of origin, their mothers were the primary providers of health instruction, information, and guidance. Few parents recalled an emphasis on health similar to the way it is today. One father explained:

In growing up...and being young...You don't think about health or nothing, you know. I just remember my parents, especially my mother, saying "you got to eat your lettuce or spinach before you leave the table." And I spent many long nights at that table!

He described things a bit differently in his wife's family of origin:

Like her mother taught her how to wash hands and this and that and to be clean and so forth. On my side now, living on a farm was a little rougher! I can't say that I was taught that way as far as washing your hands before dinner and like that...It seems like on the farm it's just a rougher atmosphere. When we got together, then her traits was carried over from her mother and so forth. It might have caused a little friction between us, you know.

His wife described her own family-of-origin experience:

Everything was spotless. Spotless!...And her house still is! You had to wash your hands. If you come to the table as a guest, she would tell you that you have to wash your hands. Everything is spotless. You know, when she had company. As soon as you hit the back door, you can smell the bleach! So, you know she had company. Any outsiders, she always puts bleach in the dishwater.

In families in which extended family members lived nearby, mothers often experi-enced role ambiguity as the mothers from the husband's or partner's family of origin continued to give them directions about how health conditions should be handled. One mother, a nurse by occupation, explained differences between her ideas and those of the paternal grandmother, whom they lived with:

Her and I have a lot of different opinions like one I can think of right off the top of my head is...She thinks suntan is healthy and I don't! I don't like (my son) out in the sun and if he is out in the sun, I like to put sunscreen on him. And she is always trying to get him to go out in the sun cause "he needs a tan...he needs a tan...you need some sun." She is always preaching to me about how I need some sun because I'm so pale, but I don't think that's healthy. I don't really want [him] out in the sun.

Mothers raised in different generations often differed on what was and was not healthy.

Reflective Thinking

As a class, discuss fathers' roles and family health. What roles do fathers play related to family health? Recall personal memories about your family-of-origin experiences. What roles did your father play in family life that were associated with health concerns? Were these more similar to or different from others in your family? What about the fathers of close friends—what did they do? What do you recall about adult male relatives and health or illness? Are there things that you recall from your childhood that your father always said or did that were related to health? If you are living in a family other than your family of origin, what roles do men play related to health? Are there any implications that can be drawn from the discussion that apply to family-focused care?

Mothers' Health

Mothers often described inequitable stress burdens, emotional fatigue, and spiritual turmoil associated with family roles and responsibilities. Close attachments to extended family meant that many mothers still had caregiver roles in their families of origin along with those in their families of procreation. Mothers described obligations to their families of origin, even when they worked, had young children, or had other responsibilities. For some mothers, stress was prolonged, and many described ongoing effects such as diminished self-esteem and self-worth. Some mothers were medically treated for depression; others described depression associated with childbirth, child-care tasks, or other caregiving roles. Some said they were depressed, and others described symptoms that identified them as at high risk for depression. Although most mothers would only seek help from the family physician, one unmarried mother actually described going for counseling and to a psychiatrist for medications to cope with her depression and sleeping difficulties. She said:

> I get myself worked up over stuff that really there is no reason to get worked up over, and it gets me down to where I don't feel like doing nothing. I think I make it hard for myself. It makes me feel like I don't want to do nothing, just be lazy and not get up and cook or not get up and take 'em [children] to the park like I should.

Another single mother said, "I have trouble with anxiety and depression and I take medication for all of this." She said that she thought the stress of being a single parent could be a reason for her feelings. Several other mothers described present problems or histories associated with alcohol and drug abuse or misuse.

Although other family members could be ill, mothers did not have the time to be ill. Although other family members were encouraged to participate in preferred activities, mothers often sacrificed their personal interests for the sake of the family. When others were relaxing, mothers often reported being occupied with caregiving tasks. Some mothers seemed to have difficulties identifying priorities and were encumbered with child-care and household tasks, work responsibilities, extended family needs, and neighborhood concerns. Mothers often reported as stressful transporting children to school and extracurricular activities and making sure that they were involved in church and other social activities. As roles and responsibilities were recounted, mothers often described feelings of endless pressures and exhaustion. Mothers repeatedly said their actions were unhealthy, but they had no concrete plans to alter the ways their households functioned or family care was provided.

Fathers' reports of stress were more likely associated with family economics, work outside of the home, or fulfilling roles as the man of the house. If fathers felt stress related to children's health concerns, they spoke less about their concerns than the mothers did. However, husbands who described caregiving roles during the terminal illnesses of their wives and tasks associated with end-of-life care reported personal and family stresses. In the families with greater economic disadvantage, unmarried mothers often discussed stressful relationships with partners who lived in the household but did not fully participate in caregiving tasks, leaving them to assume the burden of responsibility, similar to other mothers.

Mothers more often suggested that inconsistencies between health beliefs and behaviors were problems for them than fathers did. Three areas that mothers repeatedly described were weight, diet, and exercise. In the dissertation study (Denham, 1997), four mothers suggested that their spouses were overweight. However, only one described this as a personal concern, and the husband did not intend to alter his behavior. Most fathers viewed current levels of exercise as adequate; in contrast, mothers usually said that they needed to alter their behaviors and increase their activities. Children in most families did not appear overweight. The few heavier children were aware that they should eat and exercise differently, but they were usually not consistently directed by parents in these behaviors.

Most mothers believed they had been healthier before getting married and having children. They often described personal health concerns that developed subsequent to marriage or childbirth such as weight gain, inadequate exercise, little personal time, and continual stresses from role demands. One mother said that she was very healthy before marriage, exercised regularly, and ate a healthy diet. But when asked about the present, she reported, "I slipped a great deal being married. You know, you cook junk food . . . and of course, they are heavy into this meat and potato thing." She described her behaviors before and after marriage:

> I don't get the exercise I should. I mean, I just look at myself and I am thinking . . . "my gosh, this is a person who use to run everyday when I lived with my grandmother." That was when I was at my best. I ate well. I got my sleep. I rode my bike. I exercised.

This mother believed that her pregnancy 4 years earlier caused her "whole body to change to a whole different size and weight." Another mother identified her healthiest time: "For my part, it was before my kids were born." Still another said, "When I think I was the healthiest, I think it had to be . . . right before my first child!" A different mother said, "I use to exercise. When I started having kids, the exercise started going down the drain." In another interview, this mother said, "I know that I'm overweight. I wasn't even this big when I was pregnant."

Mothers were asked what the family did if she got sick. One mother responded, "I guess nobody cares! I still have to keep doing what I did before." A different mother said, "I have to do it all, I don't have time to be sick." Another mother said, "I'm not allowed to be sick. If I'm sick, I get up and function like a normal person. Basically, it's like I'm not sick!" A mother in her late 20s had been diagnosed with thyroid cancer while she was pregnant with her youngest son and had undergone treatment with radioactive iodine. She had to visit a specialist every 6 months for a cancer examination and was distressed that her family physician also wanted her to come and see him every 4 weeks. She said, "I don't know why, but every 4 weeks he wants you to have a check-up. I don't think if I'm not sick; I shouldn't have to go! Usually I don't go unless I feel bad or something like that." She reported that she had not seen her doctor for 3 months, but she was confident that everything was alright and saw little need to do follow-up care unless she experienced new symptoms.

Some mothers described trying to comply with medically prescribed regimens related to mental and physical health conditions, but others seemed to avoid taking medications. For example, one mother said, "My back was killing me yesterday and I didn't take one [Motrin]. I just kept thinking, 'Oh, I'll wait a little bit longer. I'll wait a little bit longer.' 'Cause I don't think that's good, to just keep taking those things. I don't think that's healthy!" Another mother referring to the way her doctor prescribed her medications for arthritis said:

I had a few real bad nights and I would take a half of one and then that was it! No more. If I took all he wanted me to take…In fact, when he starts writing a prescription, he'll say, "Now you will not get hooked on this." I told him years ago I don't want to get hooked on no medication because I don't want to live my life depending upon a pill or a shot. I suffer a lot of arthritis, but I would rather do that than stay stoned on medicine.

This mother, in her late 60s, was hesitant to take even small amounts of medication even when she was experiencing a great amount of discomfort. Many mothers appeared ambivalent about the medical directions they should follow for themselves or other family members. Several described neglecting their health when they were caring for others. One mother explained what happened when her husband was dying from a terminal illness:

There were days when I didn't even take my medicine. I would forget to take my medicine. My daughter-in-law would say, "Have you taken your medicine today?" I would say, "I really don't know!" I just didn't know. I was solely concentrating on him, making sure he got his medicine on time and taking care of him.

As families narrated their stories about family health, it was often obvious that a great amount of inconsistency existed in daily practices, even when mothers may have received medical care and obtained medications and directions about treatments. Mothers often described incongruity about personal health practices and related stresses. For example, mothers often said they believed a particular thing or had knowledge about something, but they described conflicting practices. Mothers, whether full-time homemakers or employed, stated that family demands left little times for themselves. A few tried to engage in a social life outside of the home, but they said stress and guilt kept them from doing things for themselves. Although mothers described characteristics of emotional and psychological well-being as part of being healthy, they often depicted a sense of hopelessness about coping with an endless list of stressful demands. One mother, a full-time homemaker said, "I feel kind of out of control! I feel almost like a puppet, my strings are being pulled one way or another at all times. I don't get to pull any of those strings." When asked who pulled the strings, she answered:

Well, part of the time it is the farm, [husband's] expectations, and three little kids' expectations. There is chicken to be put away. There is corn to be put up. There is this, that, and the other thing that needs to be done here. There is just not enough time in the day to take an hour for me.

Another mother said, "I wish I had more time for me, just time to spend by myself! Seems like I am always around somebody and I would like to be by myself sometimes, and I don't have much time for that." One mother said that she thought some counseling might be helpful in relieving some of her personal and marital stress, but she expressed reluctance to seek professional help because of what others might think.

One mother employed outside of the home described her personal situation since she and her husband had assumed responsibility for the care of two grandchildren a few years earlier:

> It's just very hard to get time to myself because we have four other grandchildren. We try to attend their ballgames. You end up almost like raising your own family. You have no time for yourself. I need an hour by myself at night. [Husband] gets upset with me because I stay up late at night, but by the time the children get to bed and you do the laundry and everything else you do . . . But, I'm getting older and I can't stay up as late as I use to! I'll get up out of bed and he doesn't understand it. It just feels good being alone.

This grandmother explained how she coped with some stress and her spouse's misunderstandings. Some mothers practiced short-term solutions to cope with stresses, but most lacked concrete plans or intentions for even changes they seemed to think would be helpful. Although mothers often described biological risks associated with family histories, few described consistently practicing health-protecting behaviors. One mother often explained about risks associated with a family history of diabetes and cardiac disease. She said, "I think because of my weight, I am more or less staring down the barrel of future problems. They concern me, but apparently not enough! I haven't lost any weight." An overweight mother discussed risks for heart problems, and although she limited her sodium intake, she rarely participated in exercise. Although mothers were aware of personal needs, they seemed more focused on the needs of others.

Conclusions about Gender and Family Health

Although many conclusions might be drawn about gender and family health, three seem especially striking. First, mothers and other women seem to be socialized within their families of origin to assume leadership in the household production of health. Although men play some roles in family health and contribute to some health tasks, they do not have primary responsibilities. Second, household tasks, caregiving roles, and role expectations often place inordinate amounts of stress on mothers and other women that may compromise their own health at times. Third, mothers often seemed unaware of alternative solutions and lacked the energy to seek them if they did not already know about them. The implications for family-focused care related to gender include assisting families to better understand parental roles and responsibilities relevant to family health and identifying ways to distribute household tasks in ways that potentiate all members' health. This means that interventions should target men and women about:

- The household production of health
- The effects of contextual systems and functional processes on health
- Ways to share roles so that processes of becoming, health, and well-being of all household members are realized

Family-focused practice should consider gender roles and responsibilities and include:

- Assessment of the cultural and ecological context that mediates family values, themes, goals, and behaviors
- Identification of expectations within the family as well as across families
- Supportive family interventions across the life course

Mothers' Roles and Family Health

Mothers as Orchestrators of Family Health

When the findings about mother's roles and responsibilities related to family health were analyzed, four roles were identified: gatekeeper, steward, sentinel, and caretender. If an analogy of an orchestra is used to understand mothers' roles, then mothers would be the conductors and family members the musicians. The musical theme would be family health. As conductors, mothers ensured that household members would readily join the chorus refrain with full vibrato, play their parts when it was time, and harmonize with others. However, mothers were more than just conductors; they also served as the rhythm section, the chorus refrain, and the pizzicato. In all three studies, mothers were similar to a percussion section that maintains consistent rhythms. They instituted changes to maintain harmonic patterns, emphasized important family themes, and encouraged solos and ensembles vital to the synchronization of the household production of health. As the chorus refrain, mothers played prominent roles in the measures of core functional processes fundamental to family health and kept the members focused on the necessary and meaningful passages that undergirded ecocultural themes. They taught new behaviors, reinforced information and skills pertinent to health needs, sought needed health information and resources, and cared for illness needs. As the pizzicato, mothers poignantly warned about risks, dangers, and safety, enforced behaviors that supported family themes and goals, and mediated discord as resources for competing priorities were instrumented. When mothers were out of sync because of inordinate stresses, coping inadequacies, or insufficient supports, then family dissonance, lack of harmony, and incongruence often occurred.

When asked how they learned to take care of family health concerns, mothers mostly described family-of-origin experiences. One mother said, "Probably just from my mom doing for us and stuff. I learned from that and other people that I know or related to me or my friends." Another mother said, "How your parents take care of you when you were sick, I think that taught me a lot! If [daughter] is sick, I basically take care of her like my Mom did me." Several mothers said that they did not recall much discussion about health or health topics when they were growing up. Mothers agreed that no formal learning about health occurred in their families, but things were mostly learned experientially over the life course.

 ## Reflective Thinking

Take some time to consider your own family history and what you recall about your own mother's roles related to family health. What were the roles of your mother? Was your mother similar to or different from those of your friends? What do you recall about other women in your family and family health? Were their actions similar to or different from those of your mother? Are there things that you recall from your childhood that your mother always said or did related to health? Were there some things that your mother did that you now find yourself repeating? What are they? If you now live in a household other than your family of origin, how has this affected your roles?

In a class discussion, relate your experiences. Make a list of the common things that most mothers did and then identify some unique differences that might be based on cultural experiences, race, ethnicity, religion, or geographic or regional differences.

Mothers as Gatekeepers

Women were gatekeepers for families' medical care and key decision makers about disease and illness care, health promotion behaviors, and the use of health information. One mother said, "I'm basically the decision maker and he agrees with me!" When asked about how she makes health decisions, a single mother said, "I don't know, I just make my decision! Whatever I feel is right." Another mother said, "It's just common sense to know that your kids sick and you can't do anything for them and you just take them to the doctor."

Mothers said that they sometimes used information learned through the media to guide decisions. Several described how they consulted with their mothers before deciding what to do. Men who expressed the greatest concerns about health issues either had education or skills in health-related fields or had recently encountered the death of a loved one, but a few exceptions were noted. Most men did not assume principal health-care roles, but women checked with them and discussed problems related to health issues. Men were most likely included in decisions about diet, children's safety, and illness care in non-emergency situations. However, mothers said they had often already decided what they intended to do and were usually informing others about their intentions rather than seeking direction.

Community informants consistently described male dominance and patriarchy in Appalachian families and said that mothers assumed prominent roles when the issues were health related. A local expert about Appalachian culture said:

> In the Appalachian culture, women seem more subservient to men, but, on the other hand, women are probably stronger. They know when to pick their battles and some of them are worth picking and others are not. Some have associated saving face with an Appalachian society and men are supposed to be the providers and have the leadership in regard to family. Some women have to work to make sure that the man saves face, although she may be the strongest person.

Men appeared willing to defer to their wives when it came to medical care, children's health-care needs, and family health. Mothers informed their spouses or partners about doctor appointments, treatment decisions, and prescribed medical regimens. Nonconfrontation was a cultural trait of these Appalachian families, the Appalachian expert said:

> We don't always confront them. We would rather not confront. And because of that you allow things to build up. I think it's a cultural thing. It's been referred to as an ethic of neutrality. It may show up in noncompetitiveness and not taking stands on issues. You know, you might take a stand on an issue back in your own home, but to come right out in public and do this . . . You don't always do that because you may be viewed in a negative light or you've just been taught that "you don't kick up a fuss." This has been used for an explanation of domestic violence . . . That people don't do well bringing out issues and confronting them, and so you just let them build . . . And then go from being very passive to very violent. In the community, you tend to know that within families! Sometimes it backfires if you use that in a positive sense that if the female should happen to expose the circumstances, sometimes the family would turn on her because she exposed something within the family.

Although a nonconfrontational stance might be true about some issues, when it came to health issues, mothers were often confrontational. Several mothers described incidents during which they sought care for children's illnesses but thought that physicians did not really listen or treatments and medications ordered were not helpful. Some mothers described how they found new doctors or went other places for care when they thought providers were ineffective. One mother had three children with chronic health-care needs and described many physician encounters during which she voiced concerns and questioned advice. She often called a local pharmacist before talking with physicians about medications. A local physician said he was often confronted when he tried to give medical instructions about health concerns, chronic problems, and risk reduction activities.

Mothers incorporated knowledge about medical services, health information, and other community resources into their decisions. When problems or concerns arose, mothers identified available options, initiated contacts to obtain information and resources, saw that children were taken to medical appointments, obtained and administered prescribed medicines, and determined when follow-up care was needed. The degree and frequency of mothers' discussion with significant others about health issues differed by family. One mother said, "I usually make all of the decisions, he just goes with what I say. I just do whatever I think is best!" A father in another family said, "Whatever she says goes." Another mother said:

> I'll ask his opinion. Actually it is that way. I'll ask his opinion on a lot of things, but it usually ends up whatever I want to do. I usually know ahead of time [what she intends to do]. I just throw in my words so that he'll know what's goin' on and if he thinks it should be done different. Then we'll talk about it.

Parents were both exposed to health information, but mothers usually paid more attention and had more interest than others. Whereas men tended to be more casual users of health information, mothers were purposeful purveyors related to specific needs. A father who was self-employed as a farmer had a television in the barn that he watched in the mornings as he milked the cows. He said he often heard health information and later casually shared it with his wife. His wife explained that his telling her about specific health information probably meant that he thought it was important and if she agreed with its significance, then she might try to incorporate it into the household. However, the husband said that he told her things but then forgot about them and seldom incorporated the new information into his own behaviors.

Mothers were interested in health topics that were directly applicable to family members and family problems. Health information viewed as helpful often focused on things such as pregnancy and childbirth, acute and chronic illnesses pertinent to members, communicable diseases, safety and protection, self-care, inherited or genetic diseases, alcoholism and substance abuse, and exercise. A few mothers also mentioned wellness lifestyles. They discussed consciously seeking information from popular magazines; television and radio; friends, families, and coworkers; food and product labels; medical experts; general reading of health-related literature; and supportive networks, agencies, or institutions. Few mothers read newspapers or gained health-related information through formal programs. When asked how health information was obtained, one mother said:

> I get a lot through the health department. There was a nutrition class through the extension office and I went through it last winter. I learned a lot of things there. You could just watch one [TV] show, like maybe the "Today Show" or whatever. You catch things, you know, in passing.

Most information was gathered informally or brought to their attention by a health-care provider.

One mother with a young son previously treated for leukemia now in remission described how she would go to the library to learn more about his disease. She said:

> Having information . . . It made me feel in control, cause you don't have no control over it. It just made me feel better 'cause like they'd [hospital staff] give you like a list of side effects and stuff to look for. If you wasn't in medical school, you wouldn't understand half those terms.

Many mothers noted that health information was obtained from physicians, nurses, clinics, and brochures they sometimes read while waiting in health-care facilities. However, obtaining information or learning about specific topics did not ensure that the information became part of family health routines, even if it might be beneficial. Mothers seemed to use an eight-step process related to their gatekeeping role and the household production of health:

1. Mothers have a purpose (or purposes) for health information or medical resources.
2. Mothers are aware that pertinent health information and medical resources exist.
3. Mothers have prior understanding or knowledge that confirms the value of new or different health information and medical resources.
4. Mothers' use of health information and medical resources is supported by member beliefs, values, and needs.
5. Mothers have some measure of communication or cooperation with other household members who support the use of health information and medical resources.
6. Mothers have access to the health information and medical resources.
7. Mothers make conscious decisions to use health information and medical resources.
8. Mothers actually use the health information and medical resources available.

🚶🚶🚶🚶 *Cooperative Learning*

Form three groups. Brainstorm about mothers' roles as gatekeepers, stewards, sentinels, and caretenders. Discuss whether these roles seem appropriate for thinking about mothers' health roles across family cultures, variations in family social status, and families with different economic conditions. Then identify the types of general health and illness information mothers might need in each of these roles if they had preschool or school-age children. Third, identify how this information might be different for teenagers. Fourth, consider the kinds of information mothers might need as children become adults and leave home. Finally, brainstorm about some ways nurses might interact with mothers in ensuring they have needed information.

Mothers as Stewards

Mothers assumed responsibility for the judicious use of resources to meet competing family health needs. Some needs were directly related to family biophysical aspects, but other needs competed for assets. Mothers acted as stewards as they monitored, dispensed, and oversaw the distribution of available resources for things such as family members, personal time, finances, health insurance, health knowledge, material goods, and access to health services. Extended family was viewed as a primary resource, and mothers often consulted them before seeking medical care or when they were uncertain about the course of action to take. Mothers learned some things germane to family health in families of origin or through more traditional forms of education, but most practical knowledge was gained through life experience in the family of procreation. One mother said, "I have to see how much resources I've got, then I make my decisions." As stewards, mothers assumed roles as overseers to see that caregiving tasks were met; this often meant they were self-sacrificing in order to provide for others' needs.

The household production of health was closely aligned with the stewardship of family resources needed to meet competing demands, and mothers were usually most responsible for decision making. A large amount of the families' economic resources was connected to diet, and a significant part of the families' income was spent for food.

Some mothers explained how they spent more or shopped less wisely when children accompanied them to the store or when their spouses did the shopping. Mothers with lower incomes who received food stamps for purchases said there was plenty of food at the beginning of the month, but selections were more limited as the month went by. Some explained how Women, Infant, and Child (WIC) coupons were used to improve their children's diets.

When unpredictable life events were met or a family faced multiple pressing demands simultaneously, it was usually the mother who made decisions about the use of resources. For instance, if families had a child with a chronic illness, mothers managed the resources to "make ends meet." Mothers often described ways financial resources were used, but they reported hesitancy about spending money on themselves because they saw this as selfishness or self-indulgence. The needs of others took priority over their personal needs. A mother with limited financial resources and several young children with chronic health problems said she seldom bought new things for herself. Her husband chided her because she refused to buy some new clothing for herself, but her response was that the children's needs were great and she felt guilty when she bought things for herself. Although many mothers indicated that they should probably think differently, they seemed powerless to make changes. Family resources were greatly impacted by the employment status of the family, but local policies, legislation, and other embedded factors were also influential.

Mothers as Sentinels

Mothers assumed roles as protectors and guardians of health and acted as sentinels as they instructed, cautioned, and warned members about illness, disease, and injury. Although fathers provided some protection for their children, especially in the areas of safety and injuries, mothers were mostly responsible. As sentinels, mothers were accountable for maintaining health; teaching and reinforcing health behaviors; and minimizing risks associated with disease, trauma, or injury. These families defined health in terms of freedom from illness and the ability to actively participate in life tasks; therefore, mothers vigilantly engaged in sentinel behaviors as they alerted, cajoled, and nagged throughout the course of the day.

Mothers' child-care roles included socializing children about expected health practices and illness responses and had roles associated with initiating, developing, and overseeing family interactions. Instructions about health behaviors appeared to be based on:

- Health beliefs and behaviors important in mothers' family of origin
- A willingness to accommodate the differences arising in the family of procreation
- Boundaries related to the involvement of extended family members and others
- The availability of health-care resources
- Personal valuing of health information

The cultural context, societal influences, local health policies, and medical service and provider availability were factors in mothers' choices.

Mothers were the primary health teachers for children and used what they knew about health to guide children in behaviors that increased health and reduced risks, but they seldom had organized plans to achieve health goals. Mothers' teaching, guiding, and counseling seemed mostly impromptu and without much premeditated planning or intention. Mothers seemed to offer information in response to children's actions, as they provided guidance about things to do and not do and corrected those who failed to complete expected tasks, ignored rules pertaining to risks, or blatantly disobeyed instructions. While conducting the family interviews, mothers were often observed correcting children when they engaged in risky or dangerous behaviors. Some mothers were vigilant in their admonitions, others were more relaxed, and some seemed completely oblivious to behaviors even when they appeared quite precarious to the author. Mothers were attentive with instructions directed to young children about self-care activities such as personal hygiene, sleep and rest, and diet. Even when children were adolescents, mothers continued to direct their behaviors and offer instructions.

Families often had many extended members living nearby, and most had regular interactions with them. Close relationships meant that mothers were aware of biological risks associated with the family's heritage and some environmental exposures. One mother identified diabetes as a family concern and said, "I am worried about sugar diabetes, because my mother died of it." Another mother said about diabetes, "It seems to affect the women in the family, that is why I hate to see granddaughters born." This same mother described her son's asthma:

> We didn't know where it was coming from and we've tracked it down to my mom's side of the family. In fact, some of her aunts died from asthma, but she was real little when they died. So, she didn't know until we got with some of the older relatives who said, "Oh yeah" [referring to the family history of asthma].

A different mother said, "My mother has high blood pressure, and she had an angina attack and she has diabetes. All these things concern me."

As mothers discussed the health of family members, they often elaborated about the intergenerational links that served as warning signs for family members. A mother described that because her husband's mother had died of leukemia at the age of 26, she had investigated her family's genealogy and discovered several deaths from leukemia. She was especially concerned about her daughter because of the high incidence of female deaths. Another mother said:

> I look at my past family history on health, things that run in the family. Like my dad's side, his parents have diabetes and his sisters have it, he [father] doesn't! My mother's side, her mother had strokes and my grandfather, his mother had a cerebral hemorrhage. On his side [father], there's like diabetes and heart problems, too. I try to keep up with that and connect with what I do and try to block it off so that the kids and me don't have these problems.

She was concerned about her 3-year-old son's risk:

> I worry about [son], 'cause [he] has had thirst. He was constantly wanting something to drink and I know that is one of the signs. I talked to his pediatrician about him and he checked him. He doesn't [have it]! They're keeping an eye on that . . . with him especially and the other kids.

When mothers spoke of health risks, they often described observing their children for symptoms, teaching them preventative activities, and encouraging pertinent risk-reducing behaviors. In many families, mothers promoted the avoidance of behaviors such as alcohol use and cigarette smoking. Mothers said that they cautioned their children about avoidance and abstinence. Although some fathers were fully supportive, children were often exposed to conflicting ideas about behaviors in families in which fathers smoked or drank alcohol.

Mothers as Caretenders

Mothers nurtured, supported, encouraged, and provided actual care to meet member needs. As the persons most responsible for the core functional processes of family health (i.e., caregiving, cathexis, celebration, change, communication, connectedness, and coordination), mothers acted as caretenders to meet family health needs. Caretending responsibilities included parenting and child care related to health, assisting chronically ill members or those with disabilities, enabling ill members to regain health, protecting others from getting sick when a members was ill, managing symptoms associated with terminal illness, and attending to end-of-life care needs. Caretending roles were also related to health promotion, disease prevention, and risk reduction and overlapped the gatekeeper, stewardship, and sentinel roles. Although mothers did not describe modeling gender roles, it seemed an unconscious behavior.

Some mothers described caretending behaviors in their families of origin that they did not want to replicate. For example, one mother with an ill sister when she was growing up said:

Where my sister had polio...Me and my brother...If she couldn't go somewhere, we couldn't go. She [her mother] didn't like people around. A few close relatives, but that was it. We weren't encouraged to have friends. We couldn't enter activities because my sister couldn't. That's why being home was an issue, because me and my brother, even if we had a fever...We wanted to go to school. We wanted to be with kids.

In a later interview, she said:

Like I said, we were sort of kept in, my brother and myself. So, we went to school no matter if we were sick or not because we wanted to be with other kids, which wasn't good for them. But staying home was never a problem because we just didn't want to.

This mother had experienced negative feelings about her mother's rules in illness care and was determined not to repeat them. She valued open relationships and encouraged family members to have friends and be involved in outside activities and welcomed interactions with outsiders.

As caretenders, mothers obtained health information, scheduled and attended members' medical appointments, purchased and administered medications, and saw that medical regimens were heeded. Mothers acted as primary caregivers with ill members, prompted boys and men to seek medical care, and encouraged follow-up and preventive care. Although fathers generally left decisions about medical care to mothers, some had strong opinions about adherence to medical treatment. One father never administered medications to the children except when he was left alone with them for short time periods. He said that he felt a great deal of anxiety about giving medicines and checked many times before administering them. He said his wife was the expert when it came to the children's health needs. Although other fathers with young children reported similar things, those fathers that were caretending for wives with terminal illnesses described how they shared responsibilities with adult children.

In another family, in which a preschool child had experienced seizures, the mother said:

This past spring and last fall....No rhyme or reason to why we had these [seizures]. There was no illness, no anything! Just play. We had EEGs done, which does show some activity. I don't think anybody believes me...That she actually had seizures. They wanted her to go on and get some medicine and put her on it and try her. [Her father] doesn't want her to go on it.

No further seizure activity had occurred, but this mother was concerned about caretending behaviors related to her daughter's needs. Her husband and other extended family members had suggested that it was unlikely that this would happen again, but she remained uncertain even after several months without any sign of recurrence.

Disease, illness events, chronic conditions, and members with disabilities required special caretending skills. Mothers often had little experience or knowledge about how to attend to concerns and sought guidance from extended family members, close friends, medical experts, and incidental media information. When members had conditions that required close attention, it was usually mothers who sat up nights or awakened at intervals to monitor events. Mothers often determined when an acute episode was over or when members could return to work, school, or play. Fathers and adult sons most often provided assistance when the illness was a terminal condition, when the ill member was male, or when the person with needs was a wife or mother.

Summary

Mothers seemed poorly prepared to assume many roles and responsibilities related to being gatekeepers, stewards, sentinels, and caretenders for their families. Family-of-origin experiences were varied, and most women entered families of procreation with limited amounts of preparation for the many tasks and decisions that became their duties. Most learning was informal and often more by chance than planned. Visits to health-care practitioners, opinions of extended family members and others, and media reports were the ways most new information was introduced to families, but it was neither systematic nor organized, and mothers were often ill prepared for the charges they inherited. Even families considered healthy often had members with chronic illnesses, disabilities, and terminal conditions that placed inordinate demands for knowledge, skills, and resources from family households.

Family-focused practices aimed at potentiating the household production of health need to address family health from ecological and life course perspectives. Individual encounters should be viewed as opportunities to provide families with information and skills pertinent to member conditions and how to optimize health behaviors. Most services and resources are presently delivered in response to episodic needs initiated by the individual with a need. Family-focused care could more effectively meet the needs of family households if it were planned based on developmental needs, population-based concerns, and community-based issues. Rather than depending on self-referral, more meaningful family-focused care could use methods of case finding and target caregiver support, availability of resources, and change processes related to incorporating health information into family routines. Family-focused practice would not only target the household production of health but also population concerns impacted by embedded contextual systems and social policy.

Q   *Critical Thinking Activity*

Form three to four groups. Each group should consider a different health condition. Perhaps one group might think about a family with a terminal illness, one a chronic illness, one a trauma incident, and one a well-functioning family. Each group should choose a recorder. Then each group should list the tasks mothers might assume related to the particular health issue and identify the kinds of health information and resources they might need. If the intended goal is to potentiate well-being for the individual and family, what proactive interventions might nurses use to intervene? After groups have explored the issues, they should share their ideas with the entire class and others should give feedback.

While the discussions occur, four students should volunteer to maintain lists on the board titled gatekeeper, sentinel, steward, and caretender. These students should listen carefully to the class discussions. As things are mentioned that fit into their category, the note takers should make notes about them. After all groups have presented their ideas, compare and contrast the fit between mothers' personal needs and maternal roles related to family health.

Test Your Knowledge

1. Describe what is meant by the idea of mothers as the orchestrators of family health and discuss the implications for family-focused care.

2. Compare and contrast mothers' roles as gatekeeper, sentinel, steward, and caretender in relation to family health.

3. Explain how family's embedded context might alter mothers' family health roles.

4. Discuss how a mother's health condition could affect the household production of health.

5. Identify ways family functioning might strengthen or threaten member roles related to family health.

6. Identify potential risks in families when mothers have a chronic illness or mental or physical disability.

7. Describe differences in nurses' ideas and family goals that might be of concern when creating a family-focused care plan.

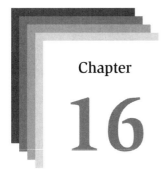

Chapter

16

Family-Focused Practice for the 21st Century

CHAPTER OBJECTIVES *At the end of this chapter, the reader will be able to:*

- Describe the effects of organizational, agency, and institutional reports on family-focused practice.
- Explain concerns educators, practitioners, and researchers might have when addressing health from a family perspective.
- Identify societal dynamics that affect family-focused practice.
- Discuss relationships between family-focused care and appropriateness, affordability, and specificity of care; safety net systems; and a population-based focus of care.

> *I am of the opinion that my life belongs to the community . . . and as long as I live, it is my privilege to do for it whatever I can. I want to be thoroughly used up when I die, for the harder I work, the more I live. I rejoice in life for its own sake. Life is no brief candle to me. It is a sort of splendid torch which I have got hold of for a moment and I want to make it burn as brightly as possible before handing it on to future generations.*
> —George Bernard Shaw

M any things beyond practitioners influence health-care practices. Organizations, agencies, and institutions not only represent societal needs but also present issues that are pertinent to the care provided. This chapter discusses some factors about the provision of health care and addresses the issues of accessibility, appropriateness, affordability, and specificity of care; safety net systems; and a population-based focus. These topics are especially pertinent for envisioning ways family-focused care might be designed to meet 21st century needs.

Reports and Recommendations from Health Organizations

To more fully understand the importance of changing traditions in health-care delivery and appreciate implications for family-focused practices, a discussion of some pressing issues pertinent to family health is provided. Despite changes in the health-care system over the past decade, the current expenditure of almost 14 percent of the nation's gross domestic product on health-care costs is expected to continue to increase over the next decade. Leadership is needed in devising policies and identifying programs, services, and health-care systems that can increase the quality and years of healthy life of all persons and eliminate health disparities. Leadership, direction, and a voice for societal concerns about health care come from many sectors of society. Organizations such as the Institute of Medicine (IOM), RAND Health, the Pew Environmental Health Commission, The Kaiser Family Foundation, the Robert Wood Johnson Foundation, and the American Nurses Association (ANA) are a few groups that reflect professional and societal response to current health-care systems and affect future policy directions. Family nurses need to be aware of the politics and policies that affect family health outcomes. This entails being politically savvy, being prepared to sit at the tables where health policies are created, and advocating for health care that best meets families' needs.

Reports from the Institute of Medicine

The IOM is a nonprofit organization initially chartered in 1970 as part of the National Academy of Sciences to work outside the government and provide guidance to legislators, health professionals, and others about scientific and medical issues. Some of the United States' leading experts serve as volunteers without compensation on various committees and bring knowledge and experience to answer complicated questions. In the past few years, the IOM has provided a number of reports that respond to health-care challenges of national and global consequence. The federal government has funded the majority of the studies, but private industry, foundations, and state and local governments have initiated others. The primary objective of the IOM is to provide timely scientific evidence that improves decision making and advises government policy, corporate sectors, health professions, and the public. Recent reports have addressed such topics as medical errors, immunization, organ procurement, Medicare reimbursement for clinical trials, smoking, public health needs, cancer care, ensuring safe food supplies, and HIV and AIDS.

In 1998, President Clinton appointed the IOM Committee on the Quality of Health Care in America to identify strategies for improving health-care delivery in the United States. In the first report, *To Err Is Human: Building a Safer Health System* (Institute of Medicine, 2000b), a general debate ensued as the public, health-care systems, and providers confronted issues about patient safety. Findings indicated that more people die each year from medical mistakes than from highway accidents, breast cancer, or

> **Box 16–1** **The Tri-Council* Response to the Institute of Medicine's Report on Medical Errors**
>
> - Nurses must be involved in evaluation, development, and implementation efforts to overcome medical errors.
> - Collection and analysis of medical error information must be done within a perspective of continuous quality improvement that focuses on building systems that support nurses, focus primarily on education and prevention, and occur in nonpunitive environments with legal protection for those reporting errors.
> - A nationwide system of data collection is needed for reporting and tracking adverse events, but the system must also include contributing organizational variables.
> - The nursing profession must foster a culture that encourages the identification and prevention of errors.
> - A research agenda is needed that identifies the root causes of errors, determines approaches for error prevention, differentiates between adverse patient outcomes caused by errors versus other causes, and discriminates between workforce and medical errors.
>
> *The Tri-Council is an alliance of four nursing organizations: The American Association of Colleges of Nursing, American Nurses Association, American Organization of Nurse Executives, and National League for Nursing.

AIDS. The report argued for a four-part plan to improve patient safety that:

1. Expands the knowledge base about errors and safety
2. Implements mechanisms to learn about and prevent errors
3. Raises oversight standards related to safety
4. Implements safe practices at the local delivery level

As a result, the Agency for Healthcare Research and Quality (AHRQ) developed a research agenda for patient safety and awarded several grants to improve the understanding of how errors can be prevented. President Clinton signed an order to initiate improvement in patient safety in federally funded health-care programs, and congressional hearings introduced legislation to increase appropriations for patient safety research. Nurses, physicians, and pharmacists work hard to be safe in practice, but errors often occur because of system failures in which demands have outstripped capacities of current delivery systems. The Tri-Council, an alliance of four nursing organizations focused on leadership, practice, and research, has provided a nursing response to the IOM report on medical errors (Box 16–1).

A major concern of the ANA 2000 House of Delegates was aimed at building safe health-care systems for informed patients (Box 16–2).

The second and latest report from the IOM, titled *Crossing the Quality Chasm: A New Health System for the 21st Century* (2001), describes a health-care system that needs reform. The findings suggest that the current system is a highly fragmented web of services that wastes resources, duplicates efforts, leaves enormous gaps in health-care coverage, and fails to build on the strengths of all health professionals. The report warns that without substantial changes, although the complexity of science and technology continue to increase, the health of the nation's citizens will not necessarily improve. The IOM committee suggested that during the next 3 to 5 years, Congress should fund new projects that focus on ways to meet needs and ensure provision of beneficial services in a timely fashion. The report proposes that the U.S. Department of Health and Human Services create new methods to monitor key areas of quality improvement (Box 16–3). The goals to achieve are to improve patients' health status and clinical outcomes, reduce costs that do not compromise quality, increase access to care, create an easier-to-use health-care system, and improve satisfaction for patients and communities (Institute of Medicine, 2001).

Box 16–2 **Building Safe Health-Care Systems for Informed Patients***

- Promote awareness among the public and policymakers about the effects of health-care system downsizing, restructuring, and reorganization that undermine the quality and safety of patient care.
- Support the following IOM recommendations:
  - Development of a National Center for Patient Safety
  - Establishment of a nationwide mandatory state-based error reporting system
  - Implementation of nonpunitive systems that do not blame individuals for reporting and analyzing errors within health-care organizations
  - Development and implementation of performance standards by regulators and accrediting agencies that require health-care institutions and systems to implement patient safety programs and processes with defined executive responsibility, including the chief executive officer and other executive personnel
  - Implementation of proven medication safety systems and practices by health-care organizations
- Promote passage of "whistle-blower" legislation that protects the essential role of nurses in efforts to correct system errors
- Promote development and implementation of policies that support:
  - Development and utilization of safe standardized procedures for the use of medical devices
  - Adequate and appropriate nurse staffing levels
  - Improved information sharing among practitioners treating the same patient
  - Continuing education and enhancement of knowledge and technical skills of practitioners
  - Demonstrated improvement of quality of care and reduction of errors through collection of data using nursing quality indicators
  - Promote nursing research on patient safety
- Continue the implementation of strategies identified in the 1998 House of Delegates action report, *Shared Accountability in Today's Work Environment.*
- Educate nurses in the science of system safety and system safety issues
- Work with the AHRQ and other organizations to make quality of care and patient safety priorities

*Actions of the ANA 2000 House of Delegates.

The IOM committee proposed that some new ideas about the uses of computer information systems and technologies should be used more effectively to address patient and system needs. The report suggests that e-mail communication with health-care professionals is a way to lower costs and speed communications. The committee advises that concerns about potential security breaches and liability risks can be minimized with proper system design and guidance of patient expectations. For example, patient

---

Box 16–3 **The Institute of Medicine's Key Areas of Quality Improvement to Monitor**

- Safe care (i.e., avoid patient injuries)
- Effective care (i.e., services based on scientific knowledge; refrain from providing services to those not likely to benefit; avoid underuse and overuse)
- Patient-centered care (i.e., provide respectful and responsive care that meets individual preferences, needs, and values in all clinical decisions)
- Timely care (i.e., reduce waits and delays)
- Efficient care (i.e., avoid waste)
- Equitable care (i.e., ensure that all care is of the same quality regardless of gender, ethnicity, geographic location, and socioeconomic status)

Source: Adapted from Institute of Medicine. Crossing the quality chasm: A new health system for the 21st century. Washington D.C., 2001.

Box 16–4   **Rules for Governing Health-Care Improvement**

- Care based on continuous healing relationships (i.e., receive care when needed; available in many forms; responsive health-care system 24 hours a day, 7 days a week; access over the Internet, by telephone, and other means in addition to face-to-face interactions)
- Customization based on patient needs and values (i.e., care system designed to meet common types of needs; able to respond to individual choices and preferences)
- The patient as the source of control (i.e., patients have information and the opportunity to exercise the degree of control they choose over health-care decisions that affect them; the health-care system accommodates differences in preferences and encourages shared decision making)
- Shared knowledge and the free flow of information (i.e., patients have unfettered access to their medical information and clinical knowledge; clinicians communicate effectively and share information with patients)
- Evidence-based decision making (i.e., care based on the best available scientific knowledge)
- Safety as a system property (i.e., patients are safe from injury caused by the health-care system)
- The need for transparency (i.e., make information available to patients and families that allows informed decisions when selecting a health plan, hospital, or clinical practice or choosing among alternative treatments; include information about the system's safety performance, evidence-based practice, and patient satisfaction)
- Anticipate needs (i.e., health system anticipates needs, rather than reacting to events)
- Continuous decrease in waste (i.e., systems should not waste resources or patient time)
- Cooperation among clinicians (i.e., active collaboration and communication among clinicians and institutions to ensure appropriate information exchanges and care coordination)

Source: Adapted from Institute of Medicine. Crossing the quality chasm: A new health system for the 21st century. Washington D.C., 2001.

---

security systems that require an authentication process can minimize risks. Although totally computerized records may not be needed in all cases, identification of the essential parts of patient records and data management to record electronically is needed, as well as some conformity in systems and languages used for data management. A nationwide effort is needed to build a technology-based infrastructure that leads to the elimination of most handwritten clinical data within the next 10 years.

Chronic conditions such as heart disease, diabetes, and asthma affect almost half of Americans and are viewed as leading causes of illness, disability, and death. The IOM reports that improving health-care conditions will require large national expenditures to identify pressing concerns but suggests that chronic conditions become the focal point of federal agencies, health-care organizations, consumers, professional disciplines, and others. According to the IOM, comprehensive systems that enable all providers to collect and access complete data about patients' conditions, medical histories, and treatment received in other settings should be considered (Box 16–4).

Immediately after the IOM (2001) report was issued, the ANA issued a press release applauding the report's assertions and recommendations. ANA President Mary Foley said: "This report reinforces what nurses across America have been saying all along: that it is the system itself that is in need of fixing, and that there is an urgent need for massive reorganization and reform of all system issues." The ANA has proposed legislation that all hospitals not only assemble data about the ongoing quality of patient care but also collect and report on the 10 nursing-sensitive quality indicators. In 1998, the ANA funded the development of a national database at the Midwest Research Institute in Kansas Missouri called the National Database of Nursing Quality Indicators. Nursing-sensitive quality indicators for acute care settings are already capturing data about evidence-based care and the outcomes most affected by nursing care (Box 16–5).

Box 16–5 **Nursing-Sensitive Quality Indicators for Acute Care Settings**

- Mix of RNs, LPNs, and unlicensed staff caring for patients in acute care settings
- Total nursing care hours provided per patient day
- Pressure ulcers
- Patient falls
- Patient satisfaction with pain management
- Patient satisfaction with educational information
- Patient satisfaction with overall care
- Patient satisfaction with nursing care
- Nosocomial infection rates
- Nurse staff satisfaction

Source: Adapted from American Nurses Association (1999). Principles for Nurse Staffing. Washington, DC: American Nurses Association.

The American Nurses' Credentialing Center has used the Magnet Recognition Program for Excellence in Nursing Services to measure nursing services and patient outcomes since 1980, when a national nursing shortage threatened and attempts were undertaken to better understand the success factors of hospitals best able to recruit and retain nurses. It is believed that this information will verify what nurses have known intuitively for decades: registered nurses make a critical and cost-effective difference in providing safe, high-quality patient care.

Implications of the Institute of Medicine Reports for Family-Focused Care

The IOM reports raise questions about inferences related to family-focused practice. The report about medication errors has specific implications for nursing educators, practitioners, and researchers. For educators, some questions might be: What do nurses need to learn about medication use in the household and ambulatory care settings that differs from more individual care provided in acute care, rehabilitation, and long-term care settings? What are the best strategies for teaching students about family safety and medication use? What do students need to learn about differences between and individual and family interventions and outcome evaluation related to safety with medications?

In family-focused practice, some questions for nurse clinicians might be: What do family members need to know about the household safety in use of medications? How can practitioners best facilitate member adherence to prescribed medical regimens that incorporates the family support to achieve intended outcomes? In what ways can nurses increase member understandings about untoward effects and risks associated with the misuse of medications?

Nurse researchers might ask: Which family routines potentiate the household production of health? What are the routine practices diverse family members use that increase medication safety? How do factors such as culture, religion, age, level of education, and poverty correlate with appropriate use of medication? Which nursing interventions contribute most to safe and effective use of medications in family households? How do the types of health-care settings where families receive medical instructions affect medication errors in family households? Issues of medication safety are also of great concerns in the daily lives of families, but little has yet been done to investigate them or consider household practices.

The IOM (2001) report about the inadequacies of current health-care systems also raises pressing questions. For instance, nurse educators should be concerned about the following questions: What do students need to learn about quality measures related to family households that differs from more institutional-focused care provision? How do teaching and learning strategies affect whether nursing students integrate family-focused thinking into meaningful interventions that produce quality outcomes? Which clinical experiences are most valuable for assisting nurses to learn about the ways multiple members integrate knowledge into behaviors across time and space?

Clinicians need to address questions related to: What needs to be done to enhance the quality of family care across multiple settings? How can nursing education better prepare clinicians for interdisciplinary practices? What skills and knowledge do family nurses who assume more autonomous roles working in and with community agencies need? How can clinicians best meet family goals and increase the household production of health in cost-effective ways so that health is appropriately impacted? In what ways can nurses collaborate and partner with the multisectorial services used by families to achieve family health? How can clinicians better anticipate family needs related to chronic illnesses? What should practitioners do to anticipate household needs and advocate for them in the health-care settings where services are sought?

Nurse researchers interested in family-focused practice also are faced with questions such as, What are the relationships between evidence-based decision making and family health outcomes? In what ways do information technologies contribute to the delivery of safe, effective, efficient, timely, equitable, and family-centered care? What are the cost, efficiency, and satisfaction associated with diverse kinds of health-care systems used to improve family health outcomes? Which technology and computer information systems are needed to ensure quality outcomes that address individual needs and capture the family household perspectives, not just those of health-care professionals, corporate goals, or legislative agendas? The questions to be investigated are endless, but they are vitally linked to the health outcomes of this new century!

RAND Health

RAND Health originated in the 1960s, when policymakers were engaged in a vigorous debate about how patients should share the costs of their medical care. In 1971, the Department of Health, Education, and Welfare (now the Department of Health and Human Services) funded the RAND Health Insurance Experiment, a 15-year, multimillion-dollar effort that still remains the largest health policy study in U.S. history. Conclusions encouraged the restructuring of private insurance and helped increase the stature of managed care. In the report titled *Taking the Pulse of Health Care in America,* a literature survey concluded that although many have blamed managed care in the past few years for the poor care found in the U.S. health-care system, empirical findings have not indicated either a substantially improved or bleaker situation than when the fee-for-service system existed. Present problems in our health-care systems related to quality care predate managed care systems. The RAND Health group found that large gaps exist for all ages across the nation between needed and received care regardless of type of health-care facility, the type of care provided, or the form of insurance used for reimbursement.

The RAND Health group has emphasized that quality of care can be improved by ensuring that technical aspects of care are competently provided and positively affect intended health outcomes, but also by ensuring that the art of care addresses issues such as patient choices or preferences and culturally sensitive delivery of services. The RAND group has suggested that poor quality of care could result from too much care, too little care, or the wrong care, but *appropriateness of care* refers to expectations that health benefits will exceed risks and *necessary care* is care that would be unethical to not provide. Over the past decade, RAND has developed many criteria for quality measurement and has emphasized that the use of clinical evaluation tools helps rationalize the allocation of health-care resources and improve decision-making processes.

Pew Environmental Health Commission

In September 2000, the Pew Environmental Health Commission at Johns Hopkins School of Public Health released a report that concluded that the United States is facing an environmental health gap. The Pew Charitable Trusts are actually seven individual charitable funds founded between 1948 and 1979 to support nonprofit activities in the areas of culture, education, the environment, health and human services, public policy, and religion. The commission suggested that the high costs associated with chronic illness can best be addressed by effective public health efforts that include the development of a Nationwide Health Tracking Network to provide communities access to information about when and where chronic diseases occur and identify links to environmental factors. Five network components are suggested:

1. Establish a nationwide baseline tracking of priority diseases and exposures (e.g., asthma, birth defects, developmental diseases, cancers, neurologic diseases, polychlorinated biphenyls [PCBs], mercury, lead, pesticides, water and air contaminants).
2. Monitor immediate health crises (e.g., heavy metal and pesticide poisonings).
3. Establish 20 state pilot programs to address regional concerns.
4. Develop a federal, state, and local rapid-response capability to investigate clusters, outbreaks, and emerging threats.
5. Support community interests and scientific research to further health tracking.

Kaiser Family Foundation

The Henry J. Kaiser Family Foundation is an independent philanthropic group that focuses on the major health-care issues facing the nation for policymakers, the media, health-care professionals, and consumers. The group's work mainly focuses on health policy, media and public education, and health. The foundation provides facts, analyses, and explanations primarily about health policy issues such as Medicaid and the uninsured, Medicare, the changing health-care marketplace, minority health, HIV, and women's health policy. The foundation operates a large program in public opinion research on health issues and conducts research on the impact of media in contemporary society. A recent study (Poverty in America, 2001) about poverty identified that only one in 10 Americans thinks that poverty or welfare is a top issue the nation should address. But when asked directly, most people think poverty is still a problem in this nation, even during prosperous times. Poverty has been inextricably linked to poor health and health risks.

The Robert Wood Johnson Foundation

The Robert Wood Johnson Foundation is a national philanthropic organization founded in 1972 and dedicated to improving the health and health care of all Americans. The grants provided by this organization have three focus areas:

1. Ensure that all Americans have access to basic health care at reasonable cost
2. Improve the care and support for people with chronic health conditions
3. Promote health and prevent disease by reducing the harm caused by substance abuse (i.e., tobacco, alcohol, and illicit drugs)

A focus of many grants awarded within the past decade has been the issues that surround end-of-life care. Recipients of grants to support training, education, research, and demonstration projects include hospitals; medical, nursing, and public schools; hospices; professional associations; research organizations; state and local agencies;

and community groups. A recent report released by the foundation titled *Health and Health Care 2010* noted that the focus of the nursing profession on the behavioral and preventive aspects of health care makes nurses the most qualified to respond to the current changes in the health-care system, a health-care arena that is placing increased attention on outpatient care and team functions. According to this report, the Bureau of Health Professions' division of nursing projects that although staffing requirements for full-time equivalent (FTE) nurses will increase by 18 percent in hospitals and ambulatory care settings by 2010, an increased number of employment opportunities will be found in nursing homes, clinics, and community health settings. Present and future needs for nurses will be in all sectors of health care, and nurses who can provide leadership in palliative, holistic, and family care will be needed.

Implications for Family-Focused Care

The implications of reports from these organizations are far reaching, impacting all societal sectors and influencing policies related to practices and services. Findings in reports have inferences for family-focused practices regardless of whether the findings relate to outcomes, economics, or quality. Family nurses need to:

- Be cognizant about organizations and reports that affect health policy
- Be advised about what reports say and the persuasiveness of their findings
- Be aware of the opposing arguments
- Be prepared to take stands on issues that affect the quality and effectiveness of family health care
- Understand federal and state initiatives and legislation influenced by corporate and private organizations as well as other interests

Family nurses are challenged to become political activists by staying current in their knowledge about things that affect family health; inform peers, professionals, families, and community partners about relevant issues; and be advocates at the tables where policies that affect family health are fashioned.

In commercial marketing, the goal is to sell a product and make a profit. However, when the goal is to broker information useful to families, the challenge and strategies may differ. Distinctions between corporate and social marketing include:

- The commercial marketplace is more aware than social markets of the resources necessary to create change.
- Commercial markets usually target a smaller scope of change than health issues.
- Environmental markets are more comprehensive from corporate perspectives and mostly fragmented from social viewpoints (Austin, 2001).

Family nurses might consider themselves information brokers to families as they relay knowledge, research findings, and empirical evidence in useful ways to consumers. Nurses will be challenged in the 21st century to identify strategies that address health issues and discover what families want and need. Research is needed that informs health-care providers and funders about why families use health information and services; how families feel about services they use or do not use; when, where, and why families use information and services; and what outcomes result from the use and disuse of services and information. Families that are more concerned about convenience than potential risks may need information and services packaged in practical ways for modern lifestyles. Greater appreciation of behaviors and needs at various developmental stages, relationships between motivation and emotions, and timely delivery of alternative services to meet a variety of needs are a few issues that need to be more critically considered.

Whether the health information relevant to family-focused care needs is targeted at policymakers, consumers, families, or individuals, the distribution plan has to be systemically integrated, appeal to broad audiences, have wide media support, be repeated over long enough periods for changes to occur, and use the benefits of interactive computer technologies and information systems. For example, childhood immunization has been a public health success story in the 20th century, with many previous life-threatening diseases eradicated or viewed as preventable through vaccines. However, new waves of concern have occurred because some parents are less fearful of the diseases being prevented and more frightened about the safety of the vaccines. Family-focused care can face the challenge of brokering information in ways that clarify issues, modify misconceptions, enable family members to make informed decisions, and provide information as needed.

Key Factors Relevant to Family-Focused Practice

Accessible Care

Families have diverse health-care needs 24 hours a day, 7 days a week. Although various needs exist, family members infrequently seek services from health-care providers. Whenever the topic of accessible care is discussed, the concerns most often described are about the availability of highly skilled and experienced personnel to meet primary health-care and specialty needs. Persons, whether young or old, who live in rural areas where hospital care is inadequate are likely to travel to more metropolitan areas to receive needed care. Those who are very old, uninsured, or recipients of Medicaid are less willing to travel elsewhere for care and are most likely to suffer from the closure of rural hospitals or limited availability of health-care providers (Basu & Cooper, 2000). These researchers studied ambulatory care conditions sensitive to primary care prevention (i.e., diabetes, asthma, hypertension) and found that key factors (e.g., severity of illness, availability of care, quality of local hospital, primary care availability, distances, insurance coverage) influenced whether care was sought locally or in another region. Younger persons, individuals with more severe illnesses, and persons who lack local hospital resources were more likely to travel for care, but older persons were less likely to travel for any reason. The number of primary care physicians was not an indicator of staying in the region for care, and the investigators concluded that physician supply might not be the most critical factor in explaining access to care in rural regions. Regional accessibility is a matter to evaluate relevant to family-focused care.

Accessible care for families might also be discussed in terms of the regional and national differences that influence providers' and families' perceptions about health, illness, and needs for health-care services. Conflict between families and providers can arise when misunderstandings about beliefs and values occur or when traditional views conflict with those of health-care providers. Although health care might be deemed accessible in terms of locating skilled practitioners or expert clinicians, care is not accessible when communication or cultural barriers get in the way. Assessments of family values, family practices, and household niches can be rudimentary in determining whether prescribed regimens result in accessible care.

Family-focused care must be provided in culturally competent ways in order to deliver quality care to minorities and others. Minorities and those on the margin of society are increasingly growing. Some predict that by the year 2035, more than 40 percent of Americans may be in this group. According to Smith and Gonzales (2000), U.S. residents speak at least 329 languages, with fewer than 60 percent of the residents in some cities speaking English. The U.S. Census Bureau estimates that the Hispanic population will increase by 113 percent and that the number of Asian-Americans will increase by 132 percent by the year 2030. Cultural competency is a fundamental concern related to accessible care. Elements of concern in encounters between nurses and clients include communication barriers, trust relationships, cultural context, and specific behaviors. Nurses need knowledge about risks, epidemiology, and treatment efficacy in diverse groups. Although the effectiveness of professional interpreters is often acknowledged, more needs to be known about relationships between cultural competency and the reduction of disparities in health-care delivery and which techniques are effective in which circumstances (Brach & Fraser, 2000).

A study by Weinick and Krauss (2000) described disadvantages faced by some Hispanic children who need health care. These disadvantages resulted from their parents' inability to speak English adequately enough to fully interact with care providers. When parents of black and Hispanic children had limited English skills or lacked knowledge about health-care systems, the children were substantially disadvantaged when compared with white children, even when differences in health insurance and socioeconomic status were taken into account. Culturally competent care can assist those from diverse racial or social groups to avoid interactions between prescribed drugs and home or folk remedies and increase treatment adherence by using client interactions and educational materials that reflect culturally specific values, attitudes, and behaviors (Brach & Fraser, 2000). A development of culturally and linguistically appropriate materials is needed by health plans and care providers to reduce barriers to effective treatment (Smith & Gonzales, 2000). Family nurses must consider accessibility in terms of services needed and obtained by not only the dominant group but also whether those who are more vulnerable are treated equitably.

Critical Thinking Activity

Create a list of cultures within the region. Identify others who might be considered vulnerable (e.g., homeless persons, homosexuals, ex-prisoners, disabled persons). After a complete list has been created, the class should form small groups. Each group should consider one or more of the cultural or vulnerable groups. Within group discussions, identify risks associated with the vulnerable group's ability to access health-care services. What specific ways might family nurses intervene to ensure that care is accessible?

Report findings back to the class and discuss the skills a family nurse should possess to be an advocate for community families to ensure that all people have equitable access to health-care services.

Appropriate Care

Access to appropriate care services is a concern associated with family-focused practice. Defining what is meant by *appropriate care* is essential. It could mean regular follow-up care related to a pregnancy, birth of a child, or care of a person with a chronic illness. Appropriateness of care might be based on whether members receive recommended screenings or whether disparate families have equal opportunity to obtain similar health-care services. Appropriateness of care might be evaluated based on whether the care conforms to empirically based guidelines, follows standards of care, or is provided by competent professionals. Many questions should be asked. Are the outcomes what were intended? Does the care address needs for caregiver support? Is the care provided in a cost-effective setting and delivered by appropriate care providers? Is the care timely? Nurses must discern whether the necessary care is received and whether care is neglected, unavailable, misused, or abused.

A variety of issues may be pertinent when trying to ascertain the appropriateness of care. For example, indicators for appropriate care may be different in rural health-care settings than urban ones. The economic capital, personnel resources, and professional expertise available in urban facilities to complete high-caliber quality improvement and quality assurance programs may be lacking in rural areas. Rural providers struggle to provide basic ambulatory care and inpatient services and may lack the sophistication of care and organizational strengths of urban areas. Expectations of accrediting bodies may need to be modified so that rural institutions can develop practical and attainable health-care quality standards (Moscovice & Rosenblatt, 2000). Although the appropriateness and quality of care received by nursing home residents may be directly related to the number of nurses employed and hours of care provided, residents' quality of life might be more greatly affected by ancillary personnel. However, even greater numbers of elderly and disabled reside in noninstitutional settings, and appropriate care for these persons might entail hands-on care for instrumental activities of daily living (e.g., chores, shopping, housework, transportation) or for activities of daily living (e.g., bathing, meals) at home. High-risk infants (e.g., those who weigh <1000 grams at birth or those who weigh 1001 to 1500 grams and require mechanical ventilation) need comprehensive follow-up care to reduce risks of complications. When high-risk infants received 24-hour access to highly experienced caregivers and a 5-day-a-week follow-up care (i.e., well-baby care, treatment for acute and chronic illnesses, routine follow-up care), 47 percent fewer died or developed life-threatening illnesses that required intensive care admission (Broyles, Tyson, & Heyne (2000). Thus, when considering the appropriateness of family-focused care, nurses must be specific about the needs evaluated.

Cost effectiveness in decisions about the appropriateness of care is an ongoing concern. An area of particular concern in the United States has to do with early detection of preinvasive and prevention of invasive cervical cancer. Women are currently encouraged to have annual Pap smears. The AHCRQ recently funded three studies to examine the effectiveness and cost effectiveness of new screening tests approved by the U.S. Food and Drug Administration to reduce false-negative results of conventional Pap smears. One study (Myers, McCrory, & Subramanian, 2000) found that new screening technologies have increased the sensitivity to uncover low-grade lesions that rarely lead to cancer but prompt further costly testing. These researchers concluded that more efficient and cost-effective screening should focus on improved specificity, decreased screening frequency, and detecting lesions more likely to become cancerous.

A second study (Sawaya, Kerlikowski, & Lee, 2000) found that after identifying a normal Pap smear result, screening every 3 years for cervical cancer rather than annually may be adequate. These investigators suggest that even though low-grade lesions were likely to be found with the usual annual screening methods, overscreening usually resulted in reports with unfounded clinical importance that led to further costly testing and procedures that increased patient anxiety.

The third study (Yabroff, Kerner, & Mandelblatt, 2000) was concerned with the return rates for follow-up after women receive a report of an abnormal diagnosis and found that a wide variance (7 to 49 percent) of women did not receive appropriate follow-up care. Reasons why women do not seek appropriate follow-up care are often associated with fear of further diagnostic procedures, financial barriers, and misunderstandings about the test results.

A meta-analysis (Yabroff et al., 2000) of cognitive, behavioral, and sociological interventions after an abnormal cervical cancer screening test result identified that cognitive interventions using telephone counseling were the most effective (24 to 31 percent compliance), behavioral interventions (e.g., patient reminders) were somewhat effective (18 percent), and sociological interventions (e.g., a videotape about abnormal Pap smears) did not increase the numbers of women going for follow-up examinations. Research findings from studies such as these show that broad ranges of knowledge are needed for making appropriate care decisions. Family-focused care requires well-informed nurses who are capable of accurately interpreting research findings and who are able to communicate this information in useful and timely ways.

Quality indicators that address care experiences with the practitioner (e.g., courtesy, information provided, technical skills, personal manners) and the organizational perspectives and systemic factors involved in the care (e.g., waiting time, staff responses, time spent with practitioner) are equally important when considering the appropriateness of care. Patient satisfaction data are becoming increasingly important as an evaluative aspect of quality care. Organizational factors outside of practitioners' control may influence the satisfaction response on survey measures unless they are carefully differentiated.

In a study (Barr, Vergun, & Barley, 2000) about patients' satisfaction related to access to care, direct physician interaction, and the overall visit, factors external to the doctor explained 36 percent of the variance in the patients' overall satisfaction with the visit and 24 percent of the variance in the quality of the encounter between the patient and the physician. Patients were especially concerned about the length of the waiting time to see the physician and the courtesy of the nonmedical staff members. Family-focused practice aimed at appropriateness of care must attend to quality indicators related to organizational and practitioner factors.

Questions about appropriateness of care choices should also consider whether individuals and families are well informed about medical choices and expected outcomes. For example, individual decisions about having back surgery can be informed and influenced by interactions with physicians or other providers. A study (Deyo, Cherkin, & Weinstein, 2000) compared the surgical decisions and outcomes of elective surgery of two different groups. One group viewed an interactive video and received an educational booklet, and the other group only received the booklet. The overall surgery rate was 22 percent lower in the group that watched the video, but the symptoms and functional outcomes at 3 months and 1 year were similar. The researchers concluded that patients who are well informed about medical choices and expected outcomes are more empowered to make appropriate decisions about their care.

In comparison, another study (Taylor, Deyo, & Ciol, 2000) investigated satisfaction with the functioning and quality of life before and 1 year after surgery for low back pain and found that 64 percent of patients reported great improvements in their quality of life and 68 percent had positive opinions about their treatment outcome. Although the levels of satisfaction are high and appear to be positive indicators of the appropriateness of care, one must be careful about assumptions. It is possible that even if the back surgery was not completed, results may have been similar. Family nurses can play critical roles and use family interventions to assist individuals and families to explore alternatives.

The appropriateness of care should also be responsive to patient and family concerns and address emotional clues, anxieties, psychological stresses, and social concerns. Physicians often miss opportunities to acknowledge patients' feelings, even when patients provide emotional clues about their medical condition or psychological concerns (Levinson, Gorawara-Bhat, & Lamb, 2000). These researchers analyzed audiotapes of randomly selected office visits to identify the frequency, nature, content, and physicians' responses to patients' feelings. About 80 percent of the clues provided by patients in primary care settings and 60 percent of clues of patients in surgical settings were emotional clues. Clues in the primary setting primarily related to social or psychological concerns (e.g., aging, loss of a family member, major life changes), and those in the surgical setting were related to anxieties about medical conditions. Findings indicated that physicians addressed emotional clues in only 38 percent of surgery patients and 21 percent of the primary care patients. One has to question whether family nurses would fare better if a similar study were conducted with them. Evidence seems to suggest that more optimum medical outcomes might occur if emotional concerns are addressed. Thus, it could be concluded that sensitive and responsive care to psychological and social clues are imperatives to appropriate family care.

Affordable Care

Affordable care is not only an issue for individuals who require care but also for care providers and financiers. Affordability is often viewed in terms of tracking care types delivered. However, significant costs are also associated with the appropriateness of care provided, whether care is inappropriate or not provided, actual costs associated with care coordination, and overlap of services or neglect of others equally or even more beneficial. Affordability might also be measured in terms of provider and family time. The needs to control health-care costs, provide affordable health-care insurance, and improve access to employment that offers health insurance continue to be of particular concern for many Americans, especially minorities and the poor. Between 1987 and 1996, health insurance remained constant for most white Americans, but gaps significantly widened for Hispanic men, who were the most likely of all minority groups to lack employment-based coverage (Monheit & Vistnes, 2000). Even when health care is available, it does not guarantee that it will meet health-care needs (Box 16–6).

Although much is known about costs associated with care, less is known about the long-term consequences of these expenses. The AHRQ began the Medical Expenditure Panel Survey (MEPS) project in March 1996. MEPS was designed to collect comprehensive data about cost and use of health care in the United States for policymakers, health-care administrators, businesses, and others aimed at improving accuracy in economic projections. According to AHRQ, in the first half of 1999, 15.8 percent of Americans, or 42.6 million people, were uninsured. A total of 32 percent of young adults ages 19 to 24 years were the most likely to be uninsured, and 13.6 percent (or 9.8 million) children younger than age 18 years were uninsured. Among persons older than age 65 years, 36 percent of Hispanics and 21 percent of blacks were uninsured compared with 14 percent of whites. Awareness of the disparities associated with health-care costs is a first step toward action, but families need advocates for policy and service changes if more appropriate care is to be available to all citizens.

Health-care expenditures have remained constant since 1987, with 1 percent of the population accounting for 27 percent of the disbursements for the noninstitutionalized population and those insured using resources far more intensively than those who are uninsured (Berk & Monheit, 2001). Is it possible that those with the greatest needs are

---

Box 16–6 | **Issues Related to the Availability of Health-Care Insurance**

- Even when some are offered insurance, they do not enroll.
- The availability of insurance does not mean that all services needed are covered.
- The availability of insurance does not imply the opportunity to choose the preferred plan, clinician, or institution.
- The availability of insurance does not ensure that a consistent source of primary care is accessible.
- The availability and accessibility of covered primary care do not imply that appropriate referrals will be made.
- The availability and accessibility of both primary care and referral services do not ensure that gaps between the quality of care that should be provided and what is delivered are addressed.

Source: Adapted from Eisenberg, JM., and Power, EJ: Transforming insurance coverage into quality health care. JAMA, 284:2100–2107, 2000.

getting the lowest levels of care? Costs associated with mental health and substance abuse have substantially increased between 1987 and 1996, but many still have unmet needs, and the high costs of psychotropic drugs may deter many from seeking help (Zuvekas, 2001). Working women ages 55 to 64 years with health problems are especially at risk because of a lack of employment-based insurance and having incomes lower than twice the poverty line (Monheit, Vistnes, & Eisenberg, 2001). Affordability in terms of family health, lifestyle behaviors, household production of health, management of chronic conditions, and caregiver support may be in sharp contrast to individual expenditures. Family-focused practitioners need to deliberate about whether what has been deemed effective care delivery for individuals is cost effective for meeting family household needs. Perhaps affordability needs to be reconsidered in terms of family. Cost–benefit analyses that measure affordability in terms of multiple member or household outcomes using life course perspectives might look quite different from individual perspectives. The 21st century will demand innovation in using economic knowledge to compare and contrast affordability and cost-effectiveness with evidence-based care outcomes.

𝕏𝕏𝕏𝕏𝕏𝕏𝕏 *Cooperative Learning*

Write three definitions of *affordable health care*. One definition should capture the family's point of view, another should identify the provider's perspective, and a final one should address the payer's viewpoint. Exchange your definitions with a classmate and have him or her provide feedback. After reviewing the critique, consider whether or not to include it in your definition.

In a class discussion, analyze the definitions. Are students' definitions more similar or different? In what ways are the elements of affordability altered when families, providers, and payers are considered separately? Is it possible to develop a single definition of affordable health care that addresses all three perspectives? If so, what would it look like? Does the concept of family-focused care alter the way affordability is conceived? If so, in what ways?

Safety Net Systems

Family-focused practice currently has two areas of concern related to safety net systems that need immediate attention. The first concern is related to the adequacy of professional care providers, and the second has to do with supports for family caregivers. A lack of professional focus on families means a limited pool of providers; the current nursing shortage with an aging workforce and forthcoming retirements need particular attention. In the past, federal programs (e.g., National Health Service Corps) provided scholarships and loan forgiveness, but a decline in these programs and a dramatic growth in state programs have been noted since the 1980s (Pathman, 2000). In 1996, 1306 physicians and 370 nurse practitioners, nurse midwives, and physician assistants were under obligation to state programs, numbers approximately equal to those of federal programs. A need exists to track, evaluate, and coordinate state, federal, and community efforts to eliminate duplication of efforts and prevent gaps in health-care services (Pathman). The Nursing Employment and Education Development Act, legislation introduced April 2001, called for innovative approaches to relieve a critical shortage in nurses and declining enrollments at nursing colleges. Consumers and politicians who are well informed about the present and future need to act in order to reverse current trends.

Another safety net concern focuses on the need for educators who can rethink nursing practice in terms of family, incorporate the knowledge and skills related to family health into the curricula, and ensure the preparation of a nursing workforce prepared to deliver family-focused care. Ways to use lifelong learning, just-in-time learning, and asynchronous strategies for continuing education will be needed to ensure that practitioners have timely updates with practice information.

The other safety net issue pertinent to family-focused care is caregiver burden. As the needs and numbers of elderly, disabled, and those with chronic illnesses grow, caregiver burden becomes an increasing concern. Who will care for the millions of relatives and friends who will need assistance in decades to come? Weuve, Boult, and Morishita (2000) studied caregivers and found that families receiving outpatient geriatric evaluation and management (17 percent) were half as likely to report an increasing caregiver burden during a 1-year follow-up visit as caregivers receiving usual care (39 percent). Where are the supports in our current systems to enable family members to be caregivers for those living into very old age with chronic illnesses and mental and physical disabilities? Family-focused practice could target the household production of health by providing family members with information, resources, and other supportive services for family care needs at various stages and for different health concerns. Neither information nor supports remain the same as the conditions change or burdens increase. Family-focused practice presents unique challenges for collaborative and comprehensive practices to assess, evaluate, and manage needs tailored to family households rather than expert perspectives. Collaborative teams consisting of consumers, family members, health professionals, social workers, institutional administrative support, and community agencies are needed to identify caregiver needs, develop cost-effective support services, and advance policies that create new funding and service agendas. Teams are not only needed to provide care management and medical treatment but also to devise information technologies that assist families with just-in-time information, counseling, assistance with advanced directives, referrals, and other interactive feedback in a timely fashion.

Population-Based Care

Nurses have been traditionally educated to provide care to individuals and consider the family as supports. Family-focused practice implies the need to think about population-based care with the family as the primary focus. Although individual care has been mostly delivered in institutional settings, family-focused care will occur more often in households, ambulatory settings, and communities. Population-based care implies thinking about families from local or regional perspectives and understanding the diversity among household populations. Urban areas may contain broad arrays of culturally diverse families, but rural regions may have far fewer. The ways families from various regions define and practice family health within their particular households and how these ways are similar to or different from those in other places is important for family-focused practice considerations. For example, in southeastern Ohio, although Appalachian families predominate, diversity still exists. Blacks and other minorities residing there may differ from other regional groups. Nurses in some counties need to know about health needs of Amish families. Furthermore, knowledge about the migrant families that live and work in a region doing seasonal farm labor is also important.

Traditional approaches to health care have not effectively reduced poverty, family and community violence, alcohol and drug abuse, preventable diseases associated with high-risk sexual behaviors, or unintended pregnancy. For example, a recent study (Klerman, Ramey, & Goldenberg, 2001) of poor minority women at risk for low-birthweight babies indicated that women receiving augmented care (i.e., educationally oriented peer groups, additional appointments, extended clinician time, other supports) did not have babies with lower birth weights than mothers receiving usual care. Although it is true that high-quality prenatal care can make a difference in pregnancy risks, perhaps greater benefits can come from family-focused practices introduced earlier and over the life course. Perhaps population-based interventions need to be targeted sooner, be broader and more inclusive in addressing family lifestyle behaviors, and extend beyond the time when risk is no longer a concern.

A series of interactive video games (i.e., smoking prevention, asthma self-management, diabetes self-management) developed by Click Health, Inc., was used in a randomized study (Liebermann, 2001) with children. Findings indicated that the children markedly increased their resolve to avoid smoking and manage either their asthma or diabetes. Family-focused practice that addresses population-based needs should use culturally and developmentally appropriate materials to address household behaviors. Broad systems of resources, creative strategies, and integrated systems are needed to address population-based problems unique to regional needs.

Specificity of Needs

A final area of concern related to family-focused practice is the specificity of needs based on things such as gender, age, race, poor minorities, disease, stage of disease, lifestyle behaviors, and disabilities. By the year 2030, it is anticipated that nearly 70 million women in the United States will be older than age 50 years, with an average life expectancy in women reaching 84.3 years by 2050 (US Department of Health and Human Services, 2000). A great concern is the adequacy of current systems to address the needs of older women, especially those most vulnerable (e.g., poor people, minority populations, chronically ill persons, the oldest-old) and those older than age 80 years. The number of women diagnosed with breast cancer and the number who die from the disease increase significantly when women are older than age 65 years. A recent study (Mandelblatt, Hadley, & Kerner, 2000) found that women age 80 years and older were undertreated by current standards and often had radiotherapy omitted after breast conservation surgery. The older women were also less likely to receive chemotherapy or be referred to a radiation oncologist than younger women, but after taking into account health and other clinical factors, they were twice as likely to receive tamoxifen as women 67 to 79 years old.

AIDS treatment in the United States has become more effective in suppressing HIV, increasing the effectiveness of the immune system, reducing morbidity, and prolonging the length of survival in HIV-infected persons, but treatment has also become more costly. A study (Anderson & Mitchell, 2000) about the use of antiretroviral drug treatment in patients in Florida living with AIDS or HIV found that men were more likely than women to receive the therapies. The investigators concluded that the survival of women could be improved if their access to antiretroviral therapies equaled that of men. Turner, Cunningham, and Duan (2000) found several reasons why patients delayed care after HIV diagnosis as having private insurance, not being sick at the time of diagnosis, being 25 years old or younger, being Hispanic or black, having been exposed to HIV through intravenous drug use, or having been tested in an anonymous or non–health-care setting. Delays between HIV diagnosis and beginning medical care are not unusual, but these delays prevent initiating therapies that might reduce serious complications and preserve the immune system's integrity.

Family-focused practice implies consideration of specificity related to illness, disease, risks, population-based concerns, prevention, and health promotion. Nurses with knowledge about the ways diversity, history, and developmental stages affect specific health issues will be far better prepared to address these needs from family perspectives.

The appropriateness and timing of interventions, as well as the duration necessary for achieving desired outcomes, may be grounded in family context and functional capacities. In other words, ascertaining the unique family context, family functional status, and family health routines relevant to the type and stage of disease will be of vital consequence when developing family health plans.

Summary

Recommendations based on analyses of health data may be interpreted differently when the care is intended to be focused on the family rather than the individual. Nurses and others interested in providing family care will be faced with ascertaining ways research findings, policy, guidelines, and standards can most optimally affect the household production of health. Leadership and innovation are needed in the 21st century for redesigning new health-care delivery systems and effectively using technology and computer information systems in practices. Continuing to target individuals may not only result in lost opportunities that impact family health but may also fail to provide individuals with more optimal outcomes. Excellence and quality in family-focused practice will require nurses who are original thinkers—nurses who are willing to choose the roads less traveled, who are risk takers valuing familiar pathways but willing to depart from them in order to forge new partnerships and alliances that address pressing family health needs. Who in the health professions is better equipped to address family health than nurses?

Test Your Knowledge

1. Describe different approaches or concerns that educators, practitioners, and researchers might have when considering the safety of care for families.

2. As a family nurse, name and describe two areas of care that might differ from a practice more focused on individuals.

3. Explain what might be meant by the appropriateness of care when practice is family focused.

4. Discuss what is meant by quality of care from a family perspective.

5. You are assigned to provide care to a Hispanic family who tells you that they have no health insurance for their school-age children. In what ways should you respond to their needs from a family-focused approach? How does this differ from the response related to individual care?

6. Identify three ways that recommendations from organizations, agencies, institutions, or professionals can affect nursing practice.

7. Although community and public health nurses often discuss population-based care, nurses who provide care to individuals seldom think in these terms. In a family-focused practice, what are two ways that a family nurse might use the concept of population-based care?

Chapter

17

Participating in Family-Focused Practice

CHAPTER OBJECTIVES *At the end of this chapter, the reader will be able to:*

- Describe what is included in family-focused practice.
- Identify the knowledge and skills needed to provide family-focused care.
- Discuss the assessment of the contextual, functional, and structural domains of family health.
- Identify strategies related to family-focused interventions.
- Explain ways to evaluate family-focused care.

Every model or system of care delivery must achieve desired patient outcomes and contribute to staff satisfaction, retention,

and productivity in an environment that is good for patients and where professionals are energized and can make a contribution.
—Maryann Fralic, PhD, RN, FAAN, Professor,
Johns Hopkins University, Nursing Leadership
for the New Millennium: Essential Knowledge
and Skills

The Family Health Model suggests that family clinicians, educators, and researchers approach practice from different perspectives than those customarily used when caring for individual clients. This chapter describes various practice dimensions related to family-focused practice and discusses concerns those working with families in embedded contextual systems need to bear in mind. Additionally, the chapter provides directions for comprehensive family health assessment of the embedded context, functional processes of interacting members, and family routines. Family assessment can occur in all three areas and produces baseline and evaluative data for designing meaningful family interventions that target family health concerns and evaluating household outcomes.

Preparing for Family-Focused Practice

Description of Family-Focused Practice

Family-focused practice uses each encounter with an individual patient or client as a means of targeting the household production of health. The family is the target or unit of care even when individuals are encountered. Assessments include the identification of interactions among multiple members and their embedded contexts relative to specific health objectives and family goals. Nurses collaborate with family members and others to provide interventions for an array of health concerns related to the biophysical, psychological, emotional, spiritual, ethical, economic, cultural, or social nature of family health and well-being across the life course. Nurses also evaluate outcomes. Family-focused practice includes focusing on families' functional, developmental, historical, temporal, and contextual dimensions. The focus of care is persons-in-context and aims to understand the ways multiple members interact to socially construct health behaviors related to family themes and goals. Family-focused practice aims to assist members to optimize resources, attain family goals, and potentiate the household production of health. Box 17–1 provides a list of assumptions about family-focused care.

Box 17–1 **Assumptions Related to Family-Focused Care**

- Nurse clinicians must have thorough knowledge about families, family context, and family functional status in order to provide family-focused care.
- Health assessments are potentially more meaningful for addressing some aspects of family health when the family context, function, and routines are included.
- Although individuals have a great deal of information about their context, they may not be able to easily describe the complex interrelationships between health and context.
- Nurses skilled in communication can assist families to provide narrative data that are useful for understanding individual and family health.
- Meaningful narrative data can be collected, interpreted, and analyzed by family nurses and used collaboratively with family members to meet family goals and achieve health outcomes.

Mauksch (1974) described the interdependence of the health of a family and its individual members as a fusion of members' unique qualities in ways that create a "family health estate." This estate is characterized by health values, habits, and risk perceptions and involves developmental processes associated with family roles and health status. "Family health is a dynamic changing relative state of well-being which includes the biological, psychological, spiritual, sociological, and culture factors of the family system" (Hanson, 2001a, p. 6) and a "holistic term referring to functional and dysfunctional families" (p. 420). Linking processes between members may positively or negatively affect internal and external member interactions, influence developmental processes and well-being, and alter health. Family health needs are often enmeshed and not easily differentiated, so practitioners must be highly skilled and knowledgeable about family dynamics.

Novice practitioners initially engaging in a family-focused practice might be overwhelmed at the complexity of care needs. Just as first encounters with the nursing process may have seemed overwhelming and difficult when first introduced as a way to think about individuals, family-focused practice presents a vast number of different tasks and concerns. New learning experiences often seem cumbersome and burdensome at first, but progressive learning allows novices to become experts. Every aspect of family assessment is not broached on every family encounter, but appraisals, interventions, and evaluations are driven by identifiable needs. Whereas individual care is mostly incident based, family-focused practice is more relationship based because the care is intended to build on past encounters over time. As nurses become more expert in family care, they gain knowledge and intuitive abilities that direct them in who, what, where, when, and how to assess and intervene.

The primary tasks of family-focused practice are similar to other nursing concerns: relieve suffering, prevent and treat illness, and promote health. However, family-focused care also includes life course and household perspectives. "Primary care that is truly family-focused uses the family unit as the basis for data gathering in assessing and meeting patient needs" (Green-Hemandez, 1999, p. 8). Family-focused care is not strategized by seeing the family as extensions of individuals; instead, it addresses actual or potential family concerns related to members. Primary care is a key aspect of family-focused care, but practitioners should not be shortsighted as they incorporate interventions related to families' embedded context.

Preparation for Becoming a Family-Focused Practitioner

Besides possessing clinical skills and a comprehensive base of knowledge relative to nursing and family practice, those practicing family-focused care must also be cognizant of what is occurring in the human population, the economics associated with the health-care industry, legislation and regulations that affect health-care policy, corporate interests, and the influences of the public and private sector. In order to be become competent family providers, nurses must be versed in the professional, political, business, and social issues that affect family health and be aware of past, present, and possible future trends. In addition to knowing about health-care systems in general, nurses need to understand the cultural diversity of the nation, region, and community where they work. Expertise in technology and computer information systems is also desirable. Nurses who choose to do family-focused practice might look at themselves as pioneers and be prepared to assume leadership in the redesign of practices and care delivery systems.

Nurses who work in family-focused care need to be comfortable working with interdisciplinary teams; collaborating with families, professionals, and others within communities; and partnering with agencies that provide family services. Family nurses must have a familiarity with a broad range of health resources for family members with common developmental needs and awareness about particular resources for unique family problems. Finally, family nurses must also be prepared to provide evidence-based practice if they are going to meet societal mandates for effective, efficient, and quality care. A family nurse specialist prepared at the graduate level should have expertise in family theories and practice associated with assessing health problems, delivering family interventions, and evaluating outcomes related to the household production of health. Some desirable characteristics for family nurses to have include:

- Possess an attitude of inquiry
- Exhibit scientific integrity
- Possess investigative skills
- Act as a team player
- Be prepared to evaluate, use, and disseminate research findings
- Participate in research studies
- Apply evidence-based outcomes in the practice setting and be prepared to champion issues related to family health policy

👫👫👫👫 *Cooperative Learning*

Write definitions that capture your perceptions about family-focused care and relationship-centered practice. Form groups of three to discuss ideas. Group members should discuss each definition separately and then identify the common themes and differences in their definitions. Develop a consensus definition of family-focused care.

In a class discussion, present the consensus definitions from all the groups and ascertain where they agree or disagree. Discuss implications of the definitions for practice and the fit with other nursing theories.

Clinician Roles and Family Advocacy

Family nurses are in unique positions to be advocates in ways that may be somewhat different from those who work with individual clients. Closer alignment with multiple members and ongoing family relationships surrounding primary care issues over the life course should increase nurses' awareness of family needs and limitations. Movement from the institutional setting to the household eliminates the isolation of particular family concerns and opens a frontier of lived reality as the practice setting. Family nurses are more apt to see access and barriers to care from a family's perspective as they strategize with members to create meaningful interventions and evaluate outcomes.

Since the late 1980s, significant changes in health-care delivery have occurred as the United States has moved from fee-for-service to managed health care. Despite the failed efforts of the Clinton administration to enact a comprehensive reform of the health-care system, incremental changes have occurred to increase some benefits for preventive care, increase access to care for children and persons with disabilities, and reduce reimbursements for some high-cost procedures. All problems have not yet been resolved, and many new troubles have surfaced. Issues still not resolved are things such as the

Patients' Bill of Rights, prescription coverage under Medicare, medical malpractice, drug review processes, and privacy and security of medical records. Other concerns center on drug costs and practices of pharmaceutical companies, abilities to get new drugs approved and available in more expeditious ways, and the rights of persons to have access to life-saving drugs even when they live in less privileged nations. Consumer protection, the right of patients to sue health plans that deny or delay benefits, and the large number of uninsured persons also continue to be concerns. Catalysts for future changes include things such as advances in biotechnology; development of new pharmaceutical agents, information technologies, and electronic commerce; and continued soaring costs. *Consumerism* implies that families are more self-reliant, knowledgeable, and interested in health-care alternatives than in the past. All of these issues are pertinent as nurses consider potential family advocacy roles.

Family advocacy may take on different venues as care delivery continues to change in the 21st century. As more care is provided in outpatient settings, how will nurses' advocacy roles be affected? What systems will be used to increase safety, reduce errors, increase quality, and decrease costs? What issues will be debated as telehealth and use of computer information systems increase? How will care provided in more autonomous settings affect liability? What are the issues related to licensure that might need to change in order to accommodate family health needs? How will demand, access, and safety be weighed across international borders? Will price controls be needed to ensure affordability for insurance payers and family consumers of health care? What costs are too formidable for the benefits achieved through innovation? What implications does the Human Genome Project have for the futures of family-focused practice? How can employers create programs that better address the household production of health (e.g., medical savings accounts, vouchers, alternative therapies)? How can practitioners better meet family health needs for the increasing numbers of poor uninsured families? Family-focused practice provides great opportunity and responsibility on nurses to understand the long- and short-term effects of changes in policy and service delivery. Although the future holds positive prospects, the potential for disparities among families may be greater than ever before.

Family-Focused Care

Hanson (2001a) defined family nursing as "the process of providing for the health care needs of families that are within the scope of nursing practice. Family health care nursing can be aimed at the family as context, the family as a whole, the family as a system, or the family as a component of society" (p. 7). Gilliss (1991c) suggested that *family as context* means that the members are sources of information about the patient or client (e.g., health history, health practices, lifestyle), but, family as unit of care, provides information about group values, supportive interactions, decision making, affective relationships, caregiving, and health habits. Family nursing should be primarily directed toward the family group rather than merely viewing them as the patient's context because the health of the family unit is both a determinant and an outcome of family care. Family-centered care is "an approach to child health care based on the assumption that the family is the child's primary source of strength and support" (Hanson, p. 420).

Assessment is an important skill learned by all nurses. Initially, assessment focuses on individuals, but this is broadened as students are taught about families, groups, and populations. Although family assessment provides baseline data, it is a reoccurring phenomenon that should occur with each nurse–client interaction as a way to evaluate the effectiveness of interventions, determine whether goals have been met, and measure

---

Box 17-2 **Goals of Family-Focused Practice**

- Collaborate with interdisciplinary teams, social institutions, community agencies, legislators, and others to achieve pertinent health outcomes related to family health and societal concerns.
- Obtain, maintain, and sustain optimal family health for diverse family populations.
- Use assessment data about contextual and functional factors to achieve national health objectives for all families.
- Assist individuals, family subsystems, and families with processes of becoming, health outcomes, and well-being throughout the life course.
- Cooperate with family members and others to construct, deconstruct, or reconstruct daily routines pertinent to the processes of becoming, health, and well-being.
- Enable multiple member households to attain potentials vital to future health outcomes.
- Teach members how to reduce risks that threaten the household production of health.
- Assist families to manage illness states when they are present.
- Support individuals, family subsystems, and families with palliative care when a member faces terminal stages.
- Identify resources that support the family's household production of health.
- Provide information, resources, education, and counseling to family members that address functional processes related to family health needs.
- Initiate and support policy and legislation that address family health needs.

---

care outcomes. The primary focus for assessment usually rests on skills learned about primary care and meeting the needs of individuals. Primary care is "recognized as the provision of integrated, accessible health care services by providers who are accountable for addressing a large majority of personal health care needs" (Singleton, Green-Hermandez, & Holzemer, 1999, p. 3). Primary care encourages the development of sustained partnerships, caring, and trust between patients, families, health-care providers, and others within the community. Singleton et al. (1999) discuss relationship-centered care as care that redefines patient–provider interactions and recognizes the value of relationships between providers, families, and communities Relationship-centered care requires:

- Partnerships that see patients as unique persons
- Practitioners who are reflective and willing to relinquish pre-existing perspectives and paternalistic views
- Technical proficiency
- Professional competence
- Interdisciplinary practice (Singleton et al.).

Family nurses have a broad array of goals to accomplish in family-focused practice (Box 17–2), but clinicians must be aware of the many potential competing family and professional goals that could be deterrents in the delivery of care.

A number of important points need to be included when thinking about what comprises family-focused practice. Although intensive assessment and evaluative measures related to families and the household niche are inextricably tied to family health, they are usually interpreted in terms of the recipients of care. Family-focused practice must also include systems effectiveness for the adequacy, accessibility, appropriateness, and affordability of care delivery. In the delivery of individual care, nurses often view patients as separate from the context and too often identify problems, conflicts, and dilemmas as if they originated from within the patient or family rather than the health-care system. It is incumbent for family nurses to examine systems from the family's perspective when outcomes are measured.

Family-Focused Care and Contextual Assessment

Family Context

Robinson (1995) described four ways to conceptualize families and care within a family. The first is to view nursing care for a single individual family member or individuals in which the individual is viewed as foreground and the family unit is perceived as the background. The second perspective is to perceive the care of an individual or a family subgroup and two or more persons with the family identified as the background or the context for the family subgroup. The third view is that of nursing a family group; in this perspective, the family is viewed as distinct, separate, and different from individual members, with the family viewed as foreground and the individual becoming the background. Finally, the nursing care of the individual and family system is a schema that invites consideration of the interactions and effects of the individual on the family and the family on the individual, with both the individual and the family system identified as the foreground. Robinson argues that this schema of family views presents a common language for nurses to discuss family practice and clarifies some understandings about the family unit. Based on this schematic, family-focused care is viewed as the fourth perspective, with the family and individual viewed as the foreground.

Contextual Assessment

A number of traditional measures have been used to assess the home environment, including the Home Observation for the Measurement of Environment (Bradley & Caldwell, 1984; Caldwell & Bradley, 1984), Family Environment Scale (Moos, Insel, & Humphrey, 1974; Moos & Moos, 1986), Family Adaptability and Cohesion Evaluation Scale (Olson, Partner, & Lavee, 1985), and Home Quality Rating Scale (Meyers, Mink, & Nihira, 1990). The Home Observation for the Measurement of Environment is an observational inventory for families of preschool children; the Family Environment Scale and the Family Adaptability and Cohesion Evaluation Scale are used to measure the psychosocial climate of the home; and the Home Quality Rating Scale is designed to assess child-rearing attitudes and family adjustment when a child has a developmental delay. These instruments are usually viewed as environmental measures, but they have mostly been used in research rather than practice to measure member interactions. The value of these family instruments is undisputed, but they may not be practical for clinical use or assessment of family context as defined in the Family Health Model.

Comprehensive assessment of the ecological context is often overlooked in health assessments of individuals and families. Identification of contextual perspectives can provide data about things that are modifiable, as well as things that are fixed, inflexible, or permanent. Contextual assessment allows nurses to differentiate among household membership, family relationships, circumstances, events, conditions, and situated systemic contexts. Data about the context can assist in family-focused practice by providing nurses with the means to identify:

- Contextual factors within the control of the family
- Contextual influences outside the control of the family
- Combinations of internal and external contextual factors that contribute to or inhibit family health, individual well-being, and members' processes of becoming

Assessment data are meaningless unless they are used in conjunction with multiple members to develop, implement, and evaluate a plan of care specific to the goals of individuals and the family.

The Family Context Assessment

The Family Context Assessment (FCA) is a comprehensive tool that can be used to gather individual and family information pertinent to family health (Appendix B). If the FCA has not previously been reviewed, then the reader might find it helpful to review it now and refer back to it as necessary. Although the FCA instrument is suggested for contextual assessment, it is possible that agencies or practice settings may want to modify this instrument, design their own tool, or use aspects of some pre-existing instruments to collect some data. It is highly unlikely that a family nurse would complete the FCA during a single visit but would instead collect some baseline information and then select the areas most pertinent to specific individual, family subsystem, or family concerns. Additional information could be collected over subsequent interactions with the same or other family members. A comprehensive assessment would take a fair amount of time to complete, but cost effectiveness and efficiency might be measured in terms of future timesaving. Use of an electronic record could make previously collected data more easily retrievable and eliminate the need to repeatedly ask the same questions unnecessarily. The nurse may collect data through a face-to-face interview or by using various computer-assisted data collection techniques (e.g., computer kiosks, the Internet, portable computers, telephone call-in) that would minimize time and economic resources.

If the FCA were constructed as an electronic file, then follow-up visits of single members or data related to multiple family members can create a continuous rather than an episodic family record. Agencies, hospitals, and institutions interested in developing electronic family records could incorporate preferred instruments already in use but link information of multiple family members into a single file. Development of an electronic database would enable the use of the file over the lifetime of an individual while retaining links to the family of origin, decreasing the collection of data previously obtained, making family-related data easily accessible, and providing ways to look at intergenerational information. As children mature and leave the family of origin, new family links could be created, but the connections to original records would be retained. An electronic record provides ways that family members could access their own information as well as the opportunity to make the data available to other health-care providers when needed. Agencies and family-focused practices could adapt the FCA to reflect the agency mission, care philosophy, standards of care, and family populations. A family database should include baseline information and be updated whenever a family nurse or other health-care provider has sequential family contact. Deciding on ways to approach the FCA would depend on things such as the purpose of the encounter, availability of family members, and expertise of the assessor. Table 17–1 provides an overview of the breadth of the contextual areas that can be assessed and can serve as a guide for data collection.

ͣͣͣͣͣͣͣ *Cooperative Learning*

Divide into four groups. Each group will look at a different aspect of the Family Context Assessment (see Fig. 17–3; Appendix A). Divide each section of the assessment tool into different areas so that two students are looking at different sections of the assessments. Identify an area to assess in each target area and write questions that might be used with families. Ask each other the questions and evaluate the usefulness of the information gathered. Consider the overall assessment data they would be collecting and ways the data might be used to develop family-focused interventions. List the ideas of the group.

In a class discussion, each group should present its findings about the data collection process and usefulness of data collected.

Table 17–1	Family Contextual Assessment		
Ecological Level	Assessment of Family Health	Planning of Family Health	Issues That Affect Family Health
Microsystem	Family member face-to-face interaction involving one another and significant others about contextual events, situations, or experiences associated with the household production of health Member characteristics Family status (e.g., education, economics, culture religion) Dyadic and triadic member interactions Individual and family health routines Neighborhood and community context Availability of health services	Care related to individual member health and illness needs, family interactions, functional status, and health routines that optimize developmental processes and well-being associated with individual and family health ▪ Six core functional processes ▪ Family health routines	Individual factors: ▪ Member biophysical ▪ Self-esteem ▪ Intelligence ▪ Motivation Family household factors: ▪ Family membership ▪ Economics ▪ Culture ▪ Religion ▪ Neighborhood Neighborhood or community factors: ▪ Schools ▪ Churches ▪ Health-care providers ▪ Recreational facilities ▪ Employment opportunities
Mesosystem	Relationships between family members and connections to others in which at least one member interacts	Peer relationships Work and play Home and school Home and church Home and neighborhood	Congruence between settings in which members interact and the household niche Levels of respect, civility, and tolerance for ambiguity of settings outside the family boundaries
Exosystem	Settings where significant decisions are made that have the potential to affect the family health of members even when the member connected to the setting does not interact in the decisions	Peer groups Parents' employment School administration Local government National policies	Effects of decisions on individual and family health Availability of supportive systems for meeting individual and family health needs
Macrosystem	Attitudes, values, ideologies, and behaviors of the larger society that organize institutional life, mandate or negate social supports, alter public policy, and define health policy	Shared societal assumptions Social policy Shared ideologies	Media messages (e.g., substance abuse, violence, nutrition, exercise) Valuing of disparate groups based upon sexuality, race, ethnicity, religion, and so on Level of marginalization of vulnerable members Individuation versus collective orientation of support and care

Genograms and Eco-maps

Genograms and eco-maps provide additional ways to collect assessment data, represent relationships important to family members, and summarize some data relevant to family health. A genogram provides a way to quickly visualize data of interest about multiple generations. A family genogram usually identifies family of origin relationships, birth dates, marital or partner relationships, occupations, offspring, deaths, and health-related data. Genograms can also be used to demonstrate the strength of attachments, conflict in relationships, and estranged and broken relationships (McGoldrick & Gerson, 1985). Eco-maps provide overviews of relationships between a family and other institutions, agencies, and persons, with variations in the connecting lines signifying the nature of the relationships. Thorough discussions about genograms and eco-maps are accessible in other nursing texts (Friedman, 1998c; Hanson, 2001b; Roth, 1989; Wright & Leahey,

2000). If a family nurse lacks experience in their use, then some time spent engaged in learning activities is suggested.

Culturally Competent Family-Focused Care

Much has already been said throughout this text about the importance of culturally competent care. Learning about culture and becoming competent in family assessment cannot be fully learned in any classroom. Although basic skills can be taught, it is through practice and experience that one realizes the full breadth needed to address unique cultural needs. Although one might be viewed as culturally competent in providing care to one cultural group, it requires great sensitivity on the part of a family nurse to discriminate his or her abilities and limitations in working within diverse cultural contexts. Family-focused care demands competence and sensitivity from practitioners as they practice and personally validate whether or not they are proficiently and equitably addressing needs. Nurses who sense their adversity toward persons of color, foreign-speaking individuals, hypochondriacs, homosexuals, welfare recipients, or others need to take remedial steps to overcome stumbling blocks if they desire to respond in culturally competent ways. It is insightful for nurses to ask themselves whether they are novices or experts in their ability to be culturally responsive to different individuals.

Family Communication

Interviewing and communication skills are necessary for collecting meaningful family data, responding to families in culturally competent ways, and developing interventions that include multiple members. Nurses learn basic communication skills for individual interactions early in their nursing education, but more advanced skills are needed for working with family subsystems, families, community groups, and interdisciplinary teams. Although nurses may be equipped to gather some data through histories and physical assessments, they may require to more fully develop communication skills relevant to family health. For instance, nurses may find themselves less comfortable or prepared to address topics in communication such as goal exploration, engagement, exploring alternative solutions, or collaboration. The third edition of the Calgary Family Assessment Model provides an excellent resource to use in conjunction with the Family Health Model because it provides specific ways to approach an interactive interview using linear and circular questions to identify family health needs (Wright & Leahey, 2000). Family-focused care commands a need for nurses who are capable communicators and able to attend to family values, perceptions, and needs. Time spent in roleplay and clinical experiences observed and discussed with faculty or preceptors can enhance family nurses' abilities to refine and optimize communication skills so that time with family members is productive and achieves intended goals.

Family-Focused Care and Functional Assessment

To fully understand the implications of family-focused care, family clinicians must not only have a thorough understanding about family context but must also be cognizant of the impact of functional processes on health. Concerns and coping with the instrumental aspects of life and activities of daily living are closely related to family members' interactive relationships. *Activities of daily living* are capacities needed by all persons to attain, maintain, and regain the usual life processes that sustain life and family health. Examples of activities of daily living include preparing meals, eating, sleeping, and exercising.

Instrumental aspects of life are the unique and specific capacities needed by individual members and families to relate to the embedded context where they live, work, and play. For example, instrumental activities might be related to communication, learning, transportation, problem solving, or physical or mental limitations. Family Functional

Assessment (FFA) should ascertain the strengths and limitations of individuals, family subsystems, and the family as a whole. Family-focused care seeks to build strong dyadic and triadic relationships within and external to the family that potentiate family strengths, minimize limitations, and optimize resource use. It is posited that strong trust and respectful relationships formed between family subsystems and nurses have great potential to positively enhance family health by creating bidirectional channels for teaching and learning. Issues related to the FFA and the core functional processes include:

- Operationalizing what members mean by health, illness, and family health
- Understanding the complexity of family dyads and triads
- Differentiating innate member traits
- Discovering relationships with networks of persons, agencies, institutions, and providers outside of the family microsystem
- Linking functional expectations with developmental stages of individual members and the family as a whole

Table 17–2 suggests the types of assessment questions to ask related to the core functional processes and provides some considerations when planning care.

Although the developmental stage may be directly linked to the context of the family, the effects of member and family status are expressed through actions, relationships, and interactions. Steinglass, Bennett, Wolin, and Reiss (1987) have provided a way to envision family development from an early, middle, and late phase perspective (Table 17–3).

In each phase, families have specific goals to accomplish and tasks that correspond to either normative or non-normative family situations. These developmental phases, goals, and tasks can provide important assessment data for nurses and other health-care practitioners as they plan care. The FFA should include assessment of families' core functional processes and family developmental stages. Family-focused care implies that data should be updated with individual and family encounters.

Communication and Family Functional Assessment

Family-focused communication related to the FFA must include opportunities to obtain multiple family perspectives, as well as those of distinct individuals comprising the household.

According to Wright and Leahey (2000), "Family functional assessment is concerned with details of how individuals actually behave in relation to one another" (p. 128). The authors describe *instrumental functioning,* or the things that regularly occur related to the usual daily activities or business of the family. In comparison, *expressive functioning* pertains to nine distinct family areas: emotional communication, verbal communication, nonverbal communication, circular communication, problem solving, roles, influence and power, beliefs, and alliances and coalitions. Instrumental and expressive issues are closely intertwined with family health concerns. For example, if the father in a family with two school-age children has just recently experienced a myocardial infarction and suffered severe cardiac damage, the family has both instrumental and expressive issues. Instrumental issues pertain to diet changes, a need to stop smoking or alter patterns of alcohol consumption, and a need to begin a rehabilitation program that includes progressive activity and exercise. Expressive issues related to roles might be:

- How is my husband's not working going to affect our ability to pay the bills?
- Who is going to help with child-care tasks while Dad is sick?
- Is Grandma going to want to come to stay with us?
- Daddy was supposed to coach our baseball game on Saturday. Who is going to do it now?
- What is the length of time that Dad is going to be off work?

Table 17-2 Using the Core Functional Processes in Family Assessment

Core Functional Processes	Assessment of the Core Functional Process	Planning for Family-Focused Care
Caregiving	Who requires care? What kinds of care are needed? What stresses are related to the caregiving activities? What are individual and family strengths and limitations? Are care needs short or long term?	Describe family priorities and goals. Identify how individual and family strengths can be maximized and limitations minimized. Ascertain which needs are usual care needs versus those that are short-term needs. Determine what supports are available.
Cathexis	What levels of attachment are identified among individuals, dyads, triads, and persons external to the family? What are the ways emotional bonds are expressed? How do family members respond to and interact with one another when they are less attached? How are attachments symbolized in the family?	Determine whether family members are mostly satisfied or dissatisfied with current patterns. Identify relationship strengths on which interventions can be built. Describe resources that might assist in meeting expressed concerns.
Celebration	How does the family celebrate itself and special times? What significant traditions do all members celebrate? What parts do various members play in family fun and ritual celebrations? What roles do culture and religion play?	Identify differences in importance of family events versus individual activities. Determine the amount of time, energy, and other resources the family wants to contribute to celebrations. Consider possible alternatives that might be of interest to members. Consider whether associated activities or roles might be distributed more effectively.
Change	What changes previously faced were viewed as having positive outcomes? How many changes has the family encountered in the past 6 months? Year? How do different members experience change?	Evaluate ways different members handle change. Differentiate between internal and external family factors that influence the change. Identify the alternatives possible in the ways for handling the change.
Communication	In what ways do members express ideas and feelings to one another? How do individuals express instrumental, spiritual, and emotional needs? What about the family? When and how does the family emphasize its beliefs, values, and expected goals?	Determine individual members' need for skills. Ascertain optimal ways for expressing valued concerns and needs for assistance. Identify family resources and build on them.
Connectedness	What are the family boundaries, and who decides what they are? What are the voices outside of the family to which members attend? How are members involved with others in the neighborhood? What are the communities of interest?	Ascertain which family boundaries assist the family in meeting goals and which create roadblocks. List resources available in the neighborhood and community. Identify areas related to diversity that are strengths and limitations for the family. Compare and contrast supports available from extended family and social networks.
Coordination	Who decides how resources are accessed and used? What are the roles of various family members? How does the family solve problems and make decisions? Whose priorities get met first?	Determine alternative modes for meeting expressed family needs. Identify options for problem solving. Determine whether important family priorities are being ignored. Describe options in ways resources might be used.

Table 17–3   **Family Goals and Developmental Tasks**

Developmental Stage	Goals to Accomplish	Normative Family Tasks	Non-normative Family Tasks
Early phase	Establish boundaries Identity formation	Have optimism about the future Develop independent free-standing system Basic rules for family functioning Loyalty to families of origin Negotiation Space distribution and use	Similar tasks to normative families Challenges and accommodations related to the non-normative issue Deciding whether non-normative issue will become the organizing principle for family themes
Middle phase	Commitment Stability	Focus on day-to-day activities Commitment to a finite number of organizing themes Commitment to stable and consistent rules Emergence of set of repetitive behaviors for organizing daily life Near the end of this phase, an inordinate amount of loss is sustained by family members and many new patterns are newly challenged	All aspects of family life become organized around the non-normative concerns and result in reinforcement and maintenance of the behaviors Family becomes fully organized to prevent the destabilizing effect of the non-normative event
Late phase	Clarification Legacy	Vacillation between shifts in family life and stabilization of family life Shift from present to future focus Focus on commonality rather than uniqueness Preserving identity and transmitting to next generation	Decide whether non-normative event will become part of the family legacy and how it will be packaged Moving away from the extreme rigidity that becomes part of life in the middle phase Risk of distortion of family identity and stability

Source: Steinglass, P, et al: The Alcoholic Family. Basic Books, New York, 1987, with permission.

Other expressive areas give rise to different sets of questions for individuals and the family.

Families are in continual transition, and these evolutions incessantly tax communication resources within families. For example, Golan (1986) said that the inability to cut loose or create meaningful distances from relationships, persons, places, or things from the past might create inherent decision-making problems when families try to make changes. Families in transition may have the inability to separate from the past, adapt to new roles or conditions, make decisions, or locate and mobilize resources for implementing decisions (Golan). Family-focused care means that nurses must communicate effectively to engage multiple members in change and interventions related to health concerns. Although traditional practices usually engage single individuals, family-focused care requires the ability to interview family members together so that interactions can be observed and interactional responses identified. Ritualization of family routines differ from family to family and also among routines in a given family (Denham, 1995). It is proposed that either very high or very low ritualization can result in family stresses that are not very conducive to family health. At one end of the continuum, high ritualization might result in obsessive-compulsive behaviors, whereas very low ritualization might result in total chaos (Fig. 17–1). The goal for family health is a more balanced level of ritualization, but characteristic behaviors have yet to be fully described in relationship to health promotion, family health, or adherence to therapeutic regimens.

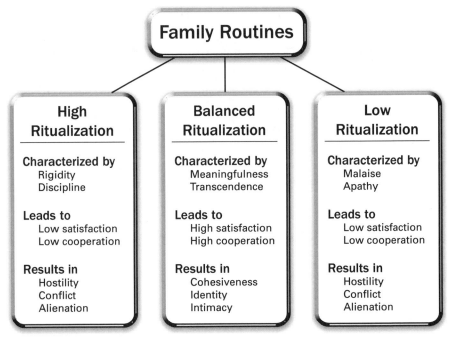

Figure 17–1 Ritualization in family routines. (From Denham, SA: Family routines: A construct for considering family health. Holistic Nursing Practice 9(4):18, 1995.)

Cooperative Learning

Divide into seven groups. Each group should focus on a different core functional processes. Select a recorder for each group. Groups should turn to Chapter 10 and review the materials that describe the core functional process they are assigned. Using Figure 17–1 as a guide, each group should identify questions they might ask individual members about themselves, about others in the family, and about the family. (If also using the Wright & Leahey, 2000 text, refer to Chapter 4.) Note whether questions address cognitive, affective, or behavioral areas. Keep lists of these questions. Describe how you would use the data collected through this assessment to develop family-focused interventions.

In a class discussion about assessment of the core functional processes, compare and contrast the kinds of information obtained with questions that address cognitive, affective, and behavioral areas. Discuss how data concerning core functional processes could be used in family-focused care.

Family-Focused Care and Family Health Routines

The functions of rituals are many, but they can all assist the family to achieve a sense of solidarity, enhance identity, regenerate commitments, and strengthen loyalties. Rituals

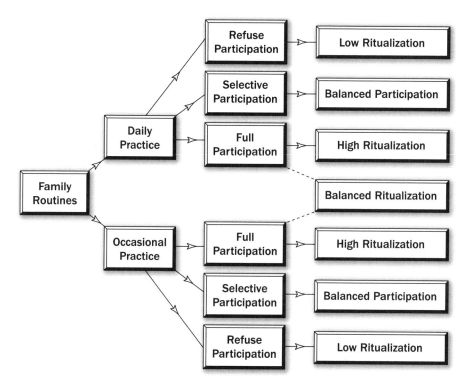

Figure 17–2 Participation in routines and level of ritualization. (From Denham, SA: Family routines: A construct for considering family health. Holistic Nursing Practice 9(4):20, 1995.)

provide order, links with traditions, and a form or structure; give families roots and wings; increase organization; and reduce chaos. Rituals can promote or diminish healing (Boyle, 1998). Families that tend toward moderation in family health routines rather than being either highly ritualized or lacking rituals may possess more resilient family health paradigms (Denham, 1995). Family routines can be characterized by degrees of ritualization and participation. Figure 17–2 provides a schematic that suggests some ways high ritualization, low ritualization, and balanced ritualization may differ.

Individuals and families differ in their levels of involvement and ritualization, ways of participation in routines, and daily or occasional practices. Various types of routines can be identified in households, including patterned behaviors, habits, rituals, individual routines, family routines, family health routines, family traditions, and family celebrations (Table 17–4). Assessment of different forms of routines can provide insight into family themes and identify practices that might be pertinent to family routines.

Rituals are often influenced by past experiences in the family of origin. Daily rituals and lifecycle rituals may be affected by different factors that may affect one's sense of self or others (Imber-Black & Roberts, 1992). It might be helpful to think about possible styles of rituals within families as:

- Minimized (i.e., few rituals that convey little sense of family identity through time)
- Interrupted (i.e., response to crisis events more important than ritual practice)

Table 17–4   **Varied Types of Routine Family Behaviors**

Types of Patterned Behavior	Definition
Patterned behaviors	Repetitive behaviors conducted by individuals and families that are mostly unconscious and interactive actions but can be recalled and discussed.
Habits	Repetitive behaviors engaged in by individuals that may have both conscious and unconscious components and either impair or promote individual well-being and processes of becoming. Habits may have special meanings for individuals and families, be difficult to alter, have links to family health routines, and create bonds with others outside the family.
Individual routines	Time-bounded routines with clear-cut beginnings and endings and a conscious awareness that a special behavior is occurring. These activities often pre-empt other behaviors; may have strong symbolic components; and are usually linked to a tradition, celebration, or special family event.
Family routines	Routines that are imbued with the meanings associated with individual routines, but they are also given special meaning and attention by multiple members. Participation involves more than a single member and may be supported by kin or extended family. Although these behaviors may be associated with symbolic meanings and special family times, they may also be organizing behaviors of the family structure.
Family health routines	Routines that include the meanings of individual and family routines but add elements of health, illness, medical or health perspectives; processes of becoming; well-being; and the holistic aspects of family related to the embedded context and core functional processes.
Family traditions	Specific recurrent behaviors with special meanings for family members. These events require special preparation and are symbolically rich events in which immediate and extended family members participate (e.g., birthdays, vacations, reunions, anniversaries).
Family celebrations	Family routines that often have a unique family quality but link the family to the larger society. These routines are rich with symbolism; involve complex preparations that involve all members; and connect the past, present, and future. Family celebrations may be culture-specific observances, religious holidays (e.g., Christmas, Passover, Kwanzaa), secular holidays (e.g., Thanksgiving, Fourth of July), or rites of passage (e.g., weddings, funerals, baptism, bar mitzvah).

- Rigid and unchanging (i.e., highly prescribed and unvarying behaviors)
- Obligatory (i.e., events are celebrated out of a sense of obligation rather than meaning)
- Imbalanced (i.e., inability to balance members' histories, legacies, and valued rituals)
- Flexible (i.e., capture and express member and family changes over time) (Imber-Black & Roberts, 1992)

Routines may differ in families, with traditional versus nontraditional divisions of labor and based on the character and changing needs of members. Primeau (2000) noted that parents must create and maintain daily routines that are sustainable and meaningful, provide opportunity to shape children's development, and meet the conflicting and competing needs of individual members. When Steinglass et al. (1987) studied structurally intact alcoholic families with reasonable occupational and economic histories, they concluded: "The impact of alcoholism on the fundamental aspects of daily life-daily routines, family rituals, family problem-solving strategies that affects many families dealing with alcoholism so profoundly as to shape the entire course of their life history" (p. 24). It is possible that other health conditions also impact routines.

Families raising children with attention deficit hyperactivity disorder were interviewed about the ways they construct daily schedules and routines. Parents scheduled times for homework, dinner, and free time after considering their children's abilities to concentrate and physiological and emotional needs as well as parental work schedules (Segal & Frank, 1998). Parents often had to change their daily routines in order to develop and use strategies that enabled children's activity competence (Segal & Frank, 1998). Some carefully scheduled and constructed family activities provide families with time and space together that are idealized family images embedded in experiences of togetherness and good relationships. When families have children with special needs, the routine times together often include sharing and providing learning opportunities.

Ludwig (1998) conducted a study of white, college-educated, unemployed, middle-class women to see how they changed their routines in later life. Findings indicated that although these women used routines to care for their well-being, they reported doing so to a lesser extent than when children lived at home or when they worked. Subjects desired more freedom as they aged, and health-care interventions should be compatible with these changing themes and routines. Although nurses have largely ignored family routines and rituals, a growing body of literature indicates that they could contribute to better family assessments and interventions.

Assessment of Family Health Routines

Families are paradoxical in that they are both resilient and fragile. The influence of time, knowledge, perceptions, experience, and events affect boundaries, values, behaviors, and social relationships. Interactions among traditions of cultural, ethnic, and spiritual origin over the life course impact accommodations to normative and non-normative life events and take on patterned characteristics. Routines may differ in patterns of rhythm, cadence, accent, quality, and meaningfulness based on various factors that need to be assessed:

- Process factors (e.g., relationships, perceptions, motivation)
- Resource factors (e.g., information, health insurance, skills, support, experience)
- Form factors (e.g., plasticity or rigidity, resilience or transitory, stable or volatile, cohesiveness or fragmented, openness or closedness)

Table 17–5 provides an overview of areas related to routines to assess when planning for health-care needs.

Daily routines provide observable expressions for families and practitioners to discuss the social construction of family health that most consistently occurs within the household niche. Planning effective care depends on the identification of high-priority family goals that are congruent with values, themes, ecocultural niches, ecocultural domains, and routines. Inclusion of the family in the assessment, planning, and evaluation processes is essential if consequential goals are to be met and meaningful outcomes achieved. Family routines have similar properties, dimensions, and variations across some families, but unique differences must be identified for effective planning, intervention, and evaluation (Table 17–6).

Interventions can be maximized when they are harmonious with other family features. Themes associated with family workload, access to health services, family economics, and response to social support are crucial factors for the development of facilitative interventions. Family-focused care implies that care providers understand that changes in tenacious behaviors are often difficult and that members overtaxed by stress, caregiver burdens, or comfortable in the safety and security of usual routine may have difficulty accommodating changes. Family care must be imparted with flexible yet comprehensive approaches that use the available resources to support members over time as accommodations are made.

Table 17–5 **Assessment and Planning Related to Family Health Routines**

Family Health Routines	Assessment of Family Routines	Planning for Family-Focused Care
Family values	What ideas, attitudes, and beliefs do members regard as meaningful? Which values do members use to guide behaviors? How do religious, cultural, and social influences affect patterned behaviors? What is the impact of popular media and current policies on family values?	Describe important member variations in values and perceptions. Differentiate between family rules and member values. Identify the contextual influences that impact the family. Identify what information and skills family members need to reconcile beliefs or perceptions with other less accepted realities.
Family themes	What are the norms of daily member interactions? What are the organizing family themes that most members ascribe? How do members regularly express relevant family themes?	Identify ways to assist family members recognize organizing themes. Describe various health-promoting ways to express a family theme. Determine ways family themes can support family health.
Ecocultural niche	How does the family household affect members' health routines? What factors in the embedded context influence family health? How do members' use of the core functional processes affect family health routines?	Identify the strengths and limitations within the household that influence family health. Describe the resources and threats in the embedded context that impact family health routines. Differentiate alternative ways the core functional processes can create meaningful family health routines.
Ecocultural domains: ▨ Caregiver roles ▨ Role relationships ▨ Child play mates ▨ Information sources ▨ Family workload ▨ Family economics ▨ Access to health services ▨ Home safety ▨ Social support ▨ Cultural influences ▨ Community influences ▨ Child care tasks	What unique ways do the ecocultural domains affect family health routines? How are family members' health routines affected differently by the domains? Are there ecocultural domains in which family routines are ineffectual?	Discuss family priorities pertaining to the ecocultural domains. Identify relationships between family health routines and the ecocultural domains. Describe the roles of various members in ecocultural domains that affect family health routines.
Family health routines: ▨ Self-care routines ▨ Safety and prevention ▨ Mental health behaviors ▨ Family care ▨ Illness care ▨ Member caregiving	What are the unique family social constructions of family rituals, traditions, and celebrations? Which perceptions about routines do members share? What is the quality of family health routines? How do members differ in their levels of routine participation? How effective are routines in helping members attain goals?	Identify the present existing routines. Describe alternative ways to create routines applicable to family health concerns. Identify ways the family has deconstructed routines and constructed new ones. List ways a specific routine might be reframed to better achieve family goals. Determine ways members can participate in optimizing family health routines.

Table 17–6   Routine Properties, Dimensions, and Variations

Routine Properties	Routine Dimensions	Routine Variations
Routine type	▪ Individual routine ▪ Family routine ▪ Family health routine ▪ Family ritual ▪ Family tradition ▪ Family celebration	▪ Ritual selection ▪ Area of ritualization ▪ Level of ritualization ▪ Beginning and endings ▪ Discreteness ▪ Focus
Regulatory behaviors	Temperamental properties: ▪ Energy level ▪ Interactional distance ▪ Behavioral range	▪ Extent across family life ▪ Importance to members ▪ Expectations over the life course ▪ Cohesiveness of family ▪ Homeostasis
Behavioral characteristics	Family identity: ▪ Rhythmicity ▪ Intensity ▪ Variability ▪ Predictability	▪ Rigidity of performance ▪ Clarity of behaviors ▪ Patterning before, after, and during ▪ Intentionality ▪ Deliberateness ▪ Affective expressiveness
Participants	▪ Who participates ▪ Rules of participation ▪ Where participation occurs ▪ Length of participation ▪ Degree of orthodoxy	▪ Role relationships ▪ Differentiated roles for children, elderly, kin or extended family, others
Meaningfulness	▪ Family values, goals, and themes ▪ Associated symbols ▪ Heritage factors	▪ Linkages to past and future ▪ Intergenerational transmission ▪ Keeper of the rituals ▪ Transcendence ▪ Legacy

𝕏 Cooperative Learning

Review the family health routines discussed in Chapter 13. Divide into groups so that several students will be working with each of the family routines. Each group should compare and contrast the assigned routine, planning, and interventions that might be associated with health promotion, chronic illness care, and end-of-life care. List assessment questions and describe interventions for each area (i.e., health promotion, chronic illness care, and end-of-life care). In a class discussion, each group should present its findings.

Communication and Family Health Routine Assessment

Family-focused care emphasizes the need to assess and plan care with multiple members, preferably building on strengths of family dyads and triads. Family Health Routine Assessments should identify agreement and disagreement about areas that impact family health, including:

▪ Rituals, traditions, and celebrations
▪ Religious beliefs and affiliations
▪ Issues surrounding race, ethnicity, and culture

- Valuing and perceptions about habits, changes in patterned behaviors, and daily routines
- Collective memory about individual and family past
- Satisfaction with present habits, patterned behaviors, and routines
- Hopes for future life course alterations

Larson (2000) suggested that eight processes associated with family orchestration exist: planning, organizing, balancing, anticipating, interpreting, forecasting, perspective shifting, and meaning making. Assessment and interventions that are germane to routines use all these processes.

Nursing care aimed at routines is more effective when interactions include a triadic perspective and include at least two family members. Doing so has the potential to obtain a broader perspective of family themes, resources, strengths, and barriers. Assessment of dyadic and triadic relationships helps determine to whom health information or interventions should be directed (Olsen, Russell, & Sprenkle, 1983; Wright & Leahey, 1994). The nurse should aim to be a neutral observer but should also be able to introduce new ideas and information germane to routines, suggest alternative ways to construct or deconstruct behaviors, and assist members to reframe attitudes and behaviors to address health concerns in accord with family themes and goals.

Family-Focused Care Maps

Family-focused care requires coordinated, comprehensive, and integrated approaches to deliver primary care that addresses unique member and family needs. Broad discussions about the usefulness of care maps exist in the literature (Bergman, 1999; Currie & Harvey, 1998; Ellrodt, Cook, Lee, Cho, Hunt, & Weingarten, 1997; Garbin, 1995; Messer & Ozmar, 1999). Care maps are useful tools for nurse practitioners, family nurses, case managers, and clinicians delivering primary care because they provide approaches to assess, plan, and evaluate quality and cost related to a variety of health-care needs. These are tools developed and used to manage clinical processes, identify potential strategies to achieve health outcomes, guide interventions, and record family responses. Care maps depend on family input and the concerns of individual members. They also include the expertise of multiple disciplines as guidelines and algorithms are created for decision making and care delivery. Care maps can be used to determine variances from policies, standards, guidelines, or protocols and evaluate the effectiveness of interventions in achieving goals. Care maps afford opportunities to consider evidence-based care from individual, family, caregiver, and practitioner perspectives and have the potential to decrease costs and increase quality measures. Care maps can be used across practitioners and settings in association with outcome and performance measures relative to family needs.

Conceptual slippage often occurs when trying to differentiate between critical pathways and clinical pathways. Critical pathways have mostly been viewed from providers' perspectives rather than those of care recipients, with quality mainly measured in terms of cost savings achieved through the avoidance of variances. Critical pathways are most often aimed at acute episodic incidents related to individuals, with little focus on family. It is posited that clinical pathways, in contrast, can use quality measures that allow for life course considerations, target family concerns, and use life course perspectives to understand the household production of health. A *clinical pathway* is a comprehensive method of planning, delivering, and monitoring care (Garbin, 1995). Clinical pathways that focus on achieving family outcomes related to member health and illness needs have not yet been developed and tested, but the concept holds a potential for family-focused practice. The use of diagnostic tools, data collection measures, algorithms, and multifoci family outcomes seem a natural fit with clinical pathways to not only consider variances and cost effectiveness but also weigh evidence related to family perceptions, satisfaction, and outcomes; error and risk reduction; standardization of practice; quality indicators; and caregiver needs. Care maps might include some aspects of clinical pathways and be useful in case management. Case management of family groups that share similar needs for clinical expertise, have comparable contextual needs, and require equivalent care management supports may benefit from the use of care maps or clinical pathways. Family nurses might use what is known about case management and clinical pathways to assume participatory roles and collaborative relationships with other care providers in the design of care maps relevant to specific health and illness foci.

Unfortunately, a scarcity of well-designed research studies that document the effective use of critical or clinical pathways in individual-focused care does little to ensure that pathways or care maps will be useful in family-focused practices. As family-focused practices are conceptualized and care is delivered, it will be vital for family nurses and nurse scientists to collaborate in the development of studies that collect assessment and outcome data in standardized ways and devise methods that lend themselves to reporting outcomes in ways that can be accessible to others. Timely dissemination and ease in access of practice outcomes, research findings, recommendations, and conclusions will enable those in family-focused practices to share the effectiveness and limitations of care strategies that are relevant to family health. Bergman (1999) suggests that knowledge dissemination has been less than effective and networks of practice sites need to be developed to share knowledge, experiences, and validation about the usefulness of guidelines. Judicious sharing about the implementation and usefulness of clinical pathways and care maps related to family-focused care will advance knowledge development and practice outcomes. Practice improvements are most likely to occur when (1) pathways and maps reflect current knowledge and practices and (2) outcomes from guidelines and care management tools are widely disseminated through practice networks and continuing education.

Thorough understandings about family context, functional core processes, and family health routines equip family nurses with a wealth of information to assist in family collaboration in devising interventions that address family health needs. Analysis of assessment data should provide evidence for decision making and may suggest treatment priorities in relationship to the health foci targeted. Planning for a family-focused care map also necessitates time spent reviewing areas related to family health, as well as priorities, goals, supports, and threats (Table 17–7).

Primary concerns of families that health-care professionals need to attend to when care maps are developed are:

- Families' beliefs, values, culture, and perceptions are respected.
- Families can define themselves as they are.
- Families are viewed as experts about themselves.
- Care and services are impartially provided in meaningful ways regardless of family disparities.
- Information, education, and counseling are supplied in ways families understand.
- Ongoing support for family needs is available even when a family's choices conflict with professional perspectives.
- Competent and ethical clinicians work in conjunction with one another to meet family needs across a variety of points of care and time.

Family Participation in Family-Focused Care Maps

As patients are being discharged from acute care centers more seriously ill, today's families are being asked to take increasingly larger responsibilities for the care of members and cope with more complex care needs. Family caregivers administer medications

Table 17–7   Planning a Family-Focused Care Map

Focal Area	Pertinent Questions	Actions to Take	Evaluation of Intervention Processes
Family priorities	What are the family priorities relevant to problems? Do members differ on priorities in significant ways? What are members' greatest concerns related to their priorities?	List the priorities in order of family importance. Discuss differences and reach consensus. Provide information, education, counseling, and resources related to the concerns.	Does priority order change over time? Do members identify differences? What additional information, education, counseling, or resources are needed?
Family goals	What does the family most want to accomplish? What strengths do members view in obtaining their goals? What do members view as the biggest obstacles to their goals?	Rank goals in order of family importance. List ways strengths can be optimized. Identify ways obstacles can be addressed.	Is time effectively used to meet goals? Are there other ways that strengths can be optimized? Are interventions to accomplish goals working? What needs to be altered?
Context concerns	Do members perceive things in similar or different ways? What boundaries affect the family? Which family dyads and triads can be used to address family goals?	Identify areas of agreement that can be built on. Provide information, resources, and supports for creating effective boundaries. List dyadic and triadic assets for achieving goals.	Do areas of agreement potentiate goal achievement? Are there things beyond the family's control that impede their ability to achieve goals? Do the family dyads and triads assist in meeting goals?
Functional concerns	What are the important member roles to consider? What is the motivation for change? Which core processes are needed to support changes?	Describe the levels of participation needed in the proposed plan. Identify rewards in meeting goals. Select interventions to address changes.	How effective and meaningful is member participation? What needs to be done to enhance motivation? Are interventions achieving the desired results?
Family health routine concerns	Which routines are most pertinent? Who will be most affected by changes in routines? What attitudes are expressed about willingness, ability, or fears about altering routines?	Describe routine aspects to be reconstructed or constructed. Discuss feelings about changes in routines. What alternatives can be considered in changing routines?	Has the prescribed regimen been incorporated into the family routine? Identify ways feelings and behaviors affect family priorities and goals Who is and is not participating in the routines?
Supports available	What things are viewed as supportive in meeting goals? Which persons outside the family are seen as supports? What resources are available?	Identify ways to incorporate supports. Find ways to include external supports. Identify, provide, or connect family with additional resources as needed.	Are there additional supports needed to achieve goals? Are persons viewed as supportive assisting in meeting goals? What resources have been used effectively, and what else is needed?
Threats present	What are the greatest threats to accomplishing goals from family and clinician perspectives? What are the actual threats? What are the perceived threats?	Discuss differences in family and clinician perspective and ways to overcome them. Describe responses to actual threats. List alternative ways for coping with perceived threats.	Are differences viewed as barriers? What alternative responses might be possible? Have effective ways been identified to reduce threats?

around the clock, monitor intravenous chemotherapy, oversee the medical needs of chronic renal patients, change sterile dressings, do urinary catheterization, respond to in-home diabetic and asthmatic emergencies, manage pumps for pain management, and operate ventilators. Additionally, families arrange care for complex care needs with multiple providers, coordinate care prescribed by multiple providers, access the Internet for medical information, make decisions about over-the-counter medications, use alternative therapies, and work with complicated insurance provider systems. Families assume pseudo-medical roles with little or no preparation and provide care similar to that which professional providers would charge significant fees.

In individual-focused medical care, clients are the recipients of care predetermined by the experts or health professionals, with little emphasis placed on their input or feedback. Inclusion of families in planning assessments, determining ways assessments will be implemented, and deciding about care and services to be provided will enhance family care. Family participation in the clinical education of nurses and other health-care professionals affords alternative perspectives. Family involvement in the development of policies and support services might offer valuable insights that are overlooked by professionals. Discussions about affordability, accessibility, and appropriateness of care might also be enhanced by the inclusion of consumer family viewpoints. The focus of programs and services aligned with family populations needs and safety net issues distinct to particular populations could improve their value. Ways to systematically obtain family feedback about care, services, and support programs are needed. Including family consumers in the design of data collection tools, determinations about ways the tools will be implemented, and the interpretations of findings could further evaluation processes and provide directions for future changes. Family input should not be viewed as a form of tokenism; rather, it should be revered as critical to family-focused practice. Greater value for the inclusion of families in all aspects of practice will come as nurse educators and others identify their importance.

👪 *Cooperative Learning*

Review a family case study. Examine the family's priorities and goals. Identify assessment questions you would ask of individuals and the family about context, function, and routines. Identify three to five questions in each area and describe the types of interventions that might be implemented. Describe ways to evaluate whether family priorities and goals are met. In a class discussion, compare your findings with those of your classmates.

Interdisciplinary Approaches to Family-Focused Care

Interdisciplinary practices that move the care focus from institutional care to family household and community context are yet to be fully developed. Family health has ubiquitous variables that demand different interventions and care. Interdisciplinary care currently administered from institutional perspectives is often shortsighted in its focus on the family. Single unidirectional interventions without consideration of the confounding and mediating factors unique to family households may be wastes of valuable health resources because the complexities of family health require systemic approaches different from those in traditional medical care.

Interdisciplinary care from family-focused perspectives is calling on new creativity, innovation, and redesign of care modalities. Many commonly cite the example of how although a half-full glass represents an optimistic perspective, a half-empty glass describes the pessimistic view. However, another viewpoint less often suggested is that there is actually twice as much glass as needed. Although questions of effectiveness and efficiency are included in discussions about outcomes and quality, careful and critical evaluation is needed to determine whether what has been accomplished is needed at all. Making care systems more effective and efficient will be relatively unproductive if, in fact, the care system never touches the real societal needs for family care services. The 21st century is clamoring for ways to develop new partnerships in which care systems are redesigned to use resources in ways that best meet the health-care needs of the world's families.

Summary

Nurses who want to provide family-focused care must build on care provided to individuals and conceptualize practice more broadly so that it includes family health care. Although some clinical or practice issues may be similar when discussing either individual or family care, many factors differ, including relationships, site of delivery, and longevity of interactions. Although technical nurses may be able to provide individual care, family-focused care is a professional scope of practice that requires specialized knowledge and skills. Baccalaureate education can provide nurses with an introduction to theories, knowledge, and skills related to family-focused care, but one becomes a specialist through graduate and doctoral studies. Family-focused care has not yet been recognized or promoted by most educators or practitioners. Significant questions yet to be answered about family-focused care include:

■ What benefits are associated with family-focused care?
■ Who will bear the cost of services, and how is care to be financed?
■ What are the options for service delivery?
■ How is family health promoted, maintained, and improved?
■ Who is responsible and competent enough to provide family care?
■ How will family-focused care alter life course and risk behaviors?
■ What social and economic policies are needed to shape family-focused practices?
■ What supports are most needed by families to increase the household production of health?

Family-focused care appears to have the potential to:

■ Respond more effectively to family rather than practitioner needs.
■ Use health-care resources to meet a broader spectrum of society's health needs.
■ Address health needs from developmental, intergenerational, and life course perspectives.
■ Integrate holistic care into each client encounter.
■ Develop collaborative interdisciplinary practices aimed at health needs.
■ Provide more effective, efficient, and robust ways to address family household perspectives.
■ Move health practice out of institutions and into community or neighborhood settings.

The Family Health Model is presented as a pragmatic argument and a dialectic to engage inquiry and discussion about the potentials inherent in moving the focus of health care from individual- to family-focused care and encourage conversations about the future of nursing practice. Nurses seem to be logical professional players who are well-prepared to assume leadership roles in present and future family-focused care and practices.

Test Your Knowledge

1. Thoroughly describe conceptual differences between individual- and family-focused care.

2. List four knowledge areas or skills that a nurse providing family-focused care might need that are different in some ways from that which individual care providers might need.

3. Identify three things that would have to change in your individual practice if you were to be able to truly provide family-focused care.

4. Describe the kinds of things a nurse would address in a Family Context Assessment.

5. Explain what a nurse would do with the data obtained after completing an FFA.

6. Identify specific concerns that the nurse might have when completing a Family Health Routines Assessment.

7. Describe how a nurse might evaluate the effectiveness of family-focused care.

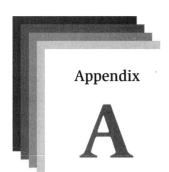

Appendix   # Glossary

A

Accommodation: Proactive social constructions made by individuals, family subsystems, and families in response to interactions within the household and larger contextual systems that contradict, threaten, or compete with accepted family norms.

Actual environment: The realized environment where individuals are present and life events occur.

Adaptation: Passive social constructions made by individuals, family subsystems, and families in response to interactions within the household and larger contextual systems that contradict, threaten, or compete with accepted family norms. It is a way to understand how actions, behaviors, and even biological responses are modulated.

Caregiving: One of the core processes important to health. A concern for other family members generated from close intimate relationships and member affections, resulting in watchful attention, thoughtfulness, and actions linked to members' development, health, and illness needs. Active accommodation to the changing needs (e.g., physical, emotional, social, contextual) of developing persons within the household niche over the life course.

Caretender: A maternal role in which the greatest responsibilities for the core processes of family health (i.e., caregiving, cathexis, celebration, change, communication, connectedness, and coordination) are assumed in order to meet daily and incidental individual and family needs related to chronic illness, caring for members with disabilities, enabling ill members to regain health, protecting members from getting sick when others are ill, nurturing members who have terminal illnesses, and attending to end-of-life care needs.

Cathexis: One of the core processes important to health. The emotional bond that develops between a developing person and those cared for as the developing person invests emotional and psychic energy in the loved one.

Celebration: One of the core processes important to health. Tangible form of shared meaning in which formal celebrations, family traditions, and family leisure are used to commemorate times, days, and events in ways that distinguish them from usual daily routines across the life course.

Change: One of the core processes important to health. A dynamic, nonlinear process that implies altering or modifying the form, direction, and outcome of the original identity by substituting alternatives.

Chronosystem: An accounting for time experienced by individuals, family subsystems, families, and others in response to the embedded context experience.

Communication: One of the core processes important to health. The primary way parents socialize children about health beliefs, values, attitudes, and behaviors and use information, knowledge, and actions applicable to individual and family health.

Connectedness: One of the core processes important to health. The ways individuals are committed and linked to family, educational, cultural, spiritual, political, social, professional, legal, economic, and commercial interests.

Coordination: One of the core processes important to health. A cooperative sharing of resources, skills, abilities, and information within a family and with the larger contextual environment to optimize individuals' health potentials, maximize the household production of health, and achieve family goals.

Core processes: The conceptual idea used to describe concepts germane to family's functional status and family health that can be targeted by nurses to enable family members to realize health potentials. These processes are caregiving, cathexis, celebration, change, communication, connectedness, and coordination.

Deconstruction: To take apart ideas, mindsets, relationships, hierarchies, and current worldviews and critique meanings, determine implications not clearly stated, and gain new insights.

Developing person: Individual from birth to death who has the potential to positively and negatively influence and be influenced by multiple environments and larger contexts over time.

Developmental niche: The household niche and multiple social, cultural, and psychological environments in which members interact on a consistent or regular basis over time that influence developing persons' well-being and processes of becoming.

Dyadic units: Interpersonal relationships between two individual family members. External dyads are initially formed with family members, but they later include others outside the family boundaries.

Ecocultural domains: Twelve categories of family life that describe the family themes germane to family identity and routines. These domains include variables imposed by contextual resources and constraints and family values, goals, and accommodations.

Ecocultural factors: Variables that are produced by the context or result from interactions within the context. They are the themes that families use to organize their daily behaviors and family health routines.

Ecocultural niche: The cultural, geographical, social, economic, and political surroundings and history (e.g., proximity of kin, health conditions imposed by the environment, stresses imposed by neighborhood conditions, employment opportunities) that influence the ways family members value themes and practice routines in their homes, households, and sociocultural environment. It is the unique ways family members perceive their traditions, value symbols, and include or exclude factors into the organization and practices of everyday life.

Ecocultural theory: Theory applicable to all cultures because it gives credence to the intense meanings of environment and assumes the family's viewpoint about goals, values, and needs. Family-constructed meanings of circumstances, proactive responses to those circumstances, and the development and components of daily routines are key aspects for analysis of family interactions.

Ecological model: A model that allows one to view human development from interaction perspectives that occur between a developing person and environmental determinants.

Ecology of human development: The progressive mutual accommodation that occurs over the life course between developing persons and changing environments. Past, present, and future household niches in which persons live and interact with their larger contextual systems mediate development processes.

Ecosystem: A subset of the larger environment with elements of wholeness and interdependent parts or "an arrangement of mutual dependencies in a population by which the whole operates as a unit and thereby maintains a viable environmental relationship" (Hawley, 1986, p. 431).

Embedded: To be embedded implies that a developing person dwells within a context in which multiple environmental actions occur. Although the interactions have consequences, the developing person may have no awareness of these relationships or effects.

Embedded family context: The ecological environments and nested relationships that affect family health over the life course.

Exosystem: One or more settings that may not directly involve the individual as an active participant but one that includes events that affect individuals and families even when they do not particiapte.

Family: A collection of individuals with a general commitment to the well-being of one another and who label themselves as family.

Family context: The multiple environments that affect and are affected by developing persons over time. All of the environments where individual members interact or larger contextual systems that have potential to act on developing persons, family subsystems, and families.

Family-focused care: Nursing care that perceives the whole family as the unit of care even when singular individuals within family households are the focus of care. Family-focused care is an interactive process in which the members, family nurse, health-care professionals, and others collaborate to devise, implement, and evaluate a plan of care specific to family needs. The family nurse collaborates with persons-in-context to identify outcomes, objectives, and strategies that address the well-being and processes of becoming relevant to developing persons, family subsystems, families, household niches, and larger contextual systems.

Family functioning: The individual and cooperative processes used by developing persons to dynamically engage with one another and their diverse environments over the life course. These interactive member processes have the potential to assist developing persons, family subsystems, and families as a whole to attain, sustain, maintain, and regain individual and family health.

Family health: A complex phenomenon that includes the complex systems, interactions, relationships, and processes with the potential to maximize the processes of becoming, enhance individual and family well-being, capitalize on the household production of health, and make the best use of contextual resources.

Family health paradigm: The ways developing persons within unique families interpret health behaviors as meaningful and elect to engage in patterned behaviors that affect health.

Family health routines: Patterns of dynamic behaviors relevant to individual and family health that are rather consistently adhered to by individuals, family subsystems, and families within a household niche and in relation to larger contextual systems.

Family household: The domicile maintained and resided in by developing members. This residence is more than merely a physical structure; it also includes the immediate surroundings; material goods; tangible and intangible family resources; and interactions between individuals, family subsystems, family, and larger contextual systems over the life course. The residence or place where individuals abide and form dyadic and triadic relationships has a potential to negate or potentiate health. The household includes the family shelter and adjoining properties, material goods possessed by the members, and the available social and economic resources.

Family identity: The dynamic ways developing members within a family microsystem view themselves and collectively interpret memories and meanings of unique affiliations and attachments to persons, places, and things.

Family leisure: Informal, usually home-based activities that have minimal costs but that provide multiple members opportunities to interact in casual, relaxed ways as they participate together (e.g., playing games, watching television or home videos, gardening, cookouts).

Family microsystem: Individuals, family subsystems, extended family members, and intergenerational relationships that characterize family as a whole. Family microsystems usually identify a household niche in which they reside and interact with larger contextual systems.

Family-to-context: Relationships that occur between a family and embedded contextual settings beyond the boundaries of the household niche.

Family traditions: Formally organized family times such as vacations, weekend getaways, family reunions, and other unique events that are characteristic of a particular family.

Formal celebrations: Prescribed events with expectations that former behaviors will be repeated and used to commemorate meaningful events tied to family identity (e.g., birthdays, anniversaries, weddings, holidays, family reunions, religious practices). They usually involve extended family members and close friends and take extensive member commitment, planning time, and cost.

Functional processes: Member interactions that potentiate, negate, threaten, mediate, and enhance individual and family health. These processes can be best understood through the dyadic and triadic interactions within families and those formed with others outside the household niche.

Gatekeeper: Mothers' role in making determinations about members' use of traditional medical care services and nontraditional health-care services; decision making about the ways medical care is used for illness, disease, and care of acute and chronic conditions; what health information is obtained; how information is used; and who and when care consultations related to member care occur.

Genogram: A model or graphic summary that depicts interests related to family health. A genogram might include family history, marriage or the joining of families, divorce or other broken relationships relevant to children, life transitions, family developmental stages, behavioral patterns of individual family members, defining characteristics of individuals, residence and patterns of household residence, parent–child relationships, connections to others outside the household, or genetic and health-related information.

Health: An adaptive state experienced by individuals as they seek opportunities and wrestle with liabilities found within themselves, the family, households, and larger contextual systems throughout the life course.

Health constraints: Forces imposed by persons, structures, or systems that impede, restrict, or inhibit the processes of becoming, health, and well-being.

Health potentials: Individual and family possibilities for optimizing individual processes of becoming and wellness states so that family health is maximized. Individual potentials are aimed at achieving characteristics such as hardiness, resilience, maturation, and individuation. Family potentials are aimed at achieving interactive processes characterized by cohesiveness, accommodation, stability, and perseverance.

Health-related behaviors: Activities, practices, routines, and habits of individuals, family subsystems, and families that are influenced by cultural beliefs, values, and knowledge that result from interactions with larger contextual systems.

Health routines: Dynamic member interactions affected by biophysical, developmental, interactional, psychosocial, spiritual, and contextual realms that have implications for the health and well-being of the members and family as a whole. Patterns of behavior, activity, or ritual relevant to health that are rather consistently adhered to for extended time periods that can usually be recalled and described by more than one family member.

Healthy family: Nurturing acts, emotional support, caring attributes, and member interactions that produce an outcome that results in individuation, unity, and identity that satisfy members' needs. The status of healthy family is dynamic, changes over the life course, and may be viewed differently when looking at various family proponents.

Helping processes: Interventions used by nurses and others to provide family-focused care that assists individuals, family subsystems, and families to enhance the functional processes used to optimize the processes of becoming, health, and well-being.

Holism: A dynamic condition or state of being experienced in multiple realms by developing persons as they struggle with complex, dichotomous, and ambiguous phenomena to attain the ephemeral state of well-being.

Household niche: The family residence that evolves over time as members adapt, accommodate, and mediate threats and resources created by member interactions and larger contextual systems. The niche includes both process (i.e., evolving, adapting, and changing) and product (i.e., uniquely contrived health patterns and routines) that potentiate or negate the household production of health.

Household production of health: "A dynamic behavioral process through which households combine their (internal) knowledge, resources, and behavioral norms and patterns with available (external) technologies, services, information, and skills to restore, maintain, and promote the health of their members" (Berman, Kendall, & Bhattacharyya, 1994, p. 2).

Isomorphism: The processes in one system influencing those in another system, resulting in functionally similar outcomes.

Macrosystem: The overarching patterned characteristics over the life course of complex interconnected contextual systems common to specific ideologies, social organization, cultures, or subcultures in which individuals and families are embedded.

Member-to-context: Relationships that occur between an individual or family subsystem and settings beyond the boundaries of the household niche.

Mesosystem: Interrelationships among two or more settings in which an individual actively participates; settings may not be physically connected, but they are not independent of one another.

Microsystem: A pattern of roles, activities, and interpersonal relationships experienced by developing persons in face-to-face interactions within specific settings that contain other family members who may be similar or have distinct characteristics. It is the principal environment where family members share meanings, objects, resources, and information. It includes interactions between individuals, subsystems, family, the household niche, the neighborhood, and the community.

Negating effects: The ability of a single or series of acts, behaviors, deeds, events, experiences, or supports to negatively influence health outcomes.

Niche: Places occupied by individuals in which they assume interdependent relationships, roles, functions, and purposes.

Ontogenic system: The complex interactive systems in which each developing person brings unique characteristics, beliefs, behaviors, and experiences to the development of other individuals within the family.

Optimize: To make as effective or functional as possible.

Person-in-context: The interactions individuals have within contextual systems that permeate family life and present ambiguous and contradictory influences integral to health.

Person-process-context: The complex individual, subsystem, family, and larger contextual system interactions that affect health over the life course.

Postmodernism: No single definition is adequate, but usually a period that goes beyond a modern era and initiates a new period in human history. This time is emergent, dynamic, and evolving and implies the acceptance of the possibility of many truths rather than a universal or absolute truth. Ideas such as multiple meanings, constructed realities, and nonlinear thinking are valued.

Potentiating effect: The ability of a single or series of acts, behaviors, deeds, events, experiences, or supports to positively influence health outcomes.

Process of becoming: An evolving holistic intrapersonal status encountered by individuals as they seek opportunities to increase well-being and overcome liabilities through interpersonal relationships and interaction with diverse contextual systems over the life course.

Provisional environment: Contextual settings beyond where one is present but including circumstances, situations, events, or surroundings that affect or have the potential to affect individuals and families.

Proximal processes: Complex reciprocal interactions between developing persons and larger contextual systems in which individuals, family subsystems, and families work, play, and live that have the potential to affect health. Proximal processes are affected by the beliefs, values, and knowledge held about the embedded context and their own abilities. Families create conversations of beliefs, values, and knowledge that serve as opportunities or threats to functional processes and health behaviors.

Reconstruction: Reordering patterns and relationships in original ways that result in fresh meanings, expanded ways of thinking, and different values. Discovery of new interpretations and explanations for what was previously thought as fixed or absolute.

Sentinel: A maternal role related to protecting individual and family health from illness, disease, and injury. Mothers are accountable for maintaining health, teaching and reinforcing health behaviors, and minimizing household and neighborhood risks associated with disease, trauma, or injury.

Social construction: Family's patterned routines that accommodate beliefs, values, goals, resources, constraints, and information about health and illness. Family processes and health behaviors respond to constructed meanings about everyday circumstances and contextual events that occur across the life course.

Spirituality: A contextual aspect defined as an innate trait of all persons that concerns connectedness to self, others, and a higher power; transcendence to places and energies beyond one's own being; and an essence of meaningfulness. Spirituality often includes religion, faith systems, sacred principles, worship, symbolic meanings, and ritual practices.

Steward: A maternal role related to the ways that family health resources are used, monitored, and dispensed to meet competing individual and family needs. Resources germane to family health include family members, personal time, finances, health insurance, health knowledge, material goods, and availability and access to needed health services.

Temporal events: Time factors that are ongoing influences on family routines as they create stress, direct choices, and influence perceptions (e.g., seasons, clock time, calendar days, traditional times, developmental stages, significant events).

Triadic units: Interpersonal relationships initially formed among three family members. External triads can also be formed when one or two family members include a person (or persons) or system outside the family boundaries.

Well-being: An optimum state of health in which opportunities have been realized, liabilities have been minimized, and the process of becoming has been maximized by individuals, family subsystems, and families.

Well families: Community families usually identified by nurses and others as "healthy" or fully functional, even when a member suffers from a chronic illness, disability, or is dying.

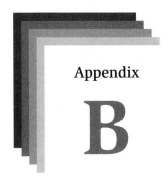

Appendix

Family Context Assessment

The initial assessment of the family context should include a comprehensive review of all aspects of the family microsystem pertinent to the family. The Family Context Assessment (FCA) includes data related to the microsystem, mesosystem, exosystem, macrosystem, and chronosystem. Time spent gathering baseline information provides family nurses with a means for comparing member and family states over the life course. In an FCA, data should be based on the presenting need for the assessment and captured for all appropriate members. Baseline information can later be compared with follow-up data so that a continuous family record can be maintained. Information collected for multiple family members has the potential to clarify complex family health relationships. Potential uses for the FCA are broad, and the purpose for gathering the information determines the areas assessed. All assessment areas are not completed on the initial visit, but data pertaining to a specific client concern directs the specifics of information collected. For example, if a client has a chronic illness, then data about the immediate caregiver should be included. Or if a family has several members with asthmatic conditions, then an environmental assessment is important. As a nurse works with a family over time, additional data can be added when assessments are completed.

The inclusion of baseline genograms, eco-grams, or both can provide excellent additions to the FCA, with modifications made or new ones drawn as the status of the family changes. The FCA can provide tools for multiple care providers from a variety of disciplines to provide input into the family record. A variety of assessment tools might be useful in gathering family data, and agencies, institutions, programs, services, and so on need to identify the data most appropriate to the care they might provide and may want to develop tools or instruments for use in the assessment process. Development of a database that electronically captures information can link multiple members into a family file. The discussion provided here is intended to provide an overview of the kinds of data that might be included in the FCA, but decisions about the appropriateness of what is collected should be guided by the intended interventions.

Family Microsystem

When considering the family microsystem, a nurse should begin by asking a few questions:

- Who are the members of the family?
- What are the relationships among the members?
- Are there members who are only residing in the household part time?
- Do some members who are considered family no longer live in the household?
- Are some extended family members viewed as immediate family members?
- Are live-in friends, partners, or relatives viewed as family members?

Are persons from past partnering relationships or marriages viewed as family members?

Which member data are appropriate for collection at this time?

Family Data

Demographic assessment data should include all persons residing within the household who are viewed as family members. These are usually persons who are either biologically or emotionally related, but they may not be persons legally recognized as family members. Data collection should also include data about persons not presently living in the household but who are still viewed as family. The charts should include all family members, listing the mother, father, children, and others in descending order of age. Dates of data collection should be noted. Some data will change over time, so a means for recording updated information should be created.

Family Name(s) _____

Members' Names	Health Insurance	Types of Insurance	Adequacy of Insurance

Members' Names	Birthplace	Current Address	Phone Number

Members' Names	Age	Gender	Race	Ethnicity	Religion

Members' Names	Family Relationship	Highest Educational Attainment	Marital Status

Members' Names	Occupation	Employed	Employer's Name	Employer's Location

Family Economic Status

This assessment is intended to gather data relevant to the families' finances to ascertain abilities and resources available to potentiate family health.

Does the family have adequate health insurance available to meet health-care needs?

Who is the primary breadwinner in the family?

Who else contributes to the family income?

Does the family receive other forms of supplemental income? What are they?

Does the family view their income as adequate to meet their needs?

■ What forms of support are available that may enable the family to meet members' needs?

■ Is the family able to manage their current income to meet their needs?

Developmental Information

This assessment is used to determine whether the developing persons within the family are acting in ways that are generally viewed as age or stage appropriate. Hanson and Boyd (1996) and Wright and Leahey (2000) provide excellent resources for developmental assessment.

Members' Names	Developmental Information	Hobbies and Interests

Health Status

Health information includes age-appropriate information. For example, information about infants and toddlers should detail immunizations; screenings; visits to physicians, dentists, and ophthalmologists; and so on. Additional health information should be obtained on an assessment form that gathers biophysical and mental health information. Well-designed instruments are available for health assessment, and appropriate tools should be identified to become part of the family database.

Cultural Assessment

Before completing an assessment, problems of language must be identified. If language barriers exist, then an interpreter should be obtained. Interpreters should be instructed to directly translate what is said without interpreting it unless asked to do so. Family nurses need to be aware of barriers related to interpretations, perceptions, slang, idioms, and colloquialisms inherent to particular regions. Deafness and hearing loss may present language barriers and flag the importance of completing a cultural assessment. Information about social organization or ways a particular culture may organize themselves (e.g., clans, castes), religious relationships to specific culture, variations in which culture affects communication patterns, attitudes about personal space, and orientation to time (e.g., present versus future orientation) may need to be assessed. A family member or a family may identify more than one relevant culture. If the person is foreign born, then assessment should identify the country of origin (e.g., a Hispanic may be from Mexico, Cuba, South America, or Spain) and differentiate the needs between American born or long settled in the nation. Cultural assessment includes values, beliefs, traditions, and routines related to the processes of becoming, health, and well-being. Many cultures have patterned behaviors associated with birth, death, child-rearing beliefs, transitional life points, diet, sexuality, disease, illness, and health. A cultural assessment tool should either be selected from existing tools or one should be created for inclusion in the database.

Father's Cultural History

Family Culture (or Cultures)	Biological Risks	Important Values	Traditional Patterns	Dietary Patterns	Health and Illness Behaviors

Mother's Cultural History

Family Culture (or Cultures)	Biological Risks	Important Values	Traditional Patterns	Dietary Patterns	Health and Illness Behaviors

Household Niche Data

Descriptive data about the family household can provide valuable information about the immediate, tangible, and intangible household where the family socially constructs their definitions and practices related to family health. What risks and benefits does the household niche present? Some examples are:

- Physical structure
- Material goods
- Immediate surroundings
- Tangible family resources
- Intangible family resources

Neighborhood Data

Understandings about the neighborhood location where the family household is located and where the members work and play can provide meaningful insights about embedded factors that are influencing family health. What things within the neighborhood have direct or indirect relationships to the household production of health? Some examples are:

- Proximal relationships
- Proximal processes

Larger Community

Information about the larger community provides an abundance of information relevant to family health that may be correlational, linked to causality, or viewed as risks and strengths. What are the relationships between the family and the community? Some examples are:

- Institutions
- Agency supports
- Employment opportunities
- Educational resources
- Health resources
- Social resources

Family Mesosystem

The family mesosystem refers to the influences experienced by family members as they interact between the family microsystem and diverse settings. Although a family may have several members, each experiences interactions, experiences, and events differently. Unique circumstances, individual interests, persons in the environment, and other contextual phenomena affect members in shared and unshared ways. Peer and family relationships, school, play, and work influence unique members, the family, and family health. Relevant questions in the following areas can provide information about individuals:

- Peer relationships (e.g., dyad and triad relationships with close kin, friendships)
- Preschool, school, and child-care processes
- Work, unemployment, and underemployment
- Play: Adult and child (e.g., regular activities, personal hobbies, vacations)
- Health-care systems (e.g., services used, relationships with providers)
- Social support systems (e.g., club or group memberships, church affiliations, formal and informal support groups)

Family Exosystem

Family health not only includes the unique characteristics and processes of the family and the interactions of its developing members but also the impact of others outside the family household. What things are occurring even when members are not present that still affect the processes of becoming, health, and well-being? Some examples are:

- Peer relationships
- Preschool and school
- Work
- Play
- Health-care systems
- Social support systems

Family Macrosystem

The macrosystem includes ideologies, social expectations, legal and moral perspectives, and cultural or subcultural traditions that affect developing persons, family households, and the social construction of family health. The macrosystem affects the reciprocal ways developing individuals treat and are treated by others outside of the family context. What things occurring in the larger environment are affecting the family and the status of its members? Some examples are:

- Social policy
- Health policy
- Public policy
- Larger environments

Chronosystem

The chronosystem refers to time elements that provide meaningful perspectives to unique individuals and families. Whether events are normative or non-normative, they have lasting member and family effects, with the potential for positive attributes (e.g., pride, celebration, positive self-esteem) or negative outcomes (e.g., remorse, sorrow, stress). What are the important historical events for various members? What are the biorhythms that influence the ways members function? How do seasons alter health patterns?

Normative events

Normative events are often highly anticipated and bound to the cultural patterns of persons within specific social contexts at given points in time. For example, those who were born in different generations; live in unique social settings; or are members of diverse religions, races, ethnicities, and cultures experience normative events in dissimilar ways. What are the shared meanings of family members related to birth, marriage, school entrance, puberty, school graduations, joining the workforce, military service, retirement, episodic illness, death in old age, and other life events? Families often have meanings and rituals associated with normative events.

Non-normative events

Non-normative events appear unexpectedly and are times for which preparedness is often lacking. These events are usually unanticipated and may significantly alter a family's life for long periods or forever. For example, non-normative events could be the birth of a child with a disability, divorce, failure to complete high school, unemployment or job inequity, relocation, winning the lottery, premature or traumatic death, and chronic illness. Members often lack rituals or routines to assist them with meaning making and may view non-normative events as threats.

Conclusions

Use of the FCA should be determined by the purposes data will serve. The assessment of areas not especially pertinent at a particular point in time should be saved for a later date. The gathering of FCA data and its analysis requires skilled practitioners who have knowledge and skills relevant to family care. Practitioners must be able to:

- Interpret the information in relation to presented problems
- Work with families to identify family health goals
- Develop and implement appropriate interventions
- Evaluate family outcomes.

Although a baseline assessment is necessary, it is expected that follow-up assessments will provide greater clarity and understanding of issues as the nurse and family collaborate in developing health plans that influence individual well-being and the household production of health.

Bibliography

Achterberg, J., Dossey, B., & Kolkmeier, L. (1994). *Rituals of healing: Using imagery for health and wellness.* New York: Bantam Books.

Ackelsberg, M., & Diamond, I. (1987). Gender and political life: New directions in political science. In B. B. Hess, & M. M. Ferree (Eds.), *Analyzing gender: A handbook of social science research* (pp. 504–525). Newbury Park, CA: Sage Publications.

Adams, R. A., Gordon, C., & Spangler, A. A. (1999). Maternal stress in caring for children with feeding disabilities: Implications for health care providers. *Journal of the American Dietetic Association, 99,* 962–966.

Alcoff, L. (1988). Cultural feminism versus post-structuralism: The identity crisis in feminist theory. *Signs, 13,* 405–436.

Allan, J. D., & Hall, B. A. (1988). Challenging the focus on technology: A critique of the medical model in a changing health care system. *Advances in Nursing Science, 10,* 22–34.

Allen, K. A., Fine, M. A., & Demo, D. H. (2000). An overview of family diversity: Controversies, questions, and values. In D. Demo, K. Allen, & M. Fine (Eds.), *Handbook of family diversity* (pp. 1–14). New York: Oxford University Press.

Allison, K. R., Adlaf, E. M., Ialomiteanu, A., et al. (1999). Predictors of health risk behaviours among young adults: Analysis of the National Population Health Survey. *Canadian Journal of Public Health, 90,* 85–89.

Amato, P. (2000). Diversity within single-parent families. In D. Demo, K. Allen, & M. Fine (Eds.), *Handbook of family diversity* (pp. 149–172). New York: Oxford University Press.

American Academy of Nursing Expert Panel on Culturally Competent Health Care. (1992). An expert panel report: Culturally competent health care. *Nursing Outlook, 40,* 277–283.

America's Children. (1999a). *Forum on child and family statistics.* http://childStats.gov.

America's Children. (1999b). *Population and family characteristics: Key national indicators of well-being.* http://www.childstats.gov/ac1999/highlight.asp.

America's Children. (2000). *America's children: Key national indicators of well-being.* http://www.childstats.gov/ac2000/highlight.asp.

American Nurses Association. (1999). *Priniciples for Nurse Staffing.* Washington, DC: American Nurses Association.

Anderson, K. H., & Mitchell, J. M. (2000). Differential access in the receipt of antiretroviral drugs for the treatment of AIDS and its implications for survival. *Archives of Internal Medicine, 160,* 3114–3120.

Anderson, K. H., & Tomlinson, P. S. (1992). The family health system as an emerging paradigmatic view for nursing. *Image: Journal of Nursing Scholarship, 24*(1), 57–63.

Antonovsky, A. (1987). *Unraveling the mystery of health: How people manage stress and stay well.* San Francisco: Jossey-Bass.

Arber, S. (1997). Comparing inequalities in women's and men's health: Britain in the 1990s. *Social Science Medicine, 44*(6), 773–787.

Artinian, B. M. (1997a). Overview of the Intersystem Model. In B. M. Artinian, & M. M. Conger (Eds.), *The Intersystem Model: Integrating theory and practice* (pp. 1–17). Thousand Oaks, CA: Sage Publications.

Artinian, B. M. (1997b). Situational sense of coherence. In B. M. Artinian, & M. M. Conger (Eds.), *The Intersystem Model: Integrating theory and practice* (pp. 18–30). Thousand Oaks, CA: Sage Publications.

Artinian, B. M., & Conger, M. M. (Eds.). (1997). *The Intersystem Model: Integrating theory and practice.* Thousand Oaks, CA: Sage Publications.

Artinian, N. T. (1991). Philosophy of science and family nursing theory development. In A. Whall, & J. Fawcett (Eds.), *Family theory development in nursing: State of the science and art* (pp. 43–54). Philadelphia: F. A. Davis Company.

Artinian, N. T. (2001). Family-focused medical-surgical nursing. In S. M. Hanson (Ed.), *Family health care nursing: Theory, practice, and research* (2nd ed., pp. 272–299). Philadelphia: F. A. Davis Company.

Astedt-Kurki, P., Hopia, H., & Vuori, A. (1999). Family health in everyday life: A qualitative study on well-being in families with children. *Journal of Advanced Nursing, 29*(3), 704–711.

Auslander, W. F., Thompson, S. J., Dreitzer, D., & Santiago, J. V. (1997). Mothers' satisfaction with medical care: Perceptions of racism, family stress, and medical outcomes in children with diabetes. *Health and Social Work, 22*(3), 190–199.

Austin, E. (2001). Profile: Sharyn Sutton, PhD. *Advances, 1,* 4.

Avant, K. C. (1988). Stressors on the childbearing family. *Journal of Obstetrical, Gynecological, and Neonatal Nursing, 17,* 179–185.

Avis, J. (1986). Feminist issues in family therapy. In F. Piercy, & D. Sprenkle (Eds.), *Family therapy sourcebook* (pp. 213–242). New York: Guilford Press.

Baber, K. M., & Allen, K. R. (1992). *Women and families: Feminist reconstructions.* New York: The Guilford Press.

Backett, K. (1992). The construction of health knowledge in middle class families. *Health Education Research, 7*(4), 497–507.

Baer, J. (1999). The effects of family structure and SES on family processes in early adolescence. *Journal of Adolescents, 22*(3), 341–354.

Bailey, D. B., & Wolery, M. (1984). *Teaching infants and preschoolers with handicaps.* Columbus, OH: Charles E. Merrill.

Ballard, N. R. (2001). Family structure, function, and process. In S.M. Hanson (Ed.), *Family health care nursing: Theory, practice, and research* (2nd ed., pp. 79–99). Philadelphia: F. A. Davis Company.

Bandura, A. (1982). The self and mechanisms of agency. In J. Suls (Ed.), *Psychological perspectives of the self* (Vol. 1, pp. 3–39). Hillsdale, NJ: Erlbaum.

Bandura, A. (1994). *Self-efficacy: The exercise of control.* New York: W.H. Freeman.

Barnard, K., Eyres, S., Lobo, M. N., & Snyder, C. (1983). An ecological paradigm for assessment and intervention. In T. B. Brazelton, & B. M. Lester (Eds.), *New approaches to developmental screening of infants* (pp. 199–218). Elsevier Science: NY.

Barnhill, L. R. (1979). Healthy family systems. *The family coordinator,* 94–100.

Barr, D., Vergun, P., & Barley, S. R. (2000). Problems in using patient satisfaction data to assess the quality of care of primary care physicians. *Journal of Clinical Outcomes Management, 7,* 19–24.

Bartley, M., Blane, D., & Montgomery, S. (1997). Health and the life course: Why safety nets matter. *British Medical Journal, 314*(7088), 1194–1196.

Basu, J., & Cooper, J. (2000). Out-of-area travel from rural and urban counties: A study of ambulatory care sensitive hospitalizations for New York State residents. *Journal of Rural Health, 16*(2), 129–138.

Bates, E., Dale, P., & Thal, D. (1995). Individual differences and their implications for theories of language development. In P. Fletcher, & B. MacWhinney (Eds.), *Handbook of child language.* Oxford, United Kingdom: Blackwell.

Bates, E., Marchman, V., Thal, D., Fenson, L., Dale, P., Reznick, J., Reilly, J., & Hartung, J. (1994). Developmental and stylistic variation in the composition of early vocabulary. *Journal of Child Language, 21*(1), 85–124.

Bateson, P. (1998). Genes, environment and the development of behavior. Novartis Found Symposium, 213, 160–170.

Baumann, S. L. (2000). Family nursing: Theory-anemic, nursing theory-deprived. *Nursing Science Quarterly, 13*(4), 285–290.

Bell, J. M. (1995). Avoiding isomorphism: A call for a different view. *Journal of Family Nursing, 1*(1), 5–7.

Bell, J. M. (1997). Levels in undergraduate family nursing education. *Journal of Family Nursing. 3*(3), 227–229.

Belsky, J. (1980). Child maltreatment: An ecological integration. *American Psychology, 35,* 320–335.

Bennett, L. A., Wolin, S. J., & McAvity, K. J. (1988). Family identity, ritual, and myth: A cultural perspective on life cycle transitions. In C. J. Falicov

(Ed.), *Family transitions: Continuity and change over the life cycle* (pp. 211–233). New York: The Guilford Press.

Bennett, L. A., Wolin, S. J., & Reiss, D. (1988). Deliberate family process: A strategy for protecting children of alcoholics. *British Journal of Addiction, 83,* 821–829.

Bennett, L. A., Wolin, S. J., Reiss, D. & Teitelbaum, M. A. (1987). Couples at risk for transmission of alcoholism: Protective influences. *Family Processes, 26*(1), 111–129.

Bergman, D. A. (1999). Evidence-based guidelines and critical pathways for quality improvement. *Pediatrics, 103*(1 suppl E), 225–232.

Berk, M. L., & Monheit, A. C. (2001). The concentration of health care expenditures revisited. *Health Affairs, 20,* 204–213.

Berkman, L. (2000). Profile. *Advances: The Robert Wood Johnson Foundation Quarterly Newsletter, 3,* 4.

Berman, P., Kendall, C., & Bhattacharyya, K. (1994). The household production of health: Integrating social science perspectives on micro-level health determinants. *Social Science Medicine, 38*(2), 205–215.

Bernheimer, L. P., Gallimore, R., & Weisner, T. S. (1990). Ecocultural theory as a context for the individual service plan. *Journal of Early Intervention, 14*(3), 219–233.

Biesecker, B. B. (1997). Psychological issues in cancer genetics. *Seminar in Oncology Nursing, 13*(2), 129–134.

Bigbee, J. L. (1992). Family stress, hardiness, and illness: A pilot study. *Family Relations, 41,* 212–217.

Billings, D. B., Norman, G., & Ledford, K. (1999). *Confronting Appalachian stereotypes: Back Talk from an American region.* Lexington, KY: The University Press of Kentucky.

Biziou, B. (1999). *The joy of ritual.* New York: Golden Books.

Black, M. M., Dubowitz, H., & Starr, R. H. (1999). African American fathers in low income, urban families: Development, behavior, and home environment of their three-year-old children. *Child Development, 70*(4), 967–978.

Blecke, J. (1990). Exploration of children's health and self-care behavior within a family context through qualitative research. *Family Relations, 39,* 284–291.

Blegan, M. A., & Tripp-Reimer, T. (1997). Implications of nursing taxonomies for middle-range theory development. *Advances in Nursing Science, 19*(3), 37–49.

Bloom, B. (1981). The effect of the home environment on children's school achievement. In B. Bloom (Ed.), *All our children learning* (pp. 89–102). New York: McGraw-Hill.

Bodenheimer, T., Lo, B., & Casalino, L. (1999). Primary care physicians should be coordinators, not gatekeepers. *Journal of the American Medical Association, 281*(21), 2045–2049.

Boland, E. A., Grey, M., Mezger, J., & Tamborlane, W. V. (1999). A summer vacation from diabetes: Evidence from a clinical trial. *Diabetes Educator, 25*(1), 31–40.

Bomar, P.J. (1990). Perspectives of family health promotion. *Family and Community Health, 12*(4), 1–11.

Bomar, P. J., & McNeely, G. (1996). Family health nursing role: Past, present, and future. In P. J.

Bomar (Ed.), *Nurses and family health promotion: Concepts, assessment, and interventions* (2nd ed., pp. 3–21). Philadelphia: W. B. Saunders Company.

Boss, P. (1988). *Family stress management.* Newbury Park, CA: Sage Publications.

Bossard, J. H., & Boll, E. S. (1950). *Rituals in family living.* Philadelphia: University of Pennsylvania Press.

Bottoroff, J. L., Steele, R., Davies, B., Garossino, C., Porterfield, P., & Shaw, M. (1998). Striving for balance: Palliative care patients' experiences of making everyday choices. *Journal of Palliative Care, 14*(1), 7–17.

Boulton, M. J., Trueman, M., Chau, C. Whithand, C. & Amatya, K. A. (1999). Concurrent and longitudinal links between friendship and peer victimization: Implications for befriending interventions. *Journal of Adolescence, 22,* 461–466.

Bowers, R. (1995). Early adolescent social and emotional development: A constructivist perspective. In M. Wavering (Ed.), *Educating young adolescents* (pp. 78–110). New York: Garland.

Bowlby, J. (1969). *Attachment and loss* (Vol. 1, Attachment). New York: Basic Books.

Bowlby, J. (1980). *Loss: Sadness and depression* (Vol. 3). New York: Basic Books.

Boyle, J. S. (1984). Indigenous caring practices in a Guatemalan colony. In M. Leininger (Ed.), *Care: The essence of nursing and health* (pp. 123–132). Thorofare, NJ: Slack.

Boyle, P. J. (1998). Ritual obligation. *The Park Ridge Center Bulletin, 5,* 2.

Boyce, W. T., Jensen, E. W., Cassel, J. C., Collier, A. M., Smith, A. H., & Ramey, C. T. (1977). Influence of life events and family routines on childhood respiratory tract illness. *Pediatrics, 60*(4), 609–615.

Brach, C., & Fraser, I. (2000). Can cultural competency reduce racial and ethnic health disparities? A review and a conceptual model. *Medical Care Research and Review, 57*(suppl 1), 181–217.

Bradley, R. H., & Caldwell, B. M. (1984). The relation of infants' home environments to achievement test performance in first grade: A follow-up study. *Child Development, 55*(3), 803–809.

Brennan, J. L., & Wamboldt, F. S. (1990). From the outside in: Examining how individuals define their experienced family. *Communication Research, 17*(4), 444–461.

Brennan, P. F., Zielstorff, R. D., Ozbolt, J. G., & Strombom, I. (1998). Setting a national research agenda in nursing informatics. *Medinfo, 9,* 1188–1191.

Bright, M. A. (1990). Therapeutic ritual: Helping families grow. *Journal of Psychosocial Nursing Mental Health Services, 28*(12), 24–29.

Brody, B. A. (1970). *Readings in the philosophy of science.* Englewood Cliffs, NJ: Prentice-Hall.

Bronfenbrenner, U. (1979). *The ecology of human development: Experiments by nature and design.* Cambridge, MA: Harvard University Press.

Bronfenbrenner, U. (1986). Ecology of the family as a context for human development: Research perspectives. *Developmental Psychology, 22,* 723–742.

Bronfenbrenner, U. (1989). Ecological systems theory. *Annuals of Child Development, 6,* 187–249.

Bronfenbrenner, U. (1995). Developmental ecology through space and time: A future perspective (pp. 619–647). In P. Moen, G. H. Elder, & K. Luscher (Eds.), *Examining lives in context.*

Washington, D.C.: American Psychological Association.

Bronfenbrenner, U., & Ceci, S. J. (1994). Nature-nurture reconceptualized in developmental perspective: A bioecological model. *Psychology Review, 101*(4), 567–586.

Brown, B. (1990). Peer groups and peer cultures. In S. Feldman, & G. Elliott (Eds.), *At the threshold: The developing adolescent* (pp.171–196). Cambridge, MA: Harvard University Press.

Brown, J. E., & Mann, L. (1990). The relationship between family structure and process variables and adolescent decision-making. *Journal of Adolescents, 13*(1), 25–37.

Broyles, R. S., Tyson, J. E, & Heyne, E. T. (2000). Comprehensive follow-up care and life threatening illnesses among high-risk infants: A randomized controlled trial. *Journal of the American Medical Association, 284,* 2070–2076.

Bubolz, M. M., & Sontag, S. (1993). Human ecology theory. In P. G. Boss, W. J. Doherty, R. LaRossa, W. R. Schumm, & S. K. Steinmetz (Eds.), *Sourcebook of family theories and methods: A contextual approach* (pp. 419–452). New York: Plenum Press.

Bulechek, G. M., & McCloskey, J. C. (1992). Defining and validating nursing interventions. *Nursing Clinics of North America, 27*(2), 289–299.

Burke, S. O., Costello, E. A., & Handley-Derry, M. (1989). Maternal stress and repeated hospitalizations of children who are physically disabled. *Children's Health Care, 18,* 82–90.

Burkett, G. (1994). Status of health in Appalachia. In R. Couto, N. Simpson, & G. Harris (Eds.), *Sowing seeds in the mountains: Community-based coalitions for cancer prevention and control* (pp. 43–60). Rockville, MD: National Cancer Institute.

Bureau of Economic Analysis. (November 26, 2000). U.S. Department of Commerce. [http://www.bea.doc.gov/bea/regional/reis/scb/svy_oh.htm].

Butler, J. P. (1999). *Gender trouble: Feminism and the subversion of identity* (10th anniversary edition). New York, NY: Routledge.

Cadoret, R. J., Leve, L. D., & Devor, E. (1997). Genetics of aggressive and violent behavior. *Psychiatric Clinics of North America, 20* (2), 301–322.

Cairns, R. B. (1972). Fighting and punishment from a developmental perspective. In J. K. Coles, & D. D. Jensen (Eds.), *Nebraska symposium on motivation* (Vol. 20, pp. 59–124). Lincoln, NB: University of Nebraska Press.

Cairns, R. B. (1976). The ontogeny and phylogeny of social behavior. In M. E. Hahn, & E. C. Simmel (Eds.), *Evolution and communicative behavior* (pp. 115–139). New York: Academic Press.

Cairns, R. B., & Cairns, B. D. (1994). *Lifelines and risks: Pathways of youth in our time.* New York: Cambridge University Press.

Cairns, R. B., & Cairns, B. D. (1995). Social ecology over time. In P. Moen, G. H. Elder, & K. Luscher (Eds.), *Examining lives in context* (pp. 397–421). Washington, D.C.: American Psychological Association.

Calderon, R. (2000). Parental involvement in deaf children's education programs as a predictor of child's language, early reading, and social-emotional development. *Journal of Deaf Studies & Deaf Education, 5*(2), 140–155.

Calderon, R., & Low, S. (1998). Early social-emotional, language, and academic development in children with hearing loss: families with and without fathers. *American Annals of the Deaf, 143*(3), 225–34.

Caldwell, B. M., & Bradley, R. H. (1984). *Home observation for measurement of the environment* (Rev. Ed.). Little Rock, AK: University of Arkansas.

Campbell, D. W. (1991). Family paradigm theory and family rituals: Implications for child and family health. *Nurse Practitioner, 16*(2), 22–26, 31.

Campbell, R. (1996). Images and identities of Appalachian women: Sorting out the impact of class, gender and cultural heritage. In P. Obermiller, *Down home, down town: Urban Appalachia today* (pp. 29–45). Dubuque, IO: Kendall/Hunt Publishing Company.

Campbell, T. L. (1986). Family's impact on health: A critical review. *Family Systems Medicine, 4*(2–3), 135–191.

Caplan, G. (1974). Support *systems and community mental health.* New York: Behavioral Publications.

Carper, B. A. (1978). Fundamental patterns of knowing in nursing, *Advances of Nursing Science, 1*(10), 13–23.

Carson, V. (1989). *Spiritual dimensions of nursing practice.* Philadelphia: W. B. Saunders Company.

Carter, B, & McGoldrick, M. (1988). *The changing family life cycle: A framework for family therapy* (2nd ed.). New York: Gardner Press.

Carter, B., & McGoldrick, M. (1999a). *The expanded family life cycle: Individual, family, and social perspectives* (3rd ed.). Boston: Allyn and Bacon.

Carter, B, & McGoldrick, M. (1999b). Overview: The expanded family life cycle (pp. 1–26). In B. Carter, & M. McGoldrick (Eds.), *The expanded family life cycle: Individual, family, and social perspectives* (3rd ed.), Boston: Allyn and Bacon.

Cattell, R. (1953). New concepts for measuring leadership in terms of groupsyntality. In D. Cartwright, & A. Zander (Eds.), *Group dynamics.* Evanston, IL: Row, Peterson, & Company.

Cavendar, A., & Beck, S. (1995). Generational change, folk medicine, and medical self-care in a rural Appalachian community. *Human Organization, 54*(2), 129–142.

Chandler, L. K., Fowler, S. A., & Lubock, R. C. (1986). Assessing family needs: The first step in providing family-focused intervention. *Diagnostique, 11,* 233–245.

Cheal, D. (1988). The ritualization of family ties. *American Behavioral Scientist, 31*(6), 632–643.

Cheal, D. (1991). *Family and the state of theory.* Toronto, Canada: University of Toronto Press.

Chen, H. (1990). *Theory-driven evaluations.* Newbury Park, CA: Sage Publications.

Chernomas, W. M. (1997). Experiencing depression: Women's perspectives in recovery. *Journal of Psychiatric Mental Health Nursing, 4*(6), 393–400.

Chinn, P. L., & Kramer, M. K. (1991). *Theory and nursing: A systematic approach* (3rd ed.). St. Louis: Mosby Year Book.

Civic, D., & Holt, V. L. (2000). Maternal depressive symptoms and child behavior problems in a nationally representative normal birthweight sample. *Journal of Maternal Child Health, 4*(4), 215–221.

Clancy, C. M., & Bierman, A. S. (2000). Quality and outcomes of care for older women with chronic disease. *Women's Health Issues, 10*(4), 178–191.

Clements, C. B., Copeland, L. G., & Loftus, M. (1990). Critical times for families with a chronically ill child. *Pediatric Nursing, 16,* 157–161, 224.

Cody, W. K. (1995). The view of family within human becoming theory. In R. R. Parse (Ed.), *Illuminations: The Human Becoming Theory in practice and research* (pp. 9–26). New York: National League for Nursing Press.

Cody, W. K. (1999). Middle-range theories: Do they foster the development of nursing science? *Nursing Science Quarterly, 12*(1), 9–14.

Cody, W. K. (2000). Parse's Human becoming school of thought and families. *Nursing Science Quarterly, 13*(4), 281–284.

Cohen, M. (1997). Helping at home: Caregivers ask for help. *Perspectives in Nursing and Health Care, 4*(4), 184–292.

Cohen, E., & Goode, T. D. (1999). *Rationale for cultural competence in primary health Care.* Washington, D.C.: National Center for Cultural Competence, George Washington University Child Development Center.

Colantonio, A. (1988). Lay concepts of health. *Health Values, 12*(5), 3–7.

Coleman, J., & Hoffer, T. (1987). *Public and private high schools: The impact of communities.* New York: Basic Books.

Conway, M. E. (1985). Toward greater specificity in defining nursing's metaparadigm. *Advances in Nursing Science, 7*(4), 73–81.

Coohey, C. (1996). Child maltreatment: Testing the social isolation hypothesis. *Child Abuse and Neglect, 20*(3), 241–254.

Coontz, S. (1992). *The way we never were.* New York: Basic Books.

Coontz, S. (1997). *The way we really are.* New York: Basic Books.

Coreil, J. (1990). The evolution of anthropology in international health. In J. Coriel, & J. D. Mull (Eds.), *Anthropology and primary health care* (pp. 3–27). Boulder, CO: Westview Press.

Coreil, J., Wilson, F., Wood, D. & Liller, K. (1998). Maternal employment and preventive child health practices. *Preventive Medicine, 27*(3), 488–492.

Cox, R. P., & Davis, L. L. (1993). Social constructivist approaches for brief, episodic, problem-focused family encounters. *Nurse Practitioner, 18*(8), 45–49.

Craft, M. J., & Willadsen, J. A. (1992). Interventions related to family. *Nursing Clinics of North America, 27*(2), 517–540.

Crittendon, P. M. (1989). Teaching maltreated children in preschool. *Topics in early childhood special education, 9*(1), 16–32.

Cross, T., Bazron, B., Dennis, K., & Isaacs, M. (1989). *Towards a culturally competent system of care* (Vol. 1). Washington, D.C.: National Technical Assistance Center for Children's Mental Health, Georgetown University Child Development Center.

Crouter, A. C., & McHale, S. M. (1993). Temporal rhythms in family life: Seasonal variation in the relation between parental work and family processes. *Developmental Psychology, 29*(2), 198–205.

Crowe, T .K. (1993). Time use of mothers with young children: The impact of a child's disability. *Developmental Medicine and Child Neurology, 35*(7), 621–630.

Crowe, T. K., VanLeit, B., & Berghmans, K. K. (2000). Mothers' perceptions of child care assistance: The impact of a child's disability. *Journal of Occupational Therapy, 54*(1), 52–58.

Crowe, T. K., VanLeit, B., Berghmans, K. K., & Mann, P. (1997). Role perceptions of mothers with young children: The impact of a child's disability. *American Journal of Occupational Therapy, 51*(8), 651–661.

Cumes-Rayner, D. P., Lucke, J. C., Singh, B., Adler, B., Lewin, T., Dunne, M., & Raphael, B. (1992). A high-risk community study of paternal alcohol consumption and adolescents' psychosocial characteristics. *Journal of Study of Alcohol, 53*(6), 626–635.

Curran, D. (1983). *Traits of a healthy family.* New York: Ballantine Books.

Curran, D. (1985). *Stress and the healthy family.* Minneapolis, MN: Winston Press.

Currie, L., & Harvey, G. (1998). Care pathways development and implementation. *Nursing Standard, 12*(30), 35–38.

Daly, K. J. (1994). *Families and time: Keeping pace in a hurried culture.* Thousand Oaks, CA: Sage Publications.

Danielson, C. B., Hamel-Bissell, B., & Winstead-Fry, P. (1993). *Families, health, & illness: Perspectives on coping and intervention.* St. Louis: Mosby Year Book.

Davies, B., & Welch, D. (1986). Motherhood and feminism: Are they compatible? The ambivalence of mothering. *Australian and New Zealand Journal of Sociology, 22*(3), 411–426.

Davis, K. (1997). *Exploring the intersection between cultural competency and managed behavioral health care policy: Implications for state and county mental health agencies.* Alexandria, VA: National Technical Assistance Center for State Mental Health Planning.

Deatrick, J. A., Brennan, D., & Cameron, M. E. (1998). Mothers with multiple sclerosis and their children: Effects of fatigue and exacerbations on maternal support. *Nursing Research, 47*(4), 205–210.

Deatrick, J. A., Knafl, K., & Walsh, M. (1998). The process of parenting a child with a disability: Normalization through accommodation. *Journal of Advanced Nursing, 13,* 15–22.

Deegan, M. J. (1998). Weaving the American ritual tapestry. In M. J. Deegan (Ed), *The American ritual tapestry: Social rules and cultural meanings* (pp. 3–17). Westport, CT: Greenwood.

de Montigny, F., Dumas, L., Bolduc, L., & Blais, S. (1997). Teaching family nursing based on conceptual models of nursing. *Journal of Family Nursing, 3*(3), 267–279.

Denham, S. A. (1995). Family routines: A construct for considering family health. *Holistic Nursing Practices, 9,* 11–23.

Denham, S. A. (1996). Family health in a rural Appalachian Ohio county. *Journal of Appalachian Studies, 2*(2), 299–310.

Denham, S. A. (1997). *An ethnographic study of family health in Appalachian microsystems.* Unpublished doctoral dissertation. Birmingham, AL: University of Alabama at Birmingham.

Denham, S. A. (1999a). The definition and practice of family health. *Journal of Family Nursing, 5,* 133–159.

Denham, S. A. (1999b). Family health: During and after death of a family member. *Journal of Family Nursing, 5*(2), 160–183.

Denham, S. A. (1999c). Family health in an economically disadvantaged population. *Journal of Family Nursing, 5,* 184–213.

Denham, S. A. (unpublished paper). Family routines: A review of the literature. *Journal of Family Nursing.*

Denton, M., & Walters, V. (1999). Gender differences in structural and behavioral determinants of health: An analysis of the social production of health. *Social Science Medicine, 48*(9), 1221–1235.

Denzin, N. K., & Lincoln, Y. S. (1994). *Handbook of qualitative research.* Thousand Oaks, CA: Sage Publications.

Deyo, R. A., Cherkin, D. C., & Weinstein, J. (2000). Involving patients in clinical decisions: Impact of an interactive video program on use of back surgery. *Medical Care, 38*(9), 959–969.

Derrida, J. (1976). *Of grammatology.* Baltimore: Johns Hopkins Press.

DeVault, M. L. (1991). *Feeding the family: The social organization of caring as a gendered work.* Chicago: University of Chicago Press.

Doherty, W. J. (1992). Linkages between family theories and primary health care. In R. J. Sawa (Ed.), *Family health care* (pp. 30–39). Newbury Park, CA: Sage Publications.

Doherty, W. J. (1997). *The intentional family: How to build family ties in our modern world.* Reading, MA: Addison-Wesley Publishing Co., Inc.

Doherty, W. J., & Campbell, T. L. (1988). *Families and health.* Newbury Park, CA: Sage Publications.

Doherty, W. J., & McCubbin, H. I. (1985). Families and health care: An emerging arena of theory, research, and clinical intervention. *Family Relations, 349,* 5–11.

Donaldson, S., & Crowley, D. (1978). The discipline of nursing. *Nursing Outlook, 26,* 113–120.

Drozda, D. J., Allen, S. R., Standiford, D. A., Turner, A. M., & McCain, G. C. (1997). Personal illness models of diabetes: Parents of preadolescents and adolescents. *Diabetes Educator, 23*(5), 550–557.

Duffy, M. E. (1988). Health promotion in the family: Current findings and directives for nursing research. *Journal of Advanced Nursing, 13,* 109–117.

Dumas, R., Lindell, A., Kercher, & Foley, M. (1999). *Nursing Tri-Council launches a movement to include a fifth vital sign for monitoring patient welfare* (ANA Task Force Report). Washington, DC: American Nurses Association.

Dunn, J., & Plomin, R. (1991). Why are siblings so different? The significance of differences in sibling experiences within the family. *Family Processes, 30*(3), 271–283.

Dupper, D. R. (1995). Moving beyond a crime-focused perspective of school violence. *Social Work in Education, 17*(2), 71–72.

Durbin, D., Darling, N., Steinberg, L., & Brown, B. (1993). Parenting style and peer group membership among European-American adolescents. *Journal of Research on Adolescence, 3,* 87–100.

Duvall, E. M., & Miller, B. C. (1985a). *Marriage and family development* (6th ed.). New York: Harper & Row.

Duvall, E. M., & Miller, B. C. (1985b). Developmental tasks: Individual and family. In E. M. Duvall, & B. C. Miller (Eds.), *Marriage and family development.* New York: Harper & Row.

Eichler, M. (1988). *Nonsexist research methods: A practical guide.* Boston: Allen & Unwin.

Eisenberg, J. M., & Power, E. J. (2000). Transforming insurance coverage into quality health care. *Journal of the American Medical Association, 284,* 2100–2107.

Elder, G. H. (1995). The life course paradigm. In P. Moen, G. H. Elder, & K. Luscher (Eds.), *Examining lives in context* (pp. 101–139). Washington, D.C.: American Psychological Association.

Ellrodt, G., Cook, D. J., Lee, J., Cho, M., Hunt, D., & Weingarten, S. (1997). Evidence-based disease management. *Journal of the American Medical Association, 278*(20), 1687–1692.

Erikson, E. (1959). Identity and the life cycle. *Psychological Issues* (No. 1). New York: International Universities Press.

Erikson, E. (1963). *Childhood and Society.* New York: W. W. Norton & Company, Inc.

Erikson, E. (1968). *Identity: Youth and crisis.* New York: Norton.

Eshelman, J. R. (1974). *The family: An introduction.* Boston: Allyn & Bacon.

Evans, R. G. (1994). Introduction. In R. G. Evans, M. L. Barer, & T. R. Marmor (Eds.), *Why are some people healthy and others not* (pp. 3–26). New York: Aldine De Gruyter.

Farrand, L. L. (1991). *Determinants of positive health behaviors in middle childhood.* Unpublished doctoral dissertation. University of Illinois at Chicago, Health Sciences Center.

Farrell, A. D., & White, K. S. (1998). Peer influences and drug use among urban adolescents: Family structure and parent-adolescent relationship as protective factors. *Journal of Consultation and Clinical Psychology, 66*(2), 248–258.

Fawcett, J. (1978). The "what" of theory development. In *Theory development: What, why, and how* (pp. 17–33). New York: National League for Nursing.

Fawcett, J. (1984). The metaparadigm of nursing: Present status and future refinements. *Image: Journal of Nursing Scholarship, 16,* 84–87.

Fawcett, J. (1993). *Analysis and evaluation of nursing theories.* Philadelphia: F. A. Davis Company.

Fawcett, J. (2000). Analysis and evaluation of contemporary nursing knowledge: *Nursing models and theories.* Philadelphia: F. A. Davis Company.

Fawcett, J., & Downs, F. S. (1992). *The relationship of theory and research* (2nd ed.). Philadelphia: F. A. Davis Company.

Fawcett, J., & Whall, A. (1991). *Family theory development in nursing: State of the science and art.* Philadelphia: F. A. Davis Company.

Feetham, S. (1990). Conceptual and methodological issues in research if families. In J. Bell, W. Watson, & L. Wright (Eds.), *The cutting edge of family nursing.* Calgary, Canada: Family Nursing Unit Publications.

Feetham, S. L. (1991). Conceptual and methodological issues in research of families. In A. L. Whall, & J. Fawcett (Eds.), *Family theory development in nursing: State of the science and art* (pp. 55–68). Philadelphia: F. A. Davis.

Fenson, L., Dale, P., Reznick, J., Bates, E., Thal, D., & Pethick, S. (1994). Variability in early communicative development. *Monographs of the Society for Research on Child Development, 59*(5, Serial No. 242).

Fernald, L. C., Ani, C., & Gardner, J. M. (1997). Aggressive behaviour in children and adolescents: A review of the effects of child and family characteristics. *West Indian Medical Journal, 46*(4), 100–103.

Field, T., Estroff, D. B., Yando, R., del Valle, C., Malphurs, J., & Hart, S. (1996). "Depressed" mothers' perceptions of infant vulnerability are related to later development. *Child Psychiatry and Human Development, 27*(1), 43–53.

Fiene, J. I. (1995). Battered women: Keeping the secret. *Journal of Women and Social Work, 10*(2), 179–193.

Fiese, B. H. (1992). Dimensions of family rituals across two generations: Relation to adolescent identity. *Family Process, 31*(2), 151–162.

Fiese, B. H. (1993). Family rituals in alcoholic and nonalcoholic households: Relations to adolescent health symptomatology and problem drinking. *Family Relations, 42,* 187–192.

Fiese, B. H. (1993a). Family rituals in the early stages of parenthood. *Journal of Marriage and the Family, 55,* 633–642.

Fiese, B. H. (1995). Family rituals. In D. Levinson (Ed.), *Encyclopedia of marriage and the family* (pp. 275–278). New York: Simon & Schuster Macmillan.

Fiese, B. H. (1997). Family context in pediatric psychology from a transactional perspective: Family rituals and stories as examples. *Journal of Pediatric Psychology, 22*(2), 183–196.

Fiese, B. H., Hooker, K. A., Kotary, L., & Schwagler, J. (1993). Family rituals in the early stages of parenthood. *Journal of Marriage and the Family, 55,* 633–642.

Fiese, B. H., & Kline, C. A. (1993). Development of the Family Ritual Questionnaire: Initial Reliability and validation studies. *Journal of Family Psychology, 6*(3), 290–299.

Fiese, B. H., & Wamboldt, F. S. (2000). Family routines and asthma management: A proposal for family-based strategies to increase treatment adherence. *Families, Systems & Health, 18*(4), 405–418.

Firestone, S. (1970). The *dialectic of sex: The case for feminist revolution.* New York: Vintage Books.

Fish, S., & Shelly, J. A. (1978). *Spiritual care: The nurse's role.* Downers Grove, IL: InterVarsity Press.

Fisher, L., & Ransom, D. C. (1990). Person-family transactions: Implications for stress and health. *Family Systems Medicine, 8*(1), 109–122.

Fleming, J., Mullen, P., & Bammer, G. (1997). A study of potential risk factors for sexual abuse in childhood. *Child Abuse and Neglect, 21*(1), 49–58.

Fletcher, K. R., & Winslow, S. A. (1991). Informal caregivers: A composite and review of needs and community resources. *Family Community Health, 14*(2), 59–67.

Fontes, L. A. (1993). Disclosures of sexual abuse by Puerto Rican children: Oppression and cultural barriers. *Journal of Sexual Abuse, 2*(1), 21–35.

Ford, F., & Herrick, J. (1974). Family rules: Family life styles. *American Journal of Orthopsychiatry, 44,* 61–69.

Forte, J. A., Franks, D. D., & Rigsby, D. (1996). Asymmetrical role-taking: Comparing battered and non-battered women. *Social Work, 41*(1), 59–73.

Franks, P., Campbell, T. L., & Shields, C. G. (1992). Social relationships and health: The relative roles of family functioning and social support. *Social Science Medicine, 34*(7), 779–788.

Fraser, M. W. (1996). Aggressive behavior in childhood and early adolescence: An ecological-developmental perspective on youth violence. *Social Work, 41*(4), 347–61.

Friedemann, M. L. (1989a). Closing the gap between grand theory and mental health practice with families: Part 1: The Framework of Systemic Organization for nursing of families and family members. *Journal of Psychiatric Nursing, 3*, 10–19.

Friedemann, M. L. (1989b). The concept of family nursing. *Journal of Advanced Nursing, 14*, 211–216.

Friedemann, M. L. (1991). An instrument to evaluate effectiveness in family functioning. *Western Journal of Nursing Research, 13*(2), 220–235.

Friedemann, M. (1995). *The framework of systemic organization: A conceptual approach to families and nursing.* Thousand Oaks, CA: Sage Publications.

Friedman, M. M. (1992). *Family nursing: Theory and practice* (3rd ed.). Norwalk, CT: Appleton & Lange.

Friedman, M. M. (1998a). *Family nursing: Research, theory & practice* (4th ed.). Stamford, CT: Appleton & Lange.

Friedman, M. M. (1998b). Family values. In M. Friedman (Ed.), *Family nursing: Research, theory & practice* (4th ed., pp. 327–349). Stamford, CN: Appleton & Lange.

Friedman, M. M. (1998c). Family identifying data: Sociocultural assessment and intervention. *Family nursing: Research, theory, and practice* (4th ed., pp. 173–212). Stamford, CN: Appleton & Lange.

Friedman, M. M., & Morgan, I. S. (1998). The family health care function. In M. Friedman (Ed.), *Family nursing: Research, theory, & practice* (4th ed., pp. 403–434). Stamford, CN: Appleton & Lange.

Gadamer, H. (1994). *Truth and method* (translated by J. Weinsheimer and G.D. Marshall). New York: Continuum.

Gale, A. (1984). Review of stress and the family. *British Journal of Psychology, 76*, 136–37.

Gale, A., & Vetere, A. (1987). Some theories of human behavior. In A. Vetere, & A. Gale (Eds.), *Ecological studies of family life* (pp. 34–63). New York: John Wiley & Sons.

Gallimore, R., Weisner, T. S., Bernheimer, L. P., Guthrie, D., & Nihira, K. (1993). Family responses to young children with developmental delays: Accommodation activity in ecological and cultural context. *American Journal of Mental Retardation, 98*(2), 185–206.

Gallimore, R., Weisner, T. S., Kaufman, S. Z., & Bernheimer, L. P. (1989). The social construction of ecocultural niches: Family accommodation of developmentally delayed children. *American Journal of Mental Retardation, 94*(3), 216–30.

Gallo, A., & Knafl, K. (1998). Parents' reports of "tricks of the trade" for managing childhood chronic illness. *Journal of the Society of Pediatric Nurses, 3*, 93–100.

Ganong, L. H. (1995). Intimate outsider or unwelcome intruder? *Journal of Family Nursing, 2*, 92–97.

Garbarino, J. (1978). *The role of schools in the human ecology of child maltreatment.* Paper submitted to 3rd Annual National Conference on Child Abuse and Neglect. New York: Best Paper Competition.

Garbarino, J. (1992). *Children and families in the social environment* (2nd ed.). Aldine DeGruyter: New York.

Garbarino, J., & Abramowitz, R. H. (1992). Sociocultural risk and opportunity. In J. Garbarino (Ed.), *Children and families in the social environment* (2nd ed., pp. 35–70). New York: Aldine DeGruyter.

Garbarino, J., Galambos, N. L., Plantz, M. C., & Kostelny, K. (1992). The territory of childhood. In J. Garbarino (Ed.), *Children and families in the social environment* (2nd ed., pp. 201–229). Aldine DeGruyter: New York.

Garbin, B. A. (1995). Introduction to clinical pathways. *Journal of Healthcare and Quality, 17*(6), 6–9.

Gelles, R. J., & Straus, M. A. (1979). Violence in the American family. *Journal of Social Issues, 35*(2), 15–39.

Gedaly-Duff, V., & Heims, M. L. (1996). Family child-health nursing. In S. M. Hanson (Ed.), *Family health care nursing: Theory, practice, and research* (2nd ed., pp. 239–265). Philadelphia: F. A. Davis Company.

Gibson, C. H. (1995). The process of empowerment in mothers of chronically ill children. *Journal of Advances in Nursing, 21*(6), 1201–1210.

Gibson, C. H. (1999). Facilitating critical reflection in mothers of chronically ill children. *Journal of Clinical Nursing, 8*(3), 305–312.

Gibson, R. L., & Hartshorne, T. S. (1996). Childhood sexual abuse and adult loneliness and network orientation. *Child Abuse and Neglect, 20*(11), 1087–1093.

Giddens, A. (1991). *Modernity and self-identity: Self and society in the late modern age.* Stanford, CA: Stanford University Press.

Gigar, J., & Davidhizar, R. (1995). *Transcultural nursing: Assessment and intervention* (2nd ed.). St. Louis: Mosby Year Book.

Gilligan, C. (1982). *In a different voice.* Cambridge, MA: Harvard University Press.

Gilliss, C. L. (1983). The family as the unit of analysis: Strategies for the nurse researcher. *Advances in Nursing Science, 5*(3), 50–59.

Gilliss, C. L. (1991a). Family nursing research, theory and practice. *Image: Journal of Nursing Scholarship, 23*, 19–22.

Gilliss, C. L. (1991b). The family as a unit of analysis: Strategies for the Nurse Researcher. In J. Fawcett, & A. Whall (Eds.), *Family theory development in nursing: State of the science and art* (pp. 197–207). Philadelphia: F. A. Davis Company.

Gilliss, C. L. (1991c). The family dimension of cardiovascular care. *CJCN, 2*(1), 3–8.

Gilliss, C. L. (1993). Family nursing research, theory, and practice. In G. D. Wegner, & R. J. Alexander (Eds.), *Readings in family nursing* (pp. 34–42). Philadelphia: J. B. Lippincott.

Gilliss, C. L., & Knafl, K. A. (1999). Nursing care of families in non-normative transitions: The state of science and practice. In A. S. Hinshaw, S. L. Feetham, & J. L. F. Shaver (Eds.), *Handbook of clinical nursing research* (251–271). Thousand Oaks, CA: Sage Publications.

Glascoe, F. P. (1997). The importance of discussing parents' concerns about development. *Ambulatory Child Health, 2*(4), 349–56.

Glass, N., & Davis, K. (1998). An emancipatory impulse: A feminist postmodern integrated turning point in nursing research. *Advances in Nursing Science, 21*(1), 43–52.

Goffman, E. (1959). *The presentation of self in everyday life.* New York: Anchor Books.

Golan, N. (1981). *Passing through transitions.* New York: The Free Press.

Golan, N. (1986). *The perilous bridge.* New York: The Free Press.

Goode, T. D., & Harrisone, S. (2000). *Eliminating health disparity: A mandate for a new research agenda.* National Center for Cultural Competence. Washington, D.C.: Georgetown University Child Development Center.

Goodnow, J. J. (1995). Differentiating among social contexts: By spatial features, forms of participation, and social contracts. In P. Moen, G. H. Elder, & K. Luscher (Eds.), *Examining lives in context* (pp. 269–301). Washington, D.C.: American Psychological Association.

Grant, L., & Fine, G. A. (1992). Sociology unleashed: Creative directions in classical ethnography. In M. D. LeCompte, W. L. Millroy, & J. Preissle (Eds.), *The handbook of qualitative research in education* (pp. 405–446). San Diego: Academic Press.

Gray, V. R., & Sergi, J. S. (1989). Family self-care. In P. Bomar (Ed.), *Nurses and family health promotion: Concepts, assessment, and interventions* (pp. 67–77). Baltimore: Williams & Wilkins.

Green, C. P. (1997). Teaching students how to "think family." *Journal of Family Nursing, 3*(3), 230–246.

Green, L. W., Kreuter, M. W., Deeds, F. G., & Partridge, K. B. (1980). *Health education planning: A diagnostic approach.* Mountain View, CA: Mayfield Publishing.

Greenberg, J. S., Seltzer, M., & Greenley, J. R. (1993). Aging parents of adults with disabilities: The gratifications and frustrations of later-life. *The Gerontological Society of America, 33,* 542–550.

Green-Hemandez, C. (1999). Family and cultural assessment measures in primary care. In Singleton, J. K., Sandowski, S. A., Green-Hernandez, C., Horvath, T. V., DiGregorio, R. V., & Holzemer, S. P. (Eds.). Primary Care (pp. 8–15). Philadelphia: J. B. Lippincott.

Grey, M. (1993). Stressors and children's health. *Journal of Pediatric Nursing, 8*(2), 85–91.

Hacking, I. (1983). *Representing and intervening.* New York: Cambridge University Press.

Haley, J. (1978). *Problem solving therapy.* San Francisco: Jossey Bass.

Hall, A. D., & Fagen, R. E. (1956). Definitions of General Systems. *The Yearbook of the Society for the Advancement of General Systems Theory, 1,* 18–28.

Hanna, D. R., & Roy, C. (2001). Roy adaptation model and perspective on the family. *Nursing Science Quarterly, 14*(1), 9–12.

Hanson, S. M. (2001a). Family health care nursing: An introduction. In S. M. Hanson (Ed.), *Family health care nursing: Theory, practice, and research* (2nd ed., pp. 3–35). Philadelphia: F. A. Davis Company.

Hanson, S. M. (2001b). Family assessment and intervention. In S. Hanson (Ed.), *Family health care nursing* (2nd ed., pp. 170–195). Philadelphia: F. A. Davis Company.

Hanson, S. M., & Boyd, S. T. (1996). Family nursing: An overview. In S. M. Hanson (Ed.), *Family health*

care nursing: Theory, practice, and research (2nd ed., pp. 5–37). Philadelphia: F. A. Davis Company.

Hanson, S. M., & Heims, M. L. (1992). Family nursing curricula in U.S. schools of nursing. *Journal of Nursing Education, 31*(7), 303–308.

Hanson, S. M., Heims, M., & Julian, D. (1992). Education for family health care professionals: Nursing as a paradigm. *Family Relations, 41,* 49–53.

Hanson, S. M., & Kaakinen, J. R. (2001). Theoretical foundations for family nursing. In S. M. Hanson (Ed.), *Family health care nursing: Theory, practice, and research* (2nd ed., pp. 37–59). Philadelphia: F. A. Davis Company.

Hanson, S. M., & Mischke, K. B. (1996). Family health assessment and intervention. In P. J. Bomar (Ed.), *Nurses and family health promotion: Concepts, assessment, and interventions* (2nd ed., pp.165–202). Philadelphia: W. B. Saunders Company.

Harding, S. (1987). *Feminism and methodology.* Bloomington, IN: Indiana University Press.

Harkness, S., & Super, C. M. (1994). The developmental niche: A theoretical framework for analyzing the household production of health. *Social Science Medicine, 38*(2), 217–226.

Harper, M. (1996). Culturally relevant health care service delivery for Appalachia. In M. Julia (Ed.), *Multi-cultural awareness in health care professions* (pp. 42–59). Needham Heights, MA: Simon & Schuster.

Hart, H., Bax, M., & Jenkins, S. (1984). Health and behavior in preschool children. *Child Care, Health and Development, 10,* 1–16.

Hartrick, G. (1995). Transforming family nursing theory: From mechanism to contextualism. *Journal of Family Nursing, 1*(2), 134–147.

Hartrick, G. A. (1996). The experience of self for women who are mothers: Implications for the unfolding of health. *Journal of Holistic Nursing, 14*(4), 316–331.

Hartrick, G. (1997). Beyond a service model of care: Health promotion and enhancement of family capacity. *Journal of Family Nursing, 3*(1), 57–69.

Hartrick, G. A. (1997b). Women who are mothers: The experience of defining self. *Health Care Women International,* 18(3), 263–277.

Hartrick, G. A., & Lindsey, A. E. (1995) The lived experience of family: A contextual approach to family nursing practice. *Journal of Family Nursing, 1*(2), 148–170.

Harvey, J. M., O'Callaghan, M. J., & Vines, B. (1997). Prevalence of maternal depression and its relationship to ADL skills in children with developmental delay. *Journal of Paediatric and Child Health, 33*(1), 42–46.

Hazler, R. J., Carney, J. V., Green, S., Powell, R. and Jolly, L. S. (1997). Areas of expert agreement on identification of school bullies and victims. *School Psychology International, 18,* 3–12.

Hawley, A. H. (1986). *Human ecology: A theoretical essay.* Chicago: The University of Chicago Press.

Heidegger, M. (1962). *Being and time* (translated by J. Macquarrie and E. Robinson). New York: Harper Row/Harper Collins.

Heidrich, S. M. (1996). Mechanisms related to psychological well-being in older women with chronic illnesses: Age and disease comparisons. *Research in Nursing and Health, 19*(3), 225–35.

Hertzman, C. (1998). The case for child development as a determinant of health. *Canadian Journal of Public Health, 89*(1), 14–21.

Hertzman, C. (1999). The biological embedding of early experience and its effects on health in adulthood. *Annals of NY Academic Science, 896,* 85–95

Hertzman, C., & Wiens, M. (1996). Child development and long-term outcomes: A population health perspective and summary of successful interventions. *Social Science Medicine, 43*(7), 1083–1095.

Higgins, L. (1991). How adequately are nurses being prepared for their health teaching role? *Australian Journal of Advances in Nursing,* 8(3), 11–14.

Higgs, P., & Jones, I. R. (1999). Evolutionary psychology and health: Confronting an evolving paradigm. *Journal of Health Service, Research, and Policy,* 4(3), 187–190.

Hilbert, G. A., Walker, M. B., & Rinehart, J. (2000). "In for the Long Haul": Responses of parents caring for children with Sturge-Weber Syndrome. *Journal of Family Nursing,* 6(2), 157–179.

Hill, R. (1949). *Families under stress.* New York: Harper & Row.

Hill, R. (1965). *Challenges and resources for family mobility: Family mobility in our dynamic society.* Ames, IA: Iowa State University.

Hoffman, L., & Lippitt, R. (1960). Measurement of family variables. In Mussen (Ed.), *Handbook of research methods in child development* (pp. 945–1014). New York: Wiley.

Hooyman, N. R., & Gonyea, J. (1995). *Feminist perspectives on family care: Policies for gender justice.* Thousand Oaks, CA: Sage Publications.

Hughes, M., Dote-Kwan, J., & Dolendo, J. (1999). Characteristics of maternal directiveness and responsiveness with young children with visual impairments. *Child Health Care Devevelopment,* 25(4), 285–298.

Humphrey, R. & Thigpen-Beck, R. (1997). Caregiver role: Ideas about feeding infants and toddlers. *Occupational Therapy Journal of Research,* 17(4), 237–263.

Imber-Black, E., & Roberts, J. (1992). *Rituals for our times.* New York: Harper Perrenial.

Institute of Medicine. (1988). *The future of public health.* Washington, D.C.: National Academy Press.

Institute of Medicine. (2000a). *Informing the future: Critical issues in health.* Washington, D.C.

Institute of Medicine. (2000b). *To err is human: Building a safer health system.* Health Care Services.

Institute of Medicine. (2001). *Crossing the quality chasm: A new health system for the 21st century.* Washington, D.C.

Isaacs, M., & Benjamin, M. (1991). *Towards a culturally competent system of care: Programs which utilize culturally competent principles* (Vol. II). Washington, D.C.: Georgetown University Child Development Center, CASSP Technical Assistance Center.

Jacobs, L. A., & Deatrick, J. A. (1999). The individual, the family, and genetic testing. *Journal of Professional Nursing,* 15(5), 313–24.

Jenkins, J. E., & Zunguze, S. T. (1998). The relationship of family structure to adolescent drug use, peer affiliation, and perception of peer acceptance of drug use. *Adolescence,* 33(132), 811–22.

Jensen E. W., James, S. A., Boyce, W. T., & Hartnett, S. A. (1983). The family routines inventory: Development and validation. *Social Science Medicine,* 1(4), 201–11.

Johnson, B. S. (2000). Mothers' perceptions of parenting children with disabilities. *Maternal Child Nursing: American Journal of Maternal-Child Nursing,* 25(3), 127–132.

Johnson, D. E. (1990). The behavioral system model for nursing. In M. E. Parker (Ed.), *Nursing theories in practice* (pp. 23–32). New York: National League for Nursing.

Johnson, M., & Maas, M. (1998). The nursing outcomes classification. *Journal of Nursing Care and Quality,* 12(5), 9–20.

Kagawa-Singer, M. (1993). Redefining health: Living with cancer. *Social Science Medicine,* 37(3), 295–304.

Kantor, D., & Lehr, W. (1975). *Inside the family: Towards a theory of family process.* San Francisco: Jossey-Bass.

Kazak, A. E. (1997). A contextual family/systems approach to pediatric psychology: Introduction to the special issue. *Journal of Pediatric Psychology,* 22(2), 141–8

Keefe, S. (1988). Appalachian family ties. In S. Keefe (Ed.), *Appalachian mental health* (pp. 24–35). Lexington, KY: The University Press of Kentucky.

Kellam, S. G., Ensminger, M. E., & Turner, R. J. (1977). Family structure and the mental health of children: Concurrent and longitudinal community-wide studies. *Archives of General Psychiatry,* 34(9), 1012–1022.

Kellegrew, D. H. (2000). Constructing daily routines: A qualitative examination of mothers with young children with disabilities. *American Journal of Occupational Therapy,* 54(3), 252–259.

Kelley, D. L., & Sequeira, D. L. (1997). Understanding family functioning in a changing America. *Communication Studies,* 48(2), 93–108.

Kelly, R. B., Zyzanski, S. J., & Alemagno, S. A. (1991). Prediction of motivation and behavior change following health promotion: Role of health beliefs, social support, and self-efficacy. *Social Science Medicine,* 32(3), 311–320.

Kelley, S. J., Yorker, B. C., & Whitley, D. (1997). To grandmother's house we go . . . and stay. Children raised in intergenerational families. *Journal of Gerontological Nursing,* 23(9), 12–20.

Keltner, B. (1990). Family characteristics of preschool social competence among Black children in a Head Start program. *Child Psychiatry and Human Development,* 21(2), 95–108.

Keltner, B. R. (1992). Family influences on child health status. *Pediatric Nursing,* 18(2), 128–131.

Keltner, B. (1994). Home environment of mothers with mental retardation. *Mental Retardation,* 32(2), 123–127.

Keltner, B., Keltner, N., & Farran, E. (1990). Family routines and conduct disorders in adolescent girls. *Western Journal of Nursing Research,* 12, 161–174.

Keltner, B., & Ramey, S. L. (1992). The family. *Current Opinion in Psychiatry,* 5, 638–644.

Keltner, B., & Ramey, S. L. (1993). Family issues. *Current Opinion in Psychiatry,* 6(5), 629–634.

Kenney, J. W. (1992). The consumer's views of health. *Journal of Advanced Nursing,* 17, 829–834.

Kerlinger, F. N. (1986). *Foundations of behavioral research*. Fort Worth, TX: Hartcourt Brace Jovanovich College Publishers.

Kim, H. S. (1987). Structuring the nursing knowledge system: A typology of four domains. *Scholarly Inquiry for Nursing Practice, 1,* 99–110.

Kim, H. S. (2000a). *The nature of theoretical thinking in nursing* (2nd ed.). New York: Springer Publishing Company.

Kim, H. S. (2000b). An integrative framework for conceptualizing clients: A proposal for a nursing perspective in the new century. *Nursing Science Quarterly, 13*(1), 37–44.

Kindlon, D., & Thompson, D. (1999). *Raising Cain: Protecting the emotional life of boys.* New York: Ballantine Books.

King, I. M. (1981). *A theory for nursing: Systems, concepts, process.* New York: Wiley.

King, I. M. (1995). A systems framework for nursing. In M. A. Frey, & C. L. Sieloff (Eds.), *Advancing King's systems framework and theory of nursing* (pp. 14–22). Thousand Oaks, CA: Sage Publications.

Kirkley, D. L. (2000). Is motherhood good for women? A feminist exploration. *Journal of Obstetrical & Gynecological Neonatal Nursing, 29*(5), 459–464.

Kleffel, D. (1991). Rethinking the environment as a domain of nursing knowledge. *Advances in Nursing Science, 14*(1), 40–51.

Klein, D.M., & White, J.M. (1996). *Family theories: An introduction.* Thousand Oaks, CA: Sage Publications.

Klerman, L., Ramey, S., & Goldenberg, R. (2001). A randomized trial of augmented prenatal care for multiple-risk, Medicaid eligible African American women. *American Journal of Public Health, 91,* 105–111.

Kohlberg, L. (1981). *The philosophy of moral development.* New York: Harper & Row.

Kohn, M. L. (1995). Social structure and personality through time and space. In P. Moen, G. H. Elder, & K. Luscher (Eds.), *Examining lives in context* (pp.141–168). Washington, D.C.: American Psychological Association.

Kohn, M. L., & Slomczynski, K. M. (1990). *Social structure and self-direction: A comparative analysis of the United States and Poland.* Oxford, United Kingdom: Basil Blackwell.

Koniak-Griffin, D., & Verzemnieks, I. (1995). The relationship between parental ratings of child behaviors, interaction, and the home environment. *Journal of Maternal Child Nursing, 23*(2), 44–56.

Krulik, T., Turner-Henson, A., Kanematsu, Y., al-Ma'aitah, R., Swan, J., & Holaday, B. (1999). Parenting stress and mothers of young children with chronic illness: A cross-cultural study. *Journal of Pediatric Nursing, 14*(2), 130–140.

Kuczynski, L., & Kochanska, G. (1995). Function and content of maternal demands: Developmental significance of early demands for competent action. *Child Development, 66*(3), 616–628.

Kuhn, T. S. (1970). *The structure of scientific revolutions* (2nd ed.). Chicago: The University of Chicago Press.

Kupersmidt, J. B., Griesler, P. C., DeRosier, M. E., Patterson, C. J., & Davis, P. W. (1995). Childhood aggression and peer relations in the context of family and neighborhood factors. *Child Development, 66*(2), 360–375.

Lackey, N., & Walker, B. L. (1998). An ecological framework for family nursing practice and research. In B. Vaughan-Cole, M. Johnson, J. Malone, & B. Walker (Eds.), *Family nursing practice* (pp. 38–48). Philadelphia: W. B. Saunders Company.

Lagerspetz, K. M. (1964). Studies on the aggressive behavior of mice. *Annales Acadamiae Scientiarum Fennicae, 131*(3, Series B), 1–131.

Lamb, M. E. (1988). The ecology of adolescent pregnancy and parenthood. In A. R. Pence (Ed.), *Ecological research with children and families* (pp. 99–121). New York: Teachers College, Columbia University.

Landesman, S., Jaccard, J., & Gunderson, V. (1991). The family environment: The combined influence of family behavior, goals, strategies, resources, and individual experiences. In M. Lewis, & S. Feinman (Eds.), *Social influences and socialization in infancy* (pp. 63–96). New York: Plenum.

Lantz, P. M., House, J. S., Lepkowski, J. M., Williams, D. R., Mero, R. P., & Chen, J. (1998). Socioeconomic factors, health behaviors, and mortality: Results from a nationally representative prospective study of US adults. *Journal of the American Medical Association, 279*(21), 1703–1708.

Larkin, H. (2000). Increasing social support: An evolving approach to better health. *Advances: The Robert Wood Johnson Foundation Quarterly Newsletter, 3,* 3.

Larson E. (1998). Reframing the meaning of disability to families: The embrace of paradox. *Social Science Medicine, 47*(7), 865–875.

Larson, E. A. (2000). The orchestration of occupation: The dance of mothers. *American Journal of Occupational Therapy, 54*(3), 269–280.

Lasky, P. A., & Eichelberger, K. M. (1985). Health-related views and self-care behaviors of young children. *Family Relations, 34,* 13–18.

Lau, R. R., Quadrel, M. J., & Hartman, K. A. (1990). Development and change of young adults' preventive health beliefs and behavior: Influence from parents and peers. *Journal of Health and Social Behavior, 31,* 240–259.

Laudan, L. (1981). A problem-solving approach to scientific progress. In I. Hacking (Ed.), *Scientific revolutions.* New York: Oxford University Press.

Lazarsfeld, P., & Menzel, H. (1969). On the relation between individuals and collective properties. In A. Etzioni (Ed.), *A sociological reader on complex organizations* (pp. 499–516). New York: Holt, Rinehart & Winston.

Leavitt, L. A. (1998). Mothers' sensitivity to infant signals. *Pediatrics, 102*(5 suppl E), 1247–1249.

Leininger, M. (1991). Selected culture care findings of diverse cultures using culture care theory and ethnomethods. In M. Leininger (Ed.), *Culture care diversity and universality: A theory of nursing* (pp. 345–371). New York: National League for nursing Press.

Leonard, B., Johnson, A., & Brust, J. (1993). Caregiving of children with disabilities: A comparison of managing "OK" and those needing more help. *Children's Health Care, 22,* 93–105.

Levinson, W., Gorawara-Bhat, R., & Lamb, J. (2000). A study of patient clues and physician responses in primary care and surgical settings. *Journal of the American Medical Association, 284*(8), 1021–1027.

Lewin, K. (1936). *Principles of topological psychology.* New York: McGraw-Hill.

Lewin, K. (1951). *Field theory in social science: Selected theoretical papers.* New York: Harper.

Lewis, M. L., Brand, K. P., Duckett, L., & Fairbanks, D. (1997). Preparing nurses for tomorrow's reality: Strategies from an honors program. *Nurse Educator, 22*(1), 12–16.

Liebermann, D. A. (2001). Management of chronic pediatric diseases with interactive games: Theory and research findings. *Journal of Ambulatory Care, 24,* 26–38.

Lightman, A. (1993). *Einstein's dreams.* New York: Pantheon Books.

Lindgren, C. L. (2000). Chronic sorrow in long-term illness across the life span. In J. Miller (Ed.), *Coping with chronic illness: Overcoming powerlessness* (3rd ed., pp.125–143). Philadelphia: F. A. Davis Company.

Loveland-Cherry, C. J. (1996). Family health promotion and health protection. In P. J. Bomar (Ed.), *Nurses and family health promotion: Concepts, assessment, and interventions* (2nd ed., pp. 22–35). Philadelphia: W. B. Saunders Company.

Lubeck, R. C., & Chandler, L. K. (1990). Organizing the home caregiving environment for infants. *Education and Treatment of Children, 13*(4), 347–363.

Ludwig, F.M. (1998). The unpackaging of routine in older women. *American Journal of Occupational Therapy, 52*(3), 168–178.

Luscher, K. (1995). *Homo interpretans*: On the relevance of perspectives, knowledge, and beliefs in the ecology of human development. In P. Moen, G. H. Elder, & K. Luscher (Eds.), *Examining lives in context* (pp. 563–597). Washington, D.C.: American Psychological Association.

Lutjens, L. R., & Horan, M. L. (1992). Nursing theory in nursing education: an educational imperative. *Journal of Professional Nursing, 8*(5), 276–281.

Maas, M. L., Johnson, M., & Moorhead, S. (1996). Classifying nursing-sensitive patient outcomes. *Image: Journal of Nursing Scholarship, 28*(4), 295–301.

MacLeod, M. L., & Farrell, P. (1994). The need for significant reform: A practice-driven approach to curriculum. *Journal of Nursing Education, 33*(5), 208–214.

Macintyre, S. (1994). Understanding the social patterning of health: The role of the social sciences. *Journal of Public Health Medicine, 16*(1), 53–59.

MacPherson, K. (1983). Feminist methods: A new paradigm for nursing research. *Advances in Nursing Science, 5*(2), 17–25.

Macran, S., Clarke, L., & Joshi, H. (1996). Women's health: Dimensions and differentials. *Social Science Medicine, 42*(9), 1203–1216.

Maden, M. F., & Wrench, D. F. (1977). Significant findings in child abuse research. *Victimology, 2*(2), 196–224.

Magnusson, D. (1988). *Individual development from an interactional perspective.* Hillsdale, NK: Erlbaum.

Mahoney, G., O'Sullivan, P., & Robinson, C. (1992). The family environments of children with disabilities: Diverse but not so different. *Topics in Early Childhood Special Education, 12,* 386–402.

Mallow, G. E., & Bechtel, G. A. (1999). Chronic sorrow: The experience of parents with children who are developmentally disabled. *Journal of Psychosocial Nursing & Mental Health Services, 37*(7), 31–5, 42–43.

Mandelblatt, J., Hadley, J., & Kerner, J. F. (2000). Patterns of breast carcinoma treatment in older women: Patient preference and clinical and physician influences. *Cancer, 89*(3), 561–573.

Marjoribanks, K. (1998). Family capital, children's individual attributes, and adolescents' aspirations: A follow-up analysis. *Journal of Psychology, 132*(3), 328–336.

Markson, S. (1998). *Family rituals as a protective factor for children with asthma.* Unpublished dissertation. Syracuse University.

Markson, S., & Fiese, B. H. (2000). Family rituals as a protective factor for children with asthma. *Journal of Pediatric Psychology, 25*(7), 471–480.

Marmot, M. G., Fuhrer, R., Ettner, S. L., Marks, N. F., Bumpass, L. L., & Ryff, C. D. (1998). *Contribution of psychosocial factors to socioeconomic differences in health. Milbank Quarterly, 76*(3), 403–448.

Maturana, H., & Varela, F. (1992). *The tree of knowledge: The biological roots of human understanding.* Boston: Shambhala Publications, Inc.

Mauksch, H. (1974). A social science basis for conceptualizing family health. *Social Science and Medicine, 8,* 521–523.

McAdoo, H. P. (1993). Ethnic families: Strengths that are found in diversity. In H. P. McAdoo (Ed.), *Family ethnicity: Strength in diversity* (pp. 3–14). Newbury Park, CA: Sage Publications.

McClanahan, S. S. (1983). Family structure and stress: A longitudinal comparison of two parent and female-headed families. *Journal of Marriage and the Family, 45,* 47–57.

McLanahan, S. S. (1985). Family structure and the reproduction of poverty. *American Journal of Sociology, 90,* 873–901.

McClearn, G. E., Vogler, G. P., & Plomin, R. (1996). Genetics and behavioral medicine. *Behavioral Medicine, 22*(3), 93–102.

McCloskey, J. C., & Bulechek, G. M. (1995). Construction and validation of a taxonomy of nursing interventions. *Medinfo, 8,* 140–143.

McCormick, J., Kirkham, S., & Hayes, V. (1998). Abstracting women: Essentialism in women's health research. *Health Care Women International, 19*(6), 495–504.

McCubbin, M. A. (1989). Family stress and family strengths: A comparison of single and two-parent families with handicapped children. *Research in Nursing and Health, 12,* 101–110.

McCubbin, M. A., & McCubbin, H. I. (1991). Family stress theory and assessment: The resiliency model of family stress, adjustment, and adaptation. In H. I. McCubbin, & A. Thompson (Eds.), *Family assessment inventories for research and practice* (pp. 3–32). Madison, WI: University of Wisconsin-Madison.

McCubbin, M. A., & McCubbin, H. I. (1993). Families coping with illness: The resiliency model of family stress, adjustment and adaptation. In C. Danielson, B. Hamel-Bissell, & P. Winstead-Fry (Eds.), *Families, health, and illness: Perspectives on coping and intervention* (pp. 21–63). St. Louis: Mosby Year Book.

McCubbin, H. I., McCubbin, M. A., Thompson, A. I., & Han, S. Y. (1999). Contextualizing family risk factors for alcoholism and alcohol abuse. *Journal of Studies on Alcohol, 13*(suppl), 75–78.

McCubbin, H. I., & Patterson, J. M. (1983). Family adaptation to crisis. In H. McCubbin, A. Cauble, & J. Patterson (Eds.), Social stress and the family (Special issue). *Marriage and Family Review, 6*(1/2), 7–27.

McFarlane, A. H., Bellissimo, A., & Norman, G. R. (1995). Family structure, family functioning and adolescent well-being: The transcendent influence of parental style. *Journal of Child Psychology and Psychiatry, 36*(5), 847–864.

McGoldrick, M., & Carter, B. (1999). Self in context: The individual life cycle in systemic perspective. In B. Carter, & M. McGoldrick (Eds.), *The expanded family life cycle: Individual, family, and social perspectives* (3rd ed., pp. 27–46). Boston: Allyn and Bacon.

McGoldrick, M., & Gerson, R. (1985). *Genograms in family assessment.* New York: W.W. Norton.

McGowan, D. E., & Artinian, B. M. (1997). The family as client. In B. M. Artinian, & M. M. Conger (Eds.), *The Intersystem Model: Integrating theory and practice* (pp. 130–154). Thousand Oaks, CA: Sage Publications.

McGowan, D. E., Delamarter, P., Schroeder, B. & Liegler, R. M. (1989). Family recreation and exercise. In P. Bomar (Ed.), *Nurses and family health promotion: Concepts, assessment, and interventions* (pp. 216–236). Baltimore: Williams & Wilkins.

McKenzie, R. (1991). Appalachian culture as reaction to uneven development: A world systems approach to regionalism. In B. Ergood, & B. Kuhre (Eds.), *Appalachia: Social context past and present* (pp. 284–289). Dubuque, IO: Kendall/Hunt Publishing Co.

McLeod, J. D., & Shanahan, M. J. (1993). Poverty, parenting, and children's mental health. *American Sociological Review, 58,* 351–366.

Mead, G. H. (1934). *Mind, self, and society.* Chicago: University of Chicago Press.

Meleis, A. I. (1991). *Theoretical nursing: Development and progress* (2nd ed.). Philadelphia: J.B. Lippincott.

Meleis, A. I. (1997). *Theoretical nursing: Development and progress* (3rd ed.). Philadelphia: J. B. Lippincott.

Messer, M., & Ozmar, B. (1999). Use of evidence-based practice management guidelines in trauma care. *International Journal of Trauma Nursing, 5*(1), 17–18.

Meyers, C. (1992). Hmong children and their families: Consideration of cultural influences in assessment. *American Journal of Occupational Therapy, 46*(8), 737–744.

Meyers, C. E., Mink, I. T., & Nihira, K. (1990). *Home quality rating scale* (Rev.). Los Angeles: University of California, Los Angeles, Department of Psychiatry and Biobehavioral Sciences.

Miller, J. F. (1986). *Development of an instrument to measure hope.* Unpublished doctoral dissertation. University of Illinois, Chicago.

Miller, J. F. (2000). Inspiring hope. In J. Miller (Ed.), *Coping with chronic illness: Overcoming powerlessness* (3rd ed., pp. 523–546). Philadelphia: F. A. Davis Company.

Miller, K. A., & Kohn, M. L. (1983). The reciprocal effects of job conditions and the intellectuality of leisure-time activities. In M. L. Kohn, & C. Schooler (Eds.), *Work and personality: An inquiry into the impact of social stratification* (pp. 217–241). Norwood, NJ: Ablex.

Minuchin, S. (1974). *Families and family therapy.* London: Tavistock.

Minuchin, S., & Fishman, H. G. (1981). *Family therapy techniques.* Cambridge, MA: Harvard University Press.

Minuchin, S., Lee, W. Y., & Simon, G. (1996). *Mastering family therapy: Journeys of growth and transformation.* New York: John Wiley & Sons.

Moen, P., & Erickson, M. A. (1995). Linked lives: A transgenerational approach to resilience. In P. Moen, G. H. Elder, & K. Luscher (Eds.), *Examining lives in context* (pp. 169–210). Washington, D.C.: American Psychological Association.

Mohr, W. K., & Naylor, M. D. (1998). Creating a curriculum for the 21st century. *Nursing Outlook, 46*(5), 206–212.

Monheit, A. C., & Vistnes, J. P. (2000). Race/ethnicity and health insurance status: 1987 and 1996. *Medical Care Research and Reviews, 57*(supplement 1), 11–35.

Monheit, A. C., Vistnes, J. P., & Eisenberg, J. M. (2001). Moving to Medicare: Trends in the health insurance status of near elderly workers, 1987–1996. *Health Affairs, 20,* 204–213.

Monk, T. H., Flaherty, J. F., Frank, E., Hoskinson, M. A., & Kupfer, D. J. (1990). The social rhythm metric: An instrument to quantify the daily rhythms of life. *Journal of Nervous and Mental Disease, 178*(2), 120–126.

Moore, S. F., & Myeroff, B. G. (1977). Secular ritual: Forms and meanings. In S. Moore, & B. Myeroff (Eds.), *Secular ritual.* Amsterdam: Van Gorcum.

Moos, R. H., Insel, P. M., & Humphrey, B. (1974). *Family environment scale.* Palo Alto, CA: Consulting Psychologist Press.

Moos, B. S., & Moos, R. H. (1986). *Family environment scale manual* (2nd ed). Palo Alto, CA: Consulting Psychologist Press.

Morris, J. A. (1999). Information and redundancy: Key concepts in understanding the genetic control of health and intelligence. *Medical Hypotheses, 53*(2), 118–123.

Morris, R. I. (1996). Preparing for the 21st century: Planning with focus groups. *Nurse Educator, 21*(6), 38–42.

Moscovice, I., & Rosenblatt, R. (2000). Quality-of-care challenges for rural health. *Journal of Rural Health, 16*(2), 168–176.

Myers, E. R., McCrory, D. C., & Subramanian, S. (2000). Setting the target for a better cervical screening test: Characteristics of a cost-effective test for cervical neoplasia screening. *Obstetrics and Gynecology, 96*(5), 645–652.

Myeroff, B. G. (1977). We don't wrap herring in a printed page: Fusions, fictions, and continuity in secular ritual. In S. Moore, & B. Myeroff (Eds.), *Secular ritual.* Amsterdam: Van Gorcum.

National Center for Health Statistics. (December, 2000). Centers for Disease Control. [http://www.cdc.gov/nchs/fastats/hexpense.html].

National Home and Hospice Care Survey. (December, 2000). Centers for Disease Control.

National Center for Health Statistics. [http://www.cdc.gov/nchs/fastats/homehosp.htm].

Nelson, D. B., & Edgil, A. E. (1998). Family dynamics in families with very low birth weight and full term infants: A pilot study. *Journal of Pediatric Nursing, 13*(2), 95–103.

Nelson, M. A. (1994). Economic impoverishment as a health risk: Methodologic and conceptual issues. *Advances in Nursing Science, 16*(3) 1–12.

Neuman, B. (1989). *The Neuman systems model.* Stamford, CN: Appleton & Lange.

Neuman, B. (1995). The *Neuman systems model* (3rd ed.). Stamford, CN: Appleton & Lange.

Newell, L. D. (1999). *A qualitative analysis of family rituals and traditions.* Unpublished dissertation.

Newman, M. A. (1983). The continuing revolution: A history of nursing science. In N.L. Chaska (Ed.), *The nursing profession: A time to speak* (pp. 385–393). New York: McGraw-Hill.

Newman, M. A. (1997). Experiencing the whole. Advances in Nursing Science, *20*(1), 34–39.

Nightengale, F. (1992). *Notes on nursing.* Philadelphia: J. B. Lippincott. (Originally published in 1860 by D. Appleton and Co.)

Nihira, K., Weisner, T. S., & Bernheimer, L. P. (1994). Ecocultural assessment in families of children with developmental delays: Construct and concurrent validities. *American Journal on Mental Retardation, 98*(5), 551–566.

Niska, K., Snyder, M., & Lia-Hoagberg, B. (1998). Family ritual facilitates adaptation to parenthood. *Public Health Nursing, 15*(5), 329–337.

Nursing Science Quarterly. (2000). Nursing theory guided by practice: A definition. *Nursing Science Quarterly, 13*(2), 177.

Oakley, A. (1981). Interviewing women: A contradiction in terms. In H. Roberts (Ed.), *Feminist research methods: Exemplary readings in the social sciences* (pp. 44–62). San Francisco: Westview Press.

O'Connor, P. J., Crabtree, B. F., & Yanoshik, M. K. (1997). Differences between diabetic patients who do and do not respond to a diabetes care intervention: A qualitative analysis. *Family Medicine, 29*(6), 42–48.

O'Farrell, T. J., & Feehan, M. (1999). Alcoholism treatment and the family: Do family and individual treatments for alcoholic adults have preventive effects for children? *Journal of Studies on Alcohol Supplement, 13,* 125–129.

O'Hear, A. (1989). *An introduction to the philosophy of science.* New York: Oxford University Press.

Ohio Job and Family Services. (October, 2000). Civilian Labor Force Estimates. [http://www.state.oh.us/odjfs/releases/unemp/ColorRateMap.pdf].

Olds, L. (1992). *Metaphors of interrelatedness: Toward a systems theory of psychology.* New York: State University of New York Press.

Olson, D. (1986). Circumplex Model VII: Validation studies and FACES III. *Family Process, 25,* 337–351.

Olson, D., McCubbin, H., Barnes, H., Larsen, A., Muxen, M., & Wilson, M. (1983). *Families: What makes them work.* Beverly Hills, CA: Sage Publications.

Olson, D., Partner, J., & Lavee, Y. (1985). *Family adaptability and cohesion evaluation scales.* St. Paul, MN: University of Minnesota, Family Social Science.

Olsen, D., Russell, C., & Sprenkle, D. (1983). Circumplex model of marital and family systems. *Family Process, 22*(1), 69–83.

Olson, D., Sprenkle, D., & Russell, C. (1979). Circumplex model of marital and family systems: Cohesion and adaptability dimensions, family types, and clinical applications. *Family Process, 18,* 3–28.

O'Neill, E. S., & Morrow, L. L. (2001). The symptom experience of women with chronic illness. *Journal of Advanced Nursing, 33*(2), 257–268.

Orem, D. (1971). *Nursing: Concepts of practice.* New York: McGraw-Hill.

Orem, D. (1995). *Nursing: Concepts of practice* (5th ed.). St. Louis: Mosby Year Book.

Palazzoli, M. S., Boscolo, L., Cecchin, G. F., & Prata, G. (1977). Family rituals a powerful tool in family therapy. *Family Process, 16*(4), 445–453.

Parad, H. J., & Caplan, G. (1965). A framework for studying family in crisis. In H. J. Parad (Ed.), *Crisis intervention: Selected readings* (pp. 55–60). New York: Family Service of America.

Parkes, C. M. (1972). *Bereavement: Studies of grief in adult life.* New York: International Universities Press.

Parse, R. R. (1981). *Man-living-health: A theory of nursing.* New York: Wiley.

Parse, R. R. (1987). Man-Living-Health theory of nursing. In R. R. Parse (Ed.), *Nursing science: Major paradigms, theories, and critiques* (pp. 159–180). Philadelphia: W. B. Saunders Company.

Parse, R. R. (1997a). The language of nursing knowledge: Saying what we mean. In I. M. King, & J. Fawcett (Eds.), *The language of nursing theory and metatheory* (pp. 73–77). Indianapolis, IN: Sigma Theta Tau International Center Nursing Press.

Parse, R. R. (1997b). The human becoming theory: The was, is, and will be. *Nursing Science Quarterly, 10,* 32–38.

Pathman, D. (2000). State scholarship, loan forgiveness, and related programs: The unheralded safety net. *Journal of the American Medical Association, 284,* 2084–2092.

Patterson, R. E., Haines, P. S., & Popkin, B. M. (1994). Health lifestyle patterns of U.S. adults. *Prevention Medicine, 23*(4), 453–460.

Patton, M. Q. (1990). *Qualitative evaluation and research methods.* Newbury Park, CA: Sage Publications.

Pearsall, P. (1990). *The power of the family: Strength, comfort, and healing.* New York: Doubleday.

Pelletier, L., Godin, G., Lepage, L., & Dussault, G. (1994). Social support received by mothers of chronically ill children. *Child Care Health Development, 20*(2), 115–131.

Pender, N. J. (1987). Health *promotion in nursing practice* (2nd ed.). Norwalk, CT: Appleton & Lange.

Pender, N. J. (1996). *Health promotion in nursing practice* (3rd ed.). Stamford, CN: Appleton & Lange.

Pender, N. J., Barkauskas, V. H., Hayman, L., Rice, V. H., & Anderson, E. T. (1992). Health promotion and disease prevention: Toward excellence in nursing practice and education. *Nursing Outlook, 40*(3), 106–112.

Pender, N. J., Walker, S. N., Sechrist, K. R., & Frank-Stromborg, M. (1990). *The health promotion model: Refinement and validation* (NR 01121). Northern Illinois University, DeKalb, IL: National

Center for Nursing Research, National Institutes of Health.

Perrin, E. C., Ayoub, C. C., & Willett, J. B. (1993). In the eyes of the beholder: Family and maternal influences on perceptions of adjustment of children with a chronic illness. *Journal of Developmental Behavior Pediatrics, 14*(2), 94–105.

Pettit, G. S. (1997). The developmental course of violence and aggression: Mechanisms of family and peer influence. *Psychiatric Clinics of North America, 20*(2), 283–299.

Piaget, J. (1971). *Science of education and the psychology of the child.* New York: Viking Press.

Piercy, M. (1976). *Women on the edge of time.* New York: Fawcett Crest.

Pike, A., & Plomin, R. (1996). Importance of non-shared environmental factors for childhood and adolescent psychopathology. *Journal of American Academy of Child and Adolescent Psychiatry, 35*(5), 560–70.

Plomin, R. (1983). Developmental behavioral genetics. *Child Development, 54*(2), 253–259.

Plomin, R. (1994). The Emanuel Miller Memorial Lecture 1993: Genetic research and identification of environmental influences. *Journal of Child Psychiatry, 35*(5), 817–834.

Plomin, R. (1995). Genetics and children's experiences in the family. *Journal of Child Psychology and Psychiatry, 36*(1), 33–68.

Pollack, W. (1998). *Real boys: Rescuing our sons from the myths of boyhood.* New York: Henry Holt and Company.

Pollitt & Hungler (1999). *Nursing research: Principles and methods* (6th ed.). New York: Lippincott.

Popper, K. (1959). *The logic of scientific discovery.* London: Hutchinson.

Popper, K. (1972). *Objective knowledge.* New York: Oxford University Press.

Poverty in America, (2002). NPR/Kaiser/Kennedy School Poll. From *http://www.nprorg/programs/specials/poll/poverty*

Power, C., Matthews, S., & Manor, O. (1996). Inequalities in self rated health in the 1958 birth cohort: Lifetime social circumstances or social mobility. *British Medical Journal, 313*(7055), 449–53.

Pratt, L. (1976). *Family structure and effective health behavior: The energized family.* Boston: Houghton Mifflin Company.

Preski, S., & Walker, L. O. (1997). Contributions of maternal identity and lifestyle to young children's adjustment. *Research in Nursing and Health, 20*(20), 107–117.

Primeau, L. (2000). Divisions of household work, routines, and child care occupations in families. *Journal of Occupational Science, 7*(1), 19–28.

Prochaska, J. O., Norcross, J. C., & Diclemente, C. C. (1994). *Changing for good.* New York: Avon Books.

Rabuzzi, K. A. (1988). *Motherself: A mythic analysis of motherhood.* Bloomington, IN: Indiana University Press.

Rahkonen, O., & Takala, P. (1998). Social differences in health and functional disability among older men and women. *International Journal of Health Services, 28*(3), 511–524.

Rahkonen, O., Lahelma, E., & Huuhka, M. (1997). Past or present? Childhood living conditions and current socioeconomic status as determinants of adult health. *Social Science Medicine, 44*(3), 327–336.

Rando, T. A. (1984). *Grief, dying, and death: Clinical interventions for caregivers.* Champaign, IL: Research Press Company.

Rando, T. A. (1993). *Treatment of complicated mourning.* Champaign, IL: Research Press.

Ransom, D. (1984). Random notes: The patient is not a dirty window. *Family Systems Medicine, 3,* 230–233.

Ransom, D. C. (1986). Research on the family in health, illness and care—State of the art. *Family Systems Medicine, 4*(2–3), 329–335.

Rappaport, R. A. (1971). Ritual, sanctity, and cybernetics. *American Anthropology, 73,* 59–76.

Ray, L. D., & Ritchie, J. (1993). Caring for chronically ill children at home: Factors that influence parents coping. *Journal of Pediatric Nursing, 8,* 217–225.

Reiss, D. (1981). *The family's construction of reality.* Cambridge, MA: Harvard University Press.

Reiss, D., & Elstein, A. S. (1971). Perceptual and cognitive resources of family members: Contrasts between families of paranoid and nonparanoid schizophrenics and nonschizophrenic psychiatric patients. *Archives of General Psychiatry, 24,* 121–134.

Reynolds, C. L. (1988). The measurement of health in nursing research. *Advances in Nursing Science, 10*(4), 23–31.

Rich, A. (1976). *Of women born: Motherhood as experience and institution.* New York: W. W. Norton.

Richards, M. M., Adams, T. D., & Hunt, S. C. (2000). Functional status and emotional well-being, dietary intake, and physical activity of severely obese subjects. *Journal of American Dietetic Association, 100*(1), 67–75.

Riesch, S. K., Coleman, R., Glowacki, J. S., & Konings, K. (1997). Understanding mothers' perceptions of what is important about themselves and parenting. *Journal of Community Health Nursing, 14*(1), 49–66.

Roberts, C. S., & Feetham, S. L. (1982). Assessing family functioning across three areas of relationships. *Nursing Research, 31,* 231–235.

Roberts, J. (1988). Setting the frame: Definitions, functions, and typology of rituals. In E. Imber-Black, J. Roberts, & E. Whiting (Eds.), *Rituals in families and family therapy* (pp. 3–46). New York: Norton.

Robinson, C. A. (1995). Unifying distinctions for nursing research with persons and families. *Journal of Family Nursing, 1*(1), 8–29.

Rodriguez, R. (1993). Violence in transience: Nursing care of battered migrant woman. *Clinical Issues in Perinatal Women's Health Nursing, 4*(3), 437–440.

Rogers, M. E. (1970). *An introduction to a theoretical basis of nursing.* Philadelphia: F. A. Davis Company.

Rogers, M. E. (1992). Nursing science and the space age. *Nursing Science Quarterly, 5,* 27–34.

Rogers, J. C., & Holloway, R. I. (1991). Family rituals and the care of individual patients. *Family Systems Medicine, 9*(3), 249–259.

Rolland, J. (1988). Model of chronic and life-threatening illness. In C. S. Chilman, E. W. Nunnally, & F. M. Cox (Eds.), *Chronic illness and disability* (pp. 17–68). Newbury Park, CA: Sage.

Rolland, J. (1993). Serious illness and disability. In F. Walsh (Ed.), *Normal family processes* (2nd ed., pp. 444–473). New York: Guilford Press.

Ross, C. E., Mirowsky, J., & Goldsteen, K. (1990). The impact of the family on health: The decade in review. *Journal of Marriage and the Family, 52,* 1059–1078.

Roth, P. (1989). Family social support. In P. Bomar (Ed.), *Nurses and family health promotion: Concepts, assessment, and interventions* (pp. 90–102). Baltimore: Williams & Wilkins.

Rowe, D. C., Jacobson, K. C., & Van den Oord, E. J. (1999). Genetic and environmental influences on vocabulary IQ: Parental education level as moderator. *Child Development, 70*(5), 1151–62.

Rosenzwig, M. R., & Schultz, T. P. (1982). The behavior of mothers as inputs to child health: The determinants of birth weight, gestation, and rate of fetal growth. In V. R. Fuchs (Ed.), *Economic aspects of health* (pp. 53–92). Chicago: University of Chicago Press.

Roy, C. (1980). The Roy adaptation model. In J. Riehl, & C. Roy (Eds.), *Conceptual models for nursing practice* (2nd ed., pp. 179–188). New York: Appleton-Century-Crofts.

Roy, C., & Andrews, H. A. (1999). *The Roy adaptation model: The definitive statement.* Norwalk, CT: Appleton & Lange.

Rutter, M. (1985a). Family and school influences on behavioural development. *Journal of Child Psychology and Psychiatry, 26*(3), 349–368.

Rutter, M. (1985b). Family and school influences on cognitive development. *Journal of Child Psychology and Psychiatry, 26*(5), 683–704.

Ryan, K. A. (1993). Mothers of adult children with schizophrenia: An ethnographic study. *Schizophrenia Research, 11*(1), 21–31.

Ryan, P. (2000). Facilitating behavior change in chronically ill persons. In J. Miller (Ed.), *Coping with chronic illness: Overcoming powerlessness* (3rd ed., pp. 481–503). Philadelphia: F. A. Davis Company.

Sachs, B., Hall, L. A., Lutenbacher, M., & Rayens, M. K. (1999). Potential for abusive parenting by rural mothers with low-birth-weight children. *Image: Journal of Nursing Scholarship, 31*(1), 21–25.

Saiki-Craighill, S. (1997). The children's sentinels: Mothers and their relationships with health professionals in the context of Japanese health care. *Social Science Medicine, 44*(3), 291–300.

Sameroff, A. J., & Fiese, B. H. (1992). Family representations of development. In I. E. Sigeland, & A. V. McGillicuddy (Eds.), *Parental belief systems* (pp. 347–369). Hillsdale, NJ: LEA.

Satir, V. (1972). *Peoplemaking.* Palo Alto, CA: Science and Behavior Books.

Sawaya, G. F., Kerlikowski, K., & Lee, N. C. (2000). Frequency of cervical smear abnormalities within 3 years of normal cytology. *Obstetrics & Gynecology, 96*(2), 219–223.

Schroeder, M., & Affara, F. (2001). The Family Nurse: Frameworks for Practice. Geneva, Switzerland: International Council of Nurses.

Schumann, D. A., & Mosley, W. H. (1994). The household production of health. *Social Science Medicine, 38*(2), 201–204.

Schuck, L. A., & Bucy, J. E. (1997). Family rituals: Implications for early intervention. *Topics in Early Childhood Special Education, 17*(4), 477–493.

Schultz, T. P. (1984). Studying the impact of household economic and community variables on child mortality. *Population Development Review, supplement 10,* 215.

Schumann, D. A., & Mosley, H. (1994). The household production of health. *Social Science Medicine, 38*(2), 201–204.

Segal, R. (1998). The construction of family occupations: A study of families with children who have attention deficit/hyperactivity disorder. *Canadian Journal of Occupational Therapy, 65*(5), 286–292.

Segal, R., & Frank, G. (1998). The extraordinary construction of ordinary experience: Scheduling daily life in families with children with attention deficit hyperactivity disorder. *Scandinavian Journal of Occupational Therapy, 5*(3), 141–147.

Segal, R., & Frank, G. (1998). The extraordinary construction of ordinary experience: Scheduling daily life in families with children with attention deficit hyperactivity disorder. *Scandinavian Journal of Occupational Therapy, 5*(3), 141–147.

Segal, R. (2000). Adaptive strategies of mothers with children with attention deficit hyperactivity disorder: Enfolding and unfolding occupations. *American Journal of Occupational Therapy, 54*(3), 300–306.

Selanders, L. C. (1998). Florence Nightingale. The evolution and social impact of feminist values in nursing. *Journal of Holistic Nursing, 16*(2), 227–243.

Seppanen, S. M., Kyngas, H. A., & Nikkonen, M. J. (1999). Coping and social support of parents with a diabetic child. *Nursing Health Sciences, 1*(1), 63–70.

Shadbolt, B. (1996). Health consequences of social-role careers for women: A life-course perspective. *Australia and New Zealand Journal of Public Health, 20*(2), 172–180.

Silva, E. B., & Smart, C. (1999). *The new family?* Thousand Oaks, CA: Sage Publications.

Silver, E. J., Bauman, L. J., Ireys, H. T. (1995). Relationships of self-esteem and efficacy to psychological distress in mothers of children with chronic physical illnesses. *Health Psychology, 14*(4), 333–340.

Silver, E. J., Stein, R. E., Dadds, M. R. (1996). Moderating effects of family structure on the relationship between physical and mental health in urban children with chronic illness. *Journal of Pediatric Psychology, 21*(1), 43–56.

Singleton, J. K., Green-Hermandez, C., & Holzemer, S. P. (1999). The structure of primary care. In Singleton, Sandowski, Green-Hernandez, Horvath, DiGregorio, & Holzemer (Eds.), *Primary Care* (pp. 3–7). Philadelphia: J. B. Lippincott.

Skolnick, A. S., & Skolnick, J. H. (1999). *Family in transition* (10th ed.). New York: Longman.

Slusarcick, A. L., & McCaig, L. F. (July 27, 2000). National Hospital Ambulatory Medical Care Survey: 1998 Outpatient Department Summary. Vital and health statistics of the Centers for Disease Control. [http://www.cdc.gov/nchs/data/ad317.pdf].

Small, C. (1995). Appalachians. In J. Gigar, & R. Davidhizar (Eds.), *Transcultural nursing: Assessment and intervention* (2nd ed., pp. 263–280). St. Louis: Mosby Year Book.

Smith, S., & Gonzales, V. (2000). All health plans need CLAMs. *Healthplan, 41*(5), 45–48.

Smith-Battle, L., & Leonard, V. W. (1998). Adolescent mothers four years later: Narratives of the self and visions of the future. *Advances in Nursing Science, 20*(3), 36–49.

Soldo, B. J., Wolf, D. A., & Agree, E. M. (1990). Family, households, and care arrangements of frail older women: A structural analysis. *Journal of Gerontology, 45*(suppl 6), 238–249.

Spitze, G., Logan, J. R., & Robinson, J. (1992). Family structure and changes in living arrangements among elderly nonmarried parents. *Journal of Gerontology, 47*(suppl 6): 289–296.

Spradley, J. P. (1979). *The ethnographic interview.* New York: Holt, Rinehart and Winston.

Spradley, J. P. (1980). *Participant observation.* New York: Holt, Rinehart & Winston.

Spruijt, E., & de Goede, M. (1997). Transitions in family structure and adolescent well-being. *Adolescence, 32*(128), 897–911.

Sprunger, L. W., Boyce, W. T., & Gaines, J. A. (1985). Family-infant congruence: Routines and rhythmicity in family adaptations to a young infant. *Child Development, 56,* 564–572.

St. John, W., & Rolls, C. (1996). Teaching family nursing: Strategies and experiences. *Journal of Advances in Nursing, 23*(1), 91–96.

St. Peter, R. F., Reed, M. C., Kemper, P., & Blumenthal, D. (1999). Changes in the scope of care provided by primary care physicians. *The New England Journal of Medicine, 341*(26), 1980–1985.

Starr, A. M. (1989). Recovery for the alcoholic family: Family systems treatment model. *Social Casework, 70,* 348–354.

Statin, H., & Magnusson, D. (1990). Pubertal development in girls. Hillsdale, NJ: Erlbaum. In P. Moen, G. H. Elder, & K. Luscher (Eds.), (pp. 423–466). *Examining lives in context* (pp. 397–421). Washington, D.C.: American Psychological Association.

Steinberg, L., Darling, N. E., & Fletcher, A. C. (1995). Authoritative parenting and adolescent adjustment: An ecological journey. In P. Moen, G. H. Elder, & K. Luscher (Eds.), *Examining lives in context* (pp. 423–466). Washington, D.C.: American Psychological Association.

Steinberg, L., Dornbusch, S. M., & Brown, B. (1992). Ethnic differences in adolescent achievement: An ecological perspective. *American Psychologist, 47,* 723–729.

Steinglass, P., Bennett, L. A., Wolin, S. J., & Reiss, D. (1987). *The alcoholic family.* New York: Basic Books.

Steinglass, P. (1992). Family systems theory and medical illness. In R. J. Sawa (Ed.), *Family health care* (pp. 18–29). Newbury Park, CA: Sage Publications.

Stephens, C. (1994). *Health belief practices of rural southern Appalachian women from an ethnographic perspective.* Unpublished doctoral dissertation, University of Alabama at Birmingham.

Stevens-Barnum, B. J. (1990). *Nursing theory: Analysis, application, evaluation* (3rd ed.). Glenview, IL: Scott, Foresman/Little, Brown Higher Education.

Stewart, M. J., Ritchie, J. A., McGrath, P., Thompson, D., & Bruce, B. (1994). Mothers of children with chronic conditions: Supportive and stressful interactions with partners and professionals regarding caregiving burdens. *Canadian Journal of Nursing Research, 26*(4), 61–82.

Straus, M. (1964). Measuring families. In H.

Christensen (Ed.), *Handbook of marriage and the family* (pp. 335–402). Chicago: Rand McNally.

Streubert, H. J., & Carpenter, D. R. (1999). *Qualitative research in nursing: Advancing the humanistic imperative* (2nd ed.). Philadelphia: J.B. Lippincott.

Stuart, M. (1991). An analysis of the concept of family. In A. Whall, & J. Fawcett (Eds.), *Family theory development in nursing: State of the science and art* (pp. 31–42). Philadelphia: F. A. Davis Company.

Super, C., & Harkness, S. (Eds.). (1980). *Anthropological perspectives on child development: New directions for child development* (No. 8). San Francisco: Jossey-Bass.

Tannen, D. (1998). *The argument culture: Stopping America's war of words.* New York: Ballantine Books.

Taylor, V. M., Deyo, R. A., & Ciol, M. (2000). Patient-oriented outcomes from low back surgery: A community-based study. *Spine, 25*(19), 2445–2452.

Techman, J. D. (2000). Diversity of family structure: Economic and social influences. In D. Demo, K. Allen, & M. Fine (Eds.), *Handbook of family diversity* (pp. 32–58). New York: Oxford University Press.

Teisler, R. C., Killian, L. M., & Gubman, G. D. (1987). Stages in family response to mental illness: An ideal type. *Psychosocial Rehabilitation Journal, 10,* 3–16.

Thibaut, J., & Kelley, H. (1959). *The social psychology of groups.* New York: Wiley.

Thomas, A., & Chess, S. (1979). *Temperament and development.* New York: Brenner/Mazel.

Thomas, H. S. (1994). Conceptual underpinnings of the family support movement. *Journal of Pediatric Health Care, 8*(2), 57–62.

Thomas, R. B. (1990). A foundation for clinical family assessment. *Children's Health Care, 19*(4), 244–250.

Thorne, S. (1990). Mothers with chronic illness: A predicament of social construction. *Health Care Women International, 11*(2), 209–221.

Thorne, S. (1993). Health belief systems in perspective. *Journal of Advanced Nursing, 18,* 1931–1941.

Thorne, S., & Patterson, B. (2000). Two decades of insider research: What we know and don't know about chronic illness experience. In J. Fitzpatrick, & J. Goeppinger (Eds.), *Annual Review of Nursing Research* (Vol. 18, pp. 3–25). New York: Springer Publishing.

Thorne. S., & Varcoe, C. (1998). The tyranny of feminist methodology in women's health research. *Health Care Women International, 19*(6), 481–493.

Tomlinson, P. S., & Anderson, K. H. (1996). Family health and the Neuman systems model. In B. Neuman (Ed.), *The Neuman Systems Model* (3rd ed., pp. 133–144). Stamford: CN: Appleton & Lange.

Tomlinson, P. S., Harbaugh, B. L., Kotchevar, J., & Swanson, C. (1995). Caregiver mental health outcomes following critical hospitalization of a child. *Issues in Mental Health Nursing, 16,* 533–545.

Tomm, W. (1994). Beyond "family models": Family as a dialogical process in a cultural household of language. *Journal of Feminist Therapy, 6*(2), 1–20.

Trost, J. (1988). Conceptualising the family. *International Sociology, 3,* 301–308.

Trost, J. (1990). We mean the same by the concept of family. *Communication Research, 17*(4), 431–443.

Turner, B. J, Cunningham, W. E., & Duan, N. (2000). Delayed medical care after diagnosis in a U.S. national probability sample of persons infected with human immunodeficiency virus. *Internal Medicine, 160,* 2614–2622.

Turner, V. (1977). Variations of a theme of liminality. In S. Moore, & B. Myeroff (Eds.), *Secular ritual.* Amsterdam: Van Gorcum.

Turner-Henson, A., Holaday, B., & Swan, J. (1992). When parenting becomes caregiving: Caring for the chronically ill child. *Family and Community Health, 15*(2), 19–30.

Uphold, C. R., & Strickland, O. L. (1989). Issues related to the unit of analysis in family nursing research. *Western Journal of Nursing Research, 11,* 405–417.

U.S. Census Bureau. (March, 1998). *Household and family characteristics.* U.S. Census Bureau Public Information Office.

U.S. Census Bureau. (March, 1998). *Supplement to the current population survey.* U.S. Census Bureau Public Information Office.

U.S. Department of Health and Human Services. (1990). *Healthy People 2000: National health promotion and disease prevention objectives* (PHS Publication No. 91–50212). Washington, D.C.: Public Health Service.

U.S. Department of Health, Education, & Welfare. (1979). *Healthy people: Surgeon general's report on health promotion and disease prevention* (PHS Publication No. 79–55071). Washington, D.C.: Public Health Service.

U.S. Department of Health and Human Services. (2000). *Healthy People 2010: Understanding and improving health.* Washington, D.C.: U.S. Department of Health and Human Services, Government Printing Office.

Van der Zalm, J. E., & Bergum, V. (2000). Hermeneutic-phenomenology: Providing living knowledge for nursing practice. *Journal of Advanced Nursing, 31*(1), 211–218.

Vaden-Kiernan, N., Ialongo, N. S., Pearson, J., & Kellam, S. (1995). Household family structure and children's aggressive behavior: A longitudinal study of urban elementary school children. *Journal of Abnormal Child Psychology, 23*(5), 553–568.

Van Manen, M. (1990). *Researching lived experience: Human science for an action sensitive pedagogy.* New York: State University of New York Press.

Van Riper, M. (2001). Factors influencing family function and the health of family members. In S. M. Hanson (Ed.), *Family health care nursing: Theory, practice, and research* (2nd ed., pp. 123–145). Philadelphia: F.A. Davis Company.

Ventura, S. J., Martin, J. A., Curtin, S. C., & Mathews, T. J. (1999). Births: Final data for 1997. *National Vital Statistics Report, 47*(18).

Vetere, A. (1987). General system theory and the family: A critical evaluation. In A. Vetere, & A. Gale (Eds.), *Ecological studies of family life* (pp. 18– 33). New York: John Wiley & Sons.

von Bertalanffy, L. (1950). The theory of open systems in physics and biology. *Science, 111,* 23–29.

von Bertalanffy, L. (1968). *General system theory.* Harmondsworth: Penguin.

Vygotsky, L. (1978). *Mind in society: The development of higher psychological processes.* Cambridge, MA: Harvard University Press.

Wachs, T. D. (1983). The use and abuse of environment in behavior-genetic research. *Child Development, 54*(2), 396–407.

Wadsworth, M. E. (1997). Health inequalities in the life course perspective. *Social Science Medicine, 44*(6), 859–869.

Walker, M., Hilbert, G., & Rinehart, J. (1999). Face-to face with Sturge-Weber syndrome. *Journal of the Society of Pediatric Nurses, 4*(2), 74–82.

Waltz, C. F., Strickland, O. L., & Lenz, E. R. (1991). *Measurement in nursing research* (2nd ed). Philadelphia: F. A. Davis Company.

Ward, G. (1997). *Postmodernism.* Chicago: NTC/ Contemporary Publishing.

Watson, J. (1985). *Nursing: The philosophy and science of caring.* Boulder, CO: Colorado Associated University Press.

Watson, J. (1988). *Nursing: Humans science and human care. A theory of nursing.* New York: National League for Nursing.

Watson, J. (1997). The theory of human caring: Retrospective and prospective. *Nursing Science Quarterly, 10,* 49–52.

Watzlawick, P., Weakland, J., & Fisch, R. (1974). *Change: Principles of problem formulation and problem resolution.* New York: W. W. Norton.

Weinart, C., & Long, K. A. (1987). Understanding the health care needs of rural families. *Family Relations, 36,* 450–455.

Weinick, R. M, & Krauss, N. A. (2000). Racial and ethnic differences in children's access to care. *American Journal of Public Health, 90,* 11–14.

Weisner, T. S. (1984). Ecocultural niches of middle childhood: A cross-cultural perspective. In W. A. Collins (Ed.), *Development during middle childhood: The years from six to twelve* (pp. 335–369). Washington, D.C.: National Academy of Science Press.

Weisner, T. S., Beizer, L., & Stolze, L. (1991). Religion and families of children with developmental delays. *American Journal of Mental Retardation, 95*(6), 647–662.

Weuve, J. L., Boult, C., & Morishita, L. (2000). The effects of outpatient geriatric evaluation and management on caregiver burden. *The Gerontologist, 40*(4), 428–436.

Whall, A. L. (1986). Introduction: Theoretical perspectives. In A. L. Whall (Ed.), *Family therapy theory for nursing: Four approaches* (pp. 1–8). Norwalk, CN: Appleton-Century-Crofts.

Whall, A. L., (1991). Family system theory: Relationship to nursing conceptual models. In J. Fawcett, & A. Whall (Eds.), *Family theory development in nursing: State of the science and art* (pp. 317–340). Philadelphia: F. A. Davis Company.

Whall, A. L., (1995). Foreword. In M. Friedemann, The *framework of systemic organization: A conceptual approach to families and nursing* (pp. vii–viii). Thousand Oaks, CA: Sage Publications.

Whall, A. L., & Fawcett, J. (1991a). The family as a focal phenomenon in nursing. In A. Whall, & J. Fawcett (Eds.), *Family theory development in nursing: State of the science and art* (pp. 7–29). Philadelphia: F. A. Davis Company.

Whall, A. L., & Fawcett, J. (1991b). Introduction. In A. Whall, & J. Fawcett (Eds.), *Family theory development in nursing: State of the science and art* (pp. 3–6). Philadelphia: F. A. Davis Company.

Whall, A. L., & Loveland-Cherry, C. J. (1993). Family unit-focused research: 1984–1991. *Annual Review of Nursing Research, 11*, 227–247.

Whitbeck, L. B. (1999). Primary socialization theory: It all begins with the family. *Substance Use and Misuse, 34*(7), 1025–1032.

White, B. (1993). *The first three years of life.* New York: Simon & Schuster.

White, K. R. (1982). The relation between socioeconomic status and academic achievement. *Psychological Bulletin, 91*, 461–481.

Whiteside, M. F. (1989). Family rituals as a key to kinship connections in remarried families. *Family Relations, 38*, 34–39.

Whiting, B. (1976). The problem of the packaged variable. In K. Riegal, & J. Meacham (Eds.), *The developing individual in a changing world: Historical and cultural issues* (Vol. 1, pp. 303–309). Netherlands: Mouton.

Whiting, B. (1980). Culture and social behavior: A model for the development of social behavior. *Ethos, 8*, 95–116.

Whiting, B., & Edwards, C. (1988). *Children of different worlds: The formation of social behavior.* Cambridge, MA: Harvard University Press.

Whiting, J., & Whiting, B. (1975). *Children of six cultures: A psychocultural analysis.* Cambridge, MA: Harvard University Press.

Wierenga, M. E., Browning, J. M., & Mahn, J. L. (1990). A descriptive study of how clients make life-style changes. *The Diabetes Educator, 16*(6), 469–473.

Winstead-Fry, P. (2000). Rogers' conceptual system and family nursing. *Nursing Science Quarterly, 13*(4), 278–280.

Wise, P. H., & Lowe, J. A. (1992). Noise or fugue: Seeking the logic of child health indicators. *Mental Retardation, 30*(6), 323–329.

Wolin, S. J., & Bennett, L. A. (1984). Family rituals. *Family Process, 23*, 401–420.

Wolin, S. J., Bennett, L. A., & Noonan, D. L. (1979). Family rituals and the recurrence of alcoholism over generations. *American Journal of Psychiatry, 136*(suppl 4B), 589–593.

Wolin, S. J., Bennett, L. A., Noonan, D. L., & Teitelbaum, M. A. (1980). Disrupted family rituals: A factor in the generational transmission of alcoholism. *Journal of Studies of Alcohol, 41*, 199–214.

Woodwell, D. A. (July 19, 2000). National Ambulatory Medical Care Survey: 1998 Outpatient Department Summary. Vital and health statistics of the Centers for Disease Control. [http://www.cdc.gov/nchs/data/ad315.pdf].

Worden, J. W. (1982). *Grief counseling and grief therapy: A handbook for the mental health practitioner.* New York: Springer Publishing Company.

World Health Organization. (1944). The Constitution of the World Health Organization. *WHO Chronicle, 1*, 29.

World Health Organization. (1986). A charter for health promotion (Ottawa charter). *Canadian Journal of Public Health, 77*, 425–430.

Wright, L. M., & Bell, J. M. (1989). A survey of family nursing education in Canadian universities. *Canadian Journal of Nursing Research, 21*(3), 50–74.

Wright, L. M., & Leahey, M. (1994). *Nurses and families: A guide to family assessment and intervention.* Philadelphia: F. A. Davis Company.

Wright, L. M., & Leahey, M. (2000). *Nurses and families: A guide to family assessment and intervention* (3rd ed.). Philadelphia: F. A. Davis Company.

Wright, L. M., Watson, W. L., & Bell, J. M. (1996). *Beliefs: The heart of healing in families and illness.* New York: Basic Books.

Yabroff, K. R., Kerner, J. F., & Mandelblatt, J. S. (2000). Effectiveness of interventions to improve follow-up after abnormal cervical cancer screening. *Preventive Medicine, 31*, 429–439.

Yin, R. K. (1994). *Case study research: Design and methods* (2nd ed.). Thousand Oaks, CA: Sage Publications.

Young, A., Taylor, S. B., & Renpenning, K. M. (2001). *Connections: Nursing Research, Theory, and Practice.* St. Louis: Mosby Year Book.

Youngblut, J. M., Brennan, P. F., & Swegart, L. A. (1994). Families with medically fragile children: An exploratory study. *Pediatric Nursing, 20*, 660–666.

Yura, H., & Torres, G. (1975). *Today's conceptual frameworks with the baccalaureate nursing programs* (NLN Pub. No. 15–1558, pp. 17–75). New York: National League for Nursing.

Zlotnick, C., & Cassanego, M. (1992). Unemployment and health. *Nursing and Health Care, 13*(2), 78–82.

Zissok, S., & Lyons, L. (1988). Grief and relationships to the deceased. *International Journal of Family Psychiatry, 9*(2), 135–146.

Zuvekas, S. H. (2001). Trends in mental health services use and spending: 1987–1996. *Health Affairs, 20*, 214–224.

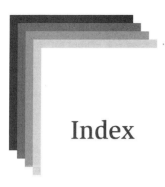

Index

An "f" following a page number indicates a figure; a "t" following a page number is a table; a "b" following a page number indicates a box.